SYNDROMES OF ATHEROSCLEROSIS

Correlations of Clinical Imaging and Pathology

Previously published:

Cardiovascular Applications of Magnetic Resonance
Edited by Gerald M. Pohost, MD

Cardiovascular Reponse to Exercise
Edited by Gerald F. Fletcher, MD

Congestive Heart Failure: Current Clinical Issues
Edited by Gemma T. Kennedy, RN, PhD,
and Michael H. Crawford, MD

Atrial Arrhythmias: State of the Art
Edited by John P. DiMarco, MD, PhD
and Eric N. Prystowsky, MD

Invasive Cardiology: Current Diagnostic
and Therapeutic Issues
Edited by George W. Vetrovec, MD
and Blase Carabello, MD

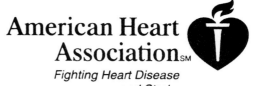

American Heart
Association℠

*Fighting Heart Disease
and Stroke*

Monograph Series

SYNDROMES OF ATHEROSCLEROSIS

Correlations of Clinical Imaging and Pathology

Edited by

Valentin Fuster, MD, PhD

*Arthur M. and Hilda A. Master Professor of Medicine
and Director, Cardiovascular Institute,
Mount Sinai Medical Center
New York, New York*

Co-edited by

The Members of the American Heart Association
Vascular Lesions Committee

**Herbert C. Stary, MD
A. Bleakley Chandler, MD
Seymour Glagov, MD
William Insull, Jr., MD
Michael E. Rosenfeld, MD
Colin J. Schwartz, MD
William D. Wagner, PhD
Robert D. Wissler, MD, PhD**

FUTURA

**Futura Publishing
Company, Inc.
Armonk, NY**

Library of Congress Cataloging-in-Publication Data
Syndromes of atherosclerosis : correlations of clinical imaging and
pathology / edited by Valentin Fuster.
    p.   cm. — (American Heart Association monograph series)
    Includes bibliographical references and index.
    ISBN 0-87993-638-X
    1. Atherosclerosis—Pathophysiology.   2. Atherosclerosis—
Imaging. I. Fuster, Valentin. II. Series.
    [DNLM: 1. Atherosclerosis—diagnosis.   2. Atherosclerosis—
pathology.   WG 550 S992 1996]
    RC692.S86   1996
    616.1'360754—dc20
    DNLM/DLC
    for Library of Congress   95-50681
                                                     CIP

The reproduction of the color illustrations in this book was made
possible by a grant from Merck and Company, Whitehouse Station,
New Jersey.

Copyright © 1996

Published by
Futura Publishing Company
135 Bedford Road
Armonk, New York 10504

LC #: 95-50681
ISBN #: 0-87993-638-X

Contributors

John J. Albers, PhD   Research Professor of Medicine and Director of Northwest Lipid Research Laboratory, Division of Metabolism, Endocrinology, and Nutrition, University of Washington School of Medicine, Seattle, Washington

John A. Ambrose, MD   Director, Cardiac Catheterization Laboratory, Mount Sinai Medical Center, New York, New York

Juan J. Badimon, PhD   Associate Professor of Medicine, Cardiovascular Institute, Mount Sinai Medical Center, New York, New York

Hisham S. Bassiouny, MD   Assistant Professor of Surgery, University of Chicago, Chicago Illinois

B. Greg Brown, MD, PhD   Professor of Medicine/Cardiology, Department of Medicine, Cardiology Division, University of Washington School of Medicine, Seattle, Washington.

Bruce H. Brundage, MD   Professor of Medicine and Radiological Sciences, UCLA School of Medicine and Chief, Division of Cardiology, Harbor-UCLA Medical Center and Scientific Director, Saint John's Cardiovascular Research Center, Torrance, California

Robert Byington, PhD   Associate Professor of Epidemiology, Department of Public Health Services, Bowman Gray School of Medicine, Winston-Salem, North Carolina

A. Bleakley Chandler, MD   Professor and Chairman, Department of Pathology, Medical College of Georgia, Augusta, Georgia

James H. Chesebro, MD   Associate Director, Cardiovascular Institute and Professor of Medicine, Mount Sinai Medical Center, New York, New York

Pim J. de Feyter, MD   Interventional Cardiologist, University Hospital Dijkzigt, Rotterdam-Erasmus University, Rotterdam, The Netherlands

Robert E. Dinsmore, MD   Department of Radiology and Cardiac Unit, General Medical Service, Massachusetts General Hospital, Boston, Massachusetts

v

Mark Doyle, PhD   Associate Professor, Department of Medicine, Division of Cardiovascular Disease, University of Alabama at Birmingham, Birmingham, Alabama

Erling Falk, MD, PhD   Professor of Cardiovascular Pathology, Skejby University Hospital, Aarhus N, Denmark

Kenneth B. Fallon, MD   Pathologist, JoEllen Smith Medical Center, New Orleans, Louisiana

Carol M. Ford, MSc   Research Associate, John P. Robarts Research Institute and Department of Medicine (Cardiology), University Hospital, University of Western Ontario, London, Ontario, Canada

Valentin Fuster, MD, PhD   Arthur M. and Hilda A. Master Professor of Medicine and Director, Cardiovascular Institute, Mount Sinai Medical Center, New York, New York

Richard Gallo, MD   Research Associate, Cardiovascular Institute, Mount Sinai Medical Center, New York, New York

Don P. Giddens, PhD   Johns Hopkins University, Baltimore, Maryland

Seymour Glagov, MD   Professor of Pathology, Department of Pathology, University of Chicago, Chicago, Illinois

Jerry Goldstone, MD   Professor of Surgery, Division of Vascular Surgery, and Vice Chair, Department of Surgery, University of California, San Francisco, San Francisco, California

Mervyn S. Gotsman, MD, FACC, FRCP.   Director, Cardiac Unit and Professor of Cardiology, Hadassah-Hebrew University Hospital and President, Israel Cardiac Society, Jerusalem, Israel

Thomas M. Grist, MD   Chief of MRI and Assistant Professor of Radiology and Assistant Professor of Medical Physics, Departments of Radiology and Medical Physics, University of Wisconsin Hospital and Clinics, Madison, Wisconsin

Yonathan Hasin, MD   Director, Coronary Care Unit (Ein Kerem) and Professor of Cardiology, Hadassah-Hebrew University Hospital, Jerusalem, Israel

Christian C. Haudenschild, MD   Head of Department of Experimental Pathology, JH Holland Laboratory, American Red Cross, Rockville, Maryland

Laura Hiltscher, ASCP   Laboratory Supervisor, University of Chicago Medical Center, Chicago, Illinois

William Insull, Jr, MD   Professor of Medicine and Pediatrics, Baylor College of Medicine and The Methodist Hospital and Director, Lipid Research Clinic, Houston, Texas

Jeffrey M. Isner, MD   Chief of Cardiovascular Research, Departments of Medicine (Cardiology), Pathology, and Biomedical Research, St. Elizabeth's Medical Center, Tufts University School of Medicine, Boston, Massachusetts

Eiji Kaneko, MD   Senior Research Fellow, Department of Pathology, University of Washington School of Medicine, Seattle, Washington

Marianne Kearney, BS   Departments of Medicine (Cardiology), Pathology, and Biomedical Research, St. Elizabeth's Medical Center, Tufts University School of Medicine, Boston, Massachusetts

Ted R. Kohler, MD   Associate Professor, Surgery, University of Washington and Chief, Vascular Surgery Division, Seattle Veterans Affairs Medical Center, Seattle, Washington

Harald Kritz, MD   Department of Nuclear Medicine, Vienna University Hospital, Vienna, Austria

Ann M. Lees, MD   Assistant Professor of Medicine, Harvard Medical School and Associate Director, Boston Heart Foundation, Cambridge, Massachusetts

Robert S. Lees, MD   Professor of Health Sciences and Technology, Harvard/MIT Division of Health Sciences and Technology, and President, Boston Heart Foundation, Cambridge, Massachusetts

Maddalena Lettino, MD   Research Associate, Cardiovascular Institute, Mount Sinai Medical Center, New York, New York

Chaim Lotan, MD, FACC   Senior Cardiologist (Senior Lecturer), Cardiology Department, Hadassah-Hebrew University Hospital, Jerusalem, Israel

Nobuhide Masawa, MD   Professor of Pathology, Dokkyo University, Japan

D. Douglas Miller, MD, FACC, FRCPC   Associate Professor of Medicine and Director of Nuclear Cardiology and Director of Cardiovascular Biology, Saint Louis University Health Sciences Center, Department of Internal Medicine, Division of Cardiology, St. Louis, Missouri

Morris Mosseri, MD   Senior Cardiologist (Senior Lecturer), Cardiology Department, Hadassah-Hebrew University Hospital, Jerusalem, Israel

Edward R. O'Brien, MD, FRCP(C)   Assistant Professor, Department of Medicine, Division of Cardiology and Director, Vascular Biology Laboratory, University of Ottawa Heart Institute, Ottawa, Ontario, Canada

J. Geoffrey Pickering, MD, PhD, FRCPC   Assistant Professor, Departments of Medicine and Medical Biophysics and Honourary Lecturer, Department of Biochemistry and Scientist, John P. Robarts Research Institute and Department of Medicine (Cardiology), University Hospital, University of Western Ontario, London, Ontario, Canada

Gerald M. Pohost, MD   Professor, Department of Medicine and Director, Division of Cardiovascular Disease, University of Alabama at Birmingham, Birmingham, Alabama

Drew Poulin, BS   Research Technician Supervisor, Department of Medicine, Cardiology Division, University of Washington School of Medicine, Seattle, Washington

Elaine W. Raines, MS   Research Professor, Department of Pathology, University of Washington School of Medicine, Seattle, Washington

S. Mitchell Rivitz, MD   Department of Radiology, Massachusetts General Hospital, Boston, Massachusetts

Margarida Rodrigues, MD   Department of Nuclear Medicine, Vienna University Hospital, Vienna, Austria

Russell Ross, PhD   Professor, Department of Pathology, University of Washington School of Medicine, Seattle, Washington

Shimon Rosenheck, MD   Senior Cardiologist (Mount Scopus) and Senior Lecturer, Cardiology Department, Hadassah-Hebrew University Hospital, Jerusalem, Israel

Yoseph Rozenman, MD, FACC   Senior Cardiologist (Lecturer), Cardiology Department, Hadassah-Hebrew University Hospital, Jerusalem, Israel

Peter N. Ruygrok, FRACP   Interventional Cardiologist, University Hospital Dijkzigt, Rotterdam, Erasmus University, Rotterdam, The Netherlands.

Yasuhiro Sakaguchi, MD   Assistant Professor of Medicine, Nara University, Japan

Steven M. Santilli, MD, PhD   Fellow, Division of Vascular Surgery, Department of Surgery, University of California, San Francisco, San Francisco, California

Colin J. Schwartz, MD, FRACP   Professor, Department of Pathology, University of Texas Health Sciences Center at San Antonio, Texas

Stephen M. Schwartz, MD, PhD   Professor of Pathology, Department of Pathology, University of Washington, School of Medicine, Seattle, Washington

Helmut Sinzinger, MD   Professor, Department of Nuclear Medicine, Vienna University Hospital, Vienna, Austria

Michael P. Skinner, MBBS, PhD, FRACP   Staff Specialist, Department of Cardiology, Division of Medicine, Westmead Hospital and Senior Lecturer, University of Sydney, Westmead, Australia

Herbert C. Stary, MD   Professor of Pathology, Louisiana State University Medical Center, New Orleans, Louisiana

James D. Stoll, MD   Internal Medicine, Louisiana State University Medical Center, New Orleans, Louisiana

Vincenzo Toschi, MD   Research Associate, Cardiovascular Institute, Mount Sinai Medical Center, New York, New York

Patrick A. Turski, MD   Chief of Neural Radiology and Professor of Radiology, Neurology and Neural Surgery, Departments of Radiology and Neurology, University of Wisconsin Hospital and Clinics, Madison, Wisconsin

Jeroen Vos, MD   Cardiologist in Training, University Hospital Dijkzigt, Rotterdam-Erasmus University, Rotterdam, The Netherlands

Matthew Wahden   Research Assistant, University of Chicago Medical Center, Chicago, Illinois

Jesse Weinberger, MD   Professor of Neurology, The Mount Sinai School of Medicine and Chief, Neurology, North General Hospital, New York, New York

A. Teddy Weiss, MD, FACC   Director, Coronary Care Unit (Mount Scopus) and Associate Professor of Cardiology, Hadassah-Hebrew University Hospital, Jerusalem, Israel

Robert W. Wissler, MD, PhD   Donald Pritzker Distinguished Service Professor, Department of Pathology and Program Director, Multicenter Cooperative Study of the Pathobiological Determinants of Atherosclerosis in Youth, University of Chicago Medical Center, Chicago, Illinois

Chengpei Xu, MD   Research Associate, University of Chicago, Chicago, Illinois

Jianfang Yin, MD   Graduate Research Assistant, Louisiana State University Medical Center, New Orleans, Louisiana

Zhongxin Yu, MD   Graduate Student, Louisiana State University Medical Center, New Orleans, Louisiana

Chun Yuan, PhD   Assistant Professor, Department of Radiology, University of Washington School of Medicine, Seattle, Washington

Christopher K. Zarins, MD   Chidester Professor of Surgery, Chief of Vascular Surgery and Acting Chairman, Department of Surgery, Stanford University Medical Center, Stanford, California

Xue-Qiao Zhao, MD   Associate Director of Quantitative Coronary Arteriography Laboratory, Department of Medicine, Cardiology Division, University of Washington School of Medicine, Seattle, Washington

Contents

Chapter 1

Coronary Artery Disease:
A Clinical-Pathological Correlation

Valentin Fuster, MD, PhD

Pathogenesis of Coronary Disease

Our understanding of the pathophysiology of coronary atherosclerosis has dramatically changed in the last few years. The mechanisms of progression of coronary atherosclerosis and plaque instability and rupture in acute coronary syndromes are now better understood.[1,2] Therapeutic strategies that will lead to coronary atherosclerosis stabilization and even regression are being pursued by many investigators.

Lesions of Atherosclerosis (Figures 1 and 2)

A new classification has been proposed to characterize atherosclerotic plaques, from fatty streak to advanced complicated lesion, by categorizing the process of plaque progression into five phases.[2] Each of these phases has been defined by a series of lesion morphological characteristics by the American Heart Association (AHA) Committee on Vascular Lesions[2a] based on a classification proposed by Stary.[3]

In Figure 1, phase 1 is represented by a small lesion of the type commonly found in individuals less than 30 years of age. Such plaques may progress over a period of years and are categorized as lesion types I, II, and III. Type I lesions consist of macrophage-

Parts of this chapter are a modification of Fuster V., Lewis A. Conner Memorial Lecture. Mechanisms leading to myocardial infarction: Insights from studies of vascular biology. *Circulation* 1994;90:2126 and Fuster V, Badimon JJ. Regression or stabilization of atherosclerosis. *Eur Heart J* 1995;16(suppl E):6–12.

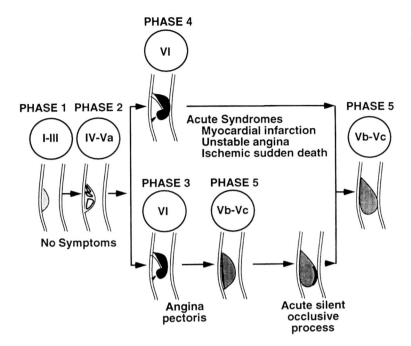

FIGURE 1. *Schematic of staging (phases and lesion morphology of the progression of coronary atherosclerosis according to gross pathological and clinical findings. (See text for details). Modified with permission from Fuster, et al.* N Engl J Med *1992;326:244 and Reference 5.*

derived foam cells that contain lipid droplets. Type II consists of both macrophages and smooth muscle cells with extracellular lipid deposits. Type III consists largely of smooth muscle cells surrounded by extracellular lipid.

Phase 2 consists of a plaque that may not necessarily be stenotic but that may have a high lipid content, and, therefore, may possibly be prone to rupture. Such a plaque represents those categorized morphologically as lesion types IV and Va. Type IV consists of a confluent cellular lesion with a great deal of extracellular lipid, whereas in type Va extracelllular lipid is found in a core that is covered by a thin fibrous cap.

Phase 2 can evolve into acute phase 3 or phase 4; either of the two can evolve into fibrotic phase 5. Phase 3 has been classified as having an acute complicated type VI lesion resulting from rupture or fissure, usually of a nonseverely stenotic type IV or Va lesion leading to the formation of a mural thrombus, which may not completely occlude the artery. As a result of the changes in geometry of the disrupted plaque and of the organization of the mural thrombus by connective tissue, this can progress to the more stenotic and fibrotic type Vb or Vc lesions of phase 5, which may manifest clinically with angina and may evolve into occlusive lesions. Because of the preceding significant stenosis and ischemia-enhancing protective collateral vessels, the final occlusion may be silent or not clinically apparent.[2] In contrast to phase 3, in the acute complicated type VI lesion of phase 4, the thrombus is occlusive with the clinical development of an acute coronary syndrome rather than being characterized by a mural thrombus. Such occlusive thrombus, if not lysed physiologically or pharmacologically, may eventually become the fibrotic or occlusive Vb or Vc lesions of phase 5.

Although this terminology initially appears complicated, Figure 1 demonstrates that this approach uses the clinical phases of plaque evolution and the pathological types of lesions described in (Figure 2), so that clinicians and investigators can share a common language and understanding of these processes.

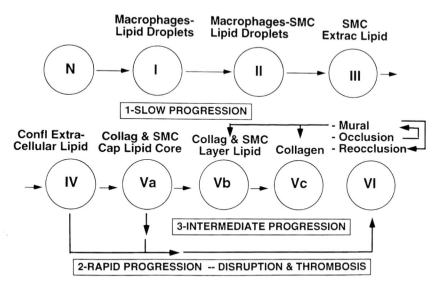

FIGURE 2. *Schematic of lesion morphology of the progression of coronary atherosclerosis according to the histopathology findings. SMC indicates smooth muscle cells. (See text for details). Modified with permission from Reference 2.*

The Dynamic Influx and Efflux of Lipoproteins in Plaque Formation (Figure 3)

In spontaneous atherosclerosis, chronic minimal injury to the arterial endothelium is caused mainly by a disturbance in the pattern of blood flow in certain parts of the arterial tree, such as bending points and areas near bifurcations.[1,2,4] In addition to local shear forces that are probably enhanced in hypertension, several other factors, including hypercholesterolemia, advanced glycosylated end products in diabetes (particularly insulin-dependent), chemical irritants in tobacco smoke, circulating vasoactive amines, immunocomplexes, and infection may potentiate chronic minimal endothelial injury, leading to accumulation of lipids and monocytes (macrophages) at these sites.[1,2,4]

The entry, accumulation, and fate of lipids and monocyte-macrophages in these early stages of atherogenesis can be divided into five phases (Figure 3).[2,5] First, most lipids deposited in the atherosclerotic lesions are derived from plasma low-density lipoproteins (LDL) that enter into the vessel wall through the injured or dysfunctional endothelium. Second, all major cell types within the vessel wall and atherosclerotic lesions can oxidize LDL, but the endothelial cell is probably critical in these very early stages of atherogenesis by mildly oxidizing LDL. Third, mildly oxidized LDL (or minimally modified LDL) may play an initial role in monocyte recruitment by inducing the expression of adhesive cell-surface glycoproteins in the endothelium. After monocytes adhere to the surface of the vessel wall, other specific molecules may attract and modify monocytes within the subendothelial space, such as a specific chemotactic protein (monocyte chemotactic protein-1) and colony-stimulating factor. After entering the vessel wall, monocytes are called macrophages. They may be responsible for converting mildly oxidized LDL into highly oxidized LDL, which bind to the scavenger receptors of macrophages and enter into the cells, converting them into foam cells. Fourth, by inhibiting the oxidation of LDL or its subsequent effects, high-density lipoproteins (HDL) may protect against excess lipid accumulation in the vessel wall. HDL may also contribute to reverse cholesterol transport or active LDL removal from the vessel wall and from the macrophage-foam cells. Finally, macrophages or foam cells, after saturation with lipid and before or after their rupture, can liberate a large number of products including cholesterol (esterified and oxidized) that can further damage the endothelium and so participate in the evolution of the atherosclerotic lesion. Thus, extracellular accumulation, at least in the very

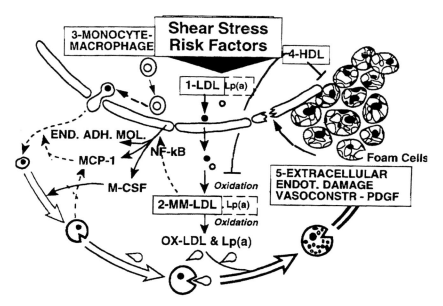

FIGURE 3. *Schematic of pathogenesis of phase I of progression: Chronic endothelial injury and risk factors—influx, accumulation, and fate of lipids and monocyte-macrophages. LDL indicates low-density lipoprotein; HDL, high-density lipoprotein; Lp(a), lipoprotein(a); OX, oxidized; END.ADH.MOL., endothelium adhesion molecule; MCP-1, monocyte chemotactic protein-1; M-CSF, monocyte-colony stimulating factor; MM, minimally modified; NF, nuclear factor; ENDOT, endothelium; VASO-CONSTR, vasonconstriction; PDGF, platelet-derived growth factor. Modified from with permission from Reference 5.*

early stages of atherogenesis, appears to be mainly caused by rupture of macrophage-foam cells or by accumulated debris resulting from cell death. Such macrophage-foam cell-liberated extracellular cholesterol esters are water soluble and form an oil-lipid crystalline phase; however, during the later phase of plaque development, the additional extracellular accumulation of free cholesterol from continued entry from the plasma results in the formation of cholesterol monohydrate crystals.

In these dynamic processes of influx and efflux of lipoproteins, it is reasonable to assume that a decrease in influx—such as by modification of risk factors and thus endothelial injury—will result in a predominance of efflux. Therefore, regression or stabilization of early atherosclerotic plaques by modification of risk factors should be theoretically possible.

The Vulnerable Lipid-Rich Plaques and the Acute Coronary Syndromes (Figures 1, 2, and 4)

The Lack of Sensitivity and Specificity of Coronary Arteriography

Although arteriography is considered the standard method of evaluating the anatomy of the epicardial coronary arteries, it lacks sensitivity and specificity. In addition, coronary arteriography is of little value in the evaluation of the microcirculation.[6]

In regard to the lack of sensitivity, several studies have concluded that coronary arteriography may underestimate the severity of coronary atherosclerosis; that is, the luminal area, as seen arteriographically, may appear to be preserved despite extensive disease of the vessel.[7] In addition, arteriography is helpful as a determinant of severity of coronary disease, but it cannot accurately predict the site of future coronary occlusion. Thus, in most patients, acute ischemic events are a complication not necessarily of severe fibrotic and calcified lesions, but rather of the disruption of the associated mildly to moderately stenotic types IV and Va lipid-rich plaques, which are often not even visible angiographically.[2,6] It is of value to consider, however, that the more severe the coronary disease at angiography, the higher the likelihood of the presence of small plaques prone to disruption.[8]

In regard to the lack of specificity, coronary arteriography cannot distinguish lipid-rich plaques, which are vulnerable to disruption, from stable more fibrotic or calcified plaques. Because of such lack of specificity of coronary arteriography, new imaging technologies are emerging with the objective of detecting these lipid-rich plaques susceptible to rupture. In addition to intravascular ultrasound, which is not yet sensitive enough,[7] it may be possible in the future to detect fatty plaques within the vascular system by high-resolution biochemical imaging techniques.

Finally, coronary arteriography cannot serve in the evaluation of the microcirculation. However, new technologies for the measurement of flow as an indirect approach to the evaluation of the microcirculation and flow reserve in humans are rapidly evolving. Technology using Doppler flow, positron emission tomography (PET), and echo-planar magnetic resonance imaging (MRI) are promising (Figure 4).

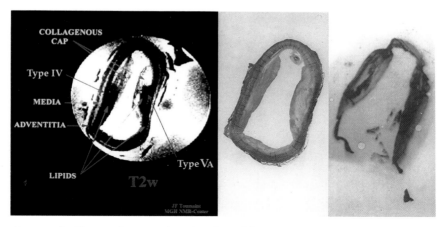

FIGURE 4. *Photomicrographs of vulnerable or unstable lesions obtained at autopsy.* **Left:** *Nuclear magnetic resonance images show two opposing lipid-rich plaques in the aorta. T2w image identifies a collagenous cap on both plaques. In the type V lesion (right), the cap completely covers the lipid core. In the type V lesion (left), the plaque is only partially covered, and infiltration of fat is more diffuse.* **Middle:** *Trichrome staining at histopathology.* **Right:** *Sudan black staining at histopathology. Reprinted with permission from Reference 2.*

Contributors to the Acute Coronary Syndromes

Plaque Disruption (Figures 1, 2, and 4)

In the process of atherogenesis and lipid accumulation, cell proliferation and extracellular matrix synthesis may be expected to be linear with time. However, angiographic studies show that the progression of coronary artery disease in humans is neither linear nor predictable. New high-grade lesions often appear in segments of artery that appeared normal only months earlier at angiographic examination. Indeed, it has become apparent that arteriographically mild coronary lesions may be associated with significant progression to severe stenosis or total occlusion.[9,10] These lesions may account for as many as two thirds of the patients in whom unstable angina or other acute coronary syndromes develop.[2,5] This unpredictable and episodic progression is likely caused by plaque disruption with subsequent thrombus formation that changes the plaque geometry, leading to intermittent plaque growth and acute occlusive coronary syndromes.[11,12] This has been confirmed by angioscopic studies performed in vivo.[13]

Recent pathological studies have revealed that such atherosclerotic plaques prone to rupture are commonly composed of a crescentic mass of lipids separated from the vessel lumen by a fibrous cap[14] (type IV and Va lesions).[2] Plaques that undergo disruption tend to be relatively soft and have a high concentration of cholesterol esters rather than free cholesterol monohydrate crystals. In addition to this rather passive phenomenon of plaque disruption, a better understanding of an active phenomenon related to macrophage activity is evolving. Thus, atherectomy specimens obtained from patients with acute coronary syndromes, including a high proportion of patients with unstable angina, revealed significantly high macrophage-rich areas compared with specimens from patients with stable angina.[15] In addition, extracts from human and rabbit atherosclerotic plaques revealed macrophages and expression of metalloproteinases that induced an increase in the breakdown of the extracellular matrix. This suggests that macrophages could be responsible for an active phenomenon of plaque disruption.[16,17]

Thrombosis (Table 1)

Disruption of a vulnerable or unstable plaque with a subsequent change in plaque geometry and thrombosis results in a type VI or complicated lesion.[2,18] Such a rapid change in the atherosclerotic plaque may result in acute occlusion with unstable angina or other acute coronary syndromes. Histopathologically, plaque fissuring comes in various shapes and sizes. The tear may be small; such tears allow blood to enter and expand the plaque but may not result in thrombus formation in the arterial lumen. The tear may be large, and the thrombus formed within the lumen may occlude the vessel;[18] such a thrombus may either be partially lysed or become replaced in the process of organization by the vascular repair response.[2,3] Of interest, an acute occlusive thrombus may be invaded by several channels and appear partially open at angiography.

At the time of coronary plaque disruption (Table 1), a number of local and systemic factors may influence the degree and duration of thrombus deposition.

TABLE 1

Thrombotic Complications of Plaque Disruption Local and Systemic Thrombogenic Risk Factors

Local Factors
   Degree of plaque disruption (ie, fissure, ulcer)
   Degree of stenosis (ie, change in geometry)
   Tissue substrate (ie, lipid-rich plaque)
   Surface of residual thrombus (ie, recurrence)
   Vasoconstriction (ie, platelets, thrombin)

Systemic Factors
   Catecholamines (ie, smoking, stress, cocaine use)
   Renin-angiotensin system (ie, DD genotype)
   Cholesterol, lipoprotein (a), and other metabolic states (ie,
      homocystinemia, diabetes)
   Fibrinogen, impaired fibrinolysis (ie, plasminogen activator inhibitor-1),
      activated platelets and clotting (ie, factor VII, thrombin generation
      [fragment 1+2], or activity [fibrinopeptide A])

High-risk indicates labile vs. fixed thrombus (unstable angina, non–Q-wave myocardial infarction, Q-wave myocardial infarction); low risk, mural thrombus (progressive). (Reproduced with permission from Reference 2.)

Vasoconstriction

Although many episodes of unstable angina and acute myocardial infarction are caused by the fissuring or disruption of plaque with superimposed thrombosis, other mechanisms that alter myocardial oxygen supply and demand must be considered. Original studies by Maseri's group that used hemodynamic, electrocardiographic, and angiographic monitoring, have suggested that coronary vasoconstriction plays an important role in the pathogenesis of ischemic heart disease[19]; more recent studies suggest a specific role in the acute coronary syndromes.[20] In the acute coronary syndromes, vasoconstriction may occur either as a response to a mildly dysfunctional endothelium near the culprit lesion or, more likely, may be a response to deep arterial damage or plaque disruption of the culprit lesion itself.

The endothelium can profoundly affect vascular tone by releasing relaxing factors such as prostacyclin[21] and endothelium-derived relaxing factor (EDRF), now known to be nitric oxide (NO),[22] and contracting factors such as endothelin-1.[23] Under physiologic conditions, EDRF appears to predominate. However, there is evidence that an alteration to the endothelium, such as occurs in early atherogenesis, particularly under the effect of atherogenic risk factors[24,25] or perhaps near the disrupted or culprit plaque in unstable angina and the other acute coronary syndromes,[20] may cause endothelial cells to generate more mediators that enhance constriction and fewer mediators that enhance dilation. The cardiovascular risk factors known to affect the epicardial coronary arteries also affect coronary microcirculatory function with a tendency for vasoconstriction that may contribute to ischemia.[25]

In acute coronary syndromes there is a predisposition for platelet-dependent and thrombin-dependent vasoconstriction at the site of plaque disruption and thrombosis that may be very significant, but transient. Thus, platelet-dependent vasoconstriction, mediated by serotonin and thromboxane A_2, and thrombin-dependent vasoconstriction[2,26] occur if the vascular wall has been significantly damaged, suggesting the direct interaction of these substances with vascular smooth muscle cells. This information, along with recent data obtained in humans after plaque damage by percutaneous transluminal coronary angioplasty, supports the angiographic observation that transient vasoconstriction often accompanies plaque disruption or fissuring and thrombosis in unstable angina and the other acute coronary syndromes.[2]

Integrated Pathogenesis of the Various Coronary Syndromes

In patients with stable coronary artery disease, angina or silent ischemia commonly results from increases in myocardial oxygen demand that outstrip the ability of stenosed coronary arteries to increase its delivery. In contrast, unstable angina, non-Q wave myocardial infarction, and Q wave infarction—on occasion these acute syndromes may also be silent—present a continuum of the disease process and are usually characterized by an abrupt reduction in coronary flow. Thus, local and systemic thrombogenic risk factors at the time of plaque disruption may modify the extent and duration of thrombus deposition and account for the variety of pathological and acute clinical manifestations (Table 1).[2]

In unstable angina, a relatively small fissuring or disruption of an atherosclerotic plaque may lead to an acute change in plaque structure and a reduction in coronary blood flow, resulting in the initiation or exacerbation of angina. Transient episodes of thrombotic vessel occlusion at the site of plaque injury may occur, leading to angina at rest.[2,26] This thrombus is usually labile and results in temporary vascular occlusion, perhaps lasting only 10 to 20 minutes. In addition, release of vasoactive substances by platelets and vasoconstriction secondary to endothelial vasodilator dysfunction may contribute to a reduction in coronary blood flow.[20,26] Overall, alterations in perfusion and myocardial oxygen supply probably account for two thirds of episodes of unstable angina; the rest may be caused by transient increases in myocardial oxygen demand.[27]

In non-Q wave myocardial infarction, more severe plaque damage results in more persistent thrombotic occlusion, perhaps lasting up to 1 hour. About one fourth of patients with non-Q wave myocardial infarction have an infarct-related vessel occluded for more than 1 hour, but the distal myocardial territory is usually supplied by collaterals.[2,28] ST segment elevation in the electrocardiogram, an early peak in plasma creatine kinase concentration, and a high rate of angiographic patency of the involved vessel in early angiograms support this idea. Resolution of vasoconstriction may also be pathogenically important in non-Q wave myocardial infarction.[2] Therefore, spontaneous thrombolysis, resolution of vasoconstriction, or the presence of collateral circulation are important in preventing the formation of Q wave myocardial infarction by limiting the duration of myocardial ischemia.

In Q wave myocardial infarction, larger plaque fissures may result in the formation of a fixed and persistent thrombus. This leads to an abrupt cessation of myocardial perfusion that lasts for longer than 1 hour, resulting in transmural necrosis of the involved myocardium. The coronary lesion responsible for the infarction is frequently only mildly to moderately stenotic, which suggests that plaque rupture with superimposed thrombus, rather than the severity of the underlying lesion, is the primary determinant of acute occlusion.[9,10] There is suggestive evidence that in patients with severe coronary stenosis, well-developed collaterals prevent or reduce the extent of infarction.[2] Indeed, in perhaps more than half of the patients, coronary occlusion, whether gradual or acute, occurs in areas of high-grade stenosis and is not evident clinically.[29]

Some cases of sudden coronary death probably involve a rapidly progressive coronary lesion in which plaque rupture and resultant thrombosis lead to ischemic and fatal ventricular arrhythmias.[30] Absence of collateral flow to the myocardium distal to the occlusion or platelet microemboli may contribute to the development of sudden ischemic death.[2]

Lipid-Modifying Arteriographic Trials of Regression and Stabilization

Conceptually, approaches toward retardation or even reversal of atherosclerotic lesions in humans for prevention of acute coronary events include better control of risk factors, such as reducing plasma cholesterol levels. Thus, it might be possible to modify the lipid-rich atherosclerotic plaques, which are more prone to rupture, preventing progression and even inducing regression by removal of fat. In trials that compare a more aggressive versus a more conservative treatment of lipid abnormalities in patients with coronary disease identified at arteriography, four important observations have been made.[31,32] 1) Progression of the disease was significantly decreased by the more aggressive approaches, but overall only minimal regression of atherosclerosis has was shown (1% to 2% decrease in degree of stenosis). 2) Despite the small degree of arteriographic regression, there was a substantial reduction in the incidence of acute cardiac events in most trials (over 50% reduction). The recent Scandinavian 4S study in a well-identified large group of patients with coronary disease and dyslipoproteinemia showed a decrease in mortality with the use of simvastatin. This landmark study with the use of an aggressive pharmacological approach supports and goes beyond the data of the regression and stabilization studies.[33] 3) Preliminarily, it appears that the effect in coronary disease progression and coronary events was also observed by modification of risk factors other than lipids. 4) It also appears that there was substantial reduction in angina in several of the studies, despite minimal or no regression of atherosclerosis.

On the basis of these observations, the following interpretation of the data is evolving.[2,31] The lack of significant regression observed on the atherosclerotic lesions seen in the arteriograms is probably because such lesions tend to be already advanced, fibrotic and less lipid-rich; therefore, they are less prone to reabsorption or to favorable remodeling. The substantial reduction in coronary events is probably related to favorable dynamics of influx and efflux of lipoproteins in the smaller lipid-rich plaques, those not necessarily visualized at arteriography, but prone to disruption and to acute events. Specifically, when high LDL cholesterol is substantially reduced therapeutically, efflux from the plaques of the liquid or sterified cholesterol and also its hydrolysis into cholesterol crystals depositing in the vessel wall predominate over the influx of LDL cholesterol. Consequently, there is a decrease in the softness of the plaque and so, presumably, in the passive phenomenon of plaque disruption previously described. Whether there is also a partial decrease in the number and activity of the macrophages and in the active phenomenon of plaque disruption is under investigation. Other effects of lipid-modifying strategies on endothelial function and in thrombogenicity—whether related to the plasma levels of LDL or to the specific agents used—are also under investigation. As discussed earlier in this section, the beneficial effects exerted by modification of risk factors other than LDL or HDL cholesterol are probably because of their influence in the entry of LDL cholesterol into the vessel wall as well as their influence in the thrombogenic complication of plaque disruption. Finally, the reduction in angina in some of the studies, despite minimal or no regression of atherosclerotic lesions in the arteriograms, possibly relates to the correction of the detrimental effect of dyslipoproteinemia and other risk factors on microvascular flow that cannot be assessed in the arteriograms.

References

1. Ross R. The pathogenesis of atherosclerosis: A perspective for the 1990s. *Nature* 1993;3262:801–808.
2. Fuster V. Mechanisms leading to myocardial infarction: Insights from studies of vascular biology. *Circulation* 1994;90:2126–2146.
2a. Stary HC, Chandler AB, Dinsmore RE, et al. A definition of advanced types of atherosclerotic lesions and a histological classification of atherosclerosis: A report from the committee on Vascular Lesions of the Council on Arteriosclerosis, American Heart Association. Arteriosler Thromb Vasc Biol 1995; 15:1512–1531.
3. Stary HC. Composition and classification of human atherosclerotic lesions. *Virch Arch Pathol Anat* 1992;421:277–290.
4. Stary HC, Chandler AB, Glagov S, et al. A definition of initial, fatty streak and intermediate lesions of atherosclerosis. A report from the Committee on Vascular Lesions of the Council on Arteriosclerosis, American Heart Association. *Circulation* 1994;89:2462–2478.
5. Steinberg D. Antioxidants and atherosclerosis: A current perspective. *Circulation* 1991;86:1420–1425.
6. Fuster V, Badimon L, Badimon JJ, et al. The pathogenesis of coronary artery disease and the acute coronary syndromes. *N Engl J Med* 1992;326:242–250; 310–318.
7. Nissen SE, Gurley JC, Grimes CL, et al. Intravascular ultrasound assessment of lumen size and wall morphology in normal subjects and patients with coronary artery disease. *Circulation* 1991;84:1087–1099.
8. Hangartner JRW, Charleston AJ, Davies MJ, et al. Morphological characteristics of clinically significant coronary artery stenosis in stable angina. *Br Heart J* 1986;56:501–508.
9. Ambrose J, Tannenbaum M, Alexpoulos D, et al. Angiographic progression of coronary artery disease and the development of myocardial infarction. *J Am Coll Cardiol* 1988;12:56–62.

10. Little WC, Constantinescu M, Applegate RJ, et al. Can coronary angiography predict the site of a subsequent myocardial infarction in patients with mild-to-moderate coronary artery disease? *Circulation* 1988;78:1157–1166.
11. Falk E. Plaque rupture with severe pre-existing stenosis precipitating coronary thrombosis: Characteristics of coronary atherosclerotic plaques underlying fatal occlusion thrombi. *Br Heart J* 1983;50:127–134.
12. Davies MJ, Richardson PD, Woolf N, et al. Risk of thrombosis in human atherosclerotic plaques: Role of extracellular lipid, macrophages and smooth muscle cell content. *Br Heart J* 1993;69:377–381.
13. Sherman CT, Litvack F, Grundfest W, et al. Coronary angioscopy in patients with unstable angina pectoris. *N Engl J Med* 1986;315:913–919.
14. Richardson RD, Davies MJ, Born GVR. Influence of plaque configuration and stress distribution on fissuring of coronary atherosclerotic plaques. *Lancet* 1989;2:941–944.
15. Moreno PR, Falk E, Palacios IF, et al. Macrophage infiltration in acute coronary syndromes: Implications for plaque rupture. *Circulation* 1994;90:775–778.
16. Galis ZS, Sukhova GK, Lark MW, et al. Increased expression of matrix metalloproteinases and matrix degrading activity in vulnerable regions of human atherosclerotic plaques. *J Clin Invest* 1994;94:2493–2503.
17. Galis ZS, Sukhova GK, Kranzhofer R, et al. Macrophage foam cells from experimental atheroma constitutively produce matrix-degrading proteinases. *Proc Natl Acad Sci USA* 1995;92:402–406.
18. DeWood MA, Spores J, Notske R, et al. Prevalence of total coronary occlusion during the early hours of transmural myocardial infarction. *N Engl J Med* 1980;303:897–902.
19. Maseri A, L'Abbate A, Baroldi, G et al. Coronary vasospasm as a possible cause of myocardial infarction: A conclusion derived from the study of preinfarction angina. *N Engl J Med* 1978;299:1271–1277.
20. Bogaty P, Hackett D, Davies G, et al. Vasoreactivity of the culprit lesion in unstable angina. *Circulation* 1994;90:5–11.
21. Moncada S, Gryglewski R, Bunting S, et al. An enzyme isolated from arteries transforms prostaglandin endoperoxides to an unstable substance that inhibits platelet aggregation. *Nature* 1976;263:663–665.
22. Furchgott RF, Zawadzki JV. The obligatory role of endothelial cells in the relaxation of arterial smooth muscle by acetylocholine. *Nature* 1980;299:372–376.
23. Yanagisawa M, Kurihara H, Kimura S, et al. A novel potent vasoconstrictor peptide produced by vascular endothelial cells. *Nature* 1988;332:411–415.
24. Egashita K, Inou T, Hirooka Y, et al. Impaired coronary blood flow response to acetylcholine in patients with coronary risk factors and proximal atherosclerotic lesions. *J Clin Invest* 1993;91:29–37.
25. Reddy KG, Nair RN, Sheehan HM, et al. Evidence that selective endothelial dysfunction may occcur in the absence of angiographic or ultrasound atherosclerosis in patients with risk factors for atherosclerosis. *J Am Coll Cardiol* 1994;23:833–843.
26. Willerson JT, Golino P, Eidt J, et al. Specific platelet mediators and unstable coronary artery lesions: Experimental evidence and potential clinical implications. *Circulation* 1989;80:198–205.

27. Braunwald E, Jones RH, Mark DB, et al. Diagnosis and managing unstable angina. *Circulation* 1994;90:6134–622.
28. DeWood MA, Stifer WF, Simpson CS, et al. Coronary arteriographic findings soon after non-Q wave myocardial infarction. *N Engl J Med* 1986;315:417–423.
29. Chesebro JH, Webster MWI, Zoldhelyi P, et al. Antithrombotic therapy and progression of coronary artery disease. *Circulation* 1992; (suppl III):III-100-III-111.
30. Falk E. Unstable angina with fatal outcome: Dynamic coronary thrombosis leading to infarction and/or sudden death: Autopsy evidence of recurrent mural thrombosis with peripheral embolization culminating in total vascular occlusion. *Circulation* 1985;71:699–708.
31. Brown ZG, Zhao XQ, Sacco DE, et al. Lipid lowering and plaque regression: New insights into prevention of plaque disruption and clinical events in coronary disease (based on FATS and other studies). *Circulation* 1993;87:1781–1791.
32. Blankenhorn DH, Hodis HN. Arterial imaging and atherosclerosis reversal. *Arterioscler Thromb* 1994;14:177–192.
33. Pedersen TR, Kjekshus J, Berg K, et al. Randomised trial of cholesterol lowering in 4,444 patients with coronary heart disease: The Scandinavian Simvastatin Survival Study (4S). *Lancet* 1994;344:1383–1389.

Chapter 2

Coronary Atherosclerotic Disease:
Pathological Background

Colin J. Schwartz, MD
and A. Bleakley Chandler, MD

Introduction

The category disorders of the coronary circulation comprises two clinical syndromes: angina pectoris (dolor) and myocardial infarction along with their variants.[1] The relation of these disorders to obstructive disease of the coronary arteries remained an enigma for centuries. The first definitive clinical description of effort angina is attributed to William Heberden (1818),[2] but he had no idea of the underlying cause. Although a severe degree of coronary artery disease had already been described at necropsy in association with the symptoms of angina pectoris, it was Jenner and Parry who suggested that the symptoms of angina pectoris might be related to disease of the coronary arteries. In his monograph on heart disease, Terence East (1957)[3] cites Jenner on the importance of the coronary arteries: " . . . the heart must suffer from their not being able fully to perform their duties." Jenner also continued with a prophetic remark: "[S]hould it be admitted that this is the cause of the disease, I fear the medical world may seek in vain for a remedy." The passage of some 200 years has seen considerable progress. Parry (1799), as cited by Sir Thomas Lewis (1932),[4] agreed with Jenner on the pathological basis of angina pectoris and the likely significance of an inadequate coronary circulation. Although early emphasis was on the extent of coronary artery disease, it is of interest that as long ago as 1867, Brunton[5] believed that angina pectoris resulted from coronary artery spasm, thus unwittingly anticipating the potential importance of the L-arginine nitric oxide pathway and the

From: Fuster V, (ed.) *Syndromes of Atherosclerosis: Correlations of Clinical Imaging and Pathology.* Armonk, NY: Futura Publishing Company, Inc.: © 1996.

endothelins in regulating coronary artery vasomotor reactivity in selected cases of angina. Even in the mid-20th century, however, coronary artery spasm was considered by one distinguished Oxford physician as " . . . a diagnosis of the destitute." Such problems notwithstanding, the functional relations between the state of the coronary arteries and the myocardium received little attention. Patients dying with angina pectoris were variously categorized as having either myocardial fatty change or a chronic myocarditis. It was the landmark observations of Weigert in 1880[6] that first and clearly established the critically important relations between massive coagulation necrosis of heart muscle and occlusive coronary artery disease. Subsequently, it was shown that the end result or healing of acute myocardial coagulation necrosis is a reparative or replacement fibrosis. Over the ensuing years there has been much dissent as to the role of occlusive thrombosis in the pathogenesis of myocardial infarction, due in no small measure to equating cases of sudden unexpected cardiac death, so-called subendocardial infarction, and full thickness or transmural (Q wave) infarction. It was only in 1974 that the causal role of thrombotic occlusion in the genesis of acute myocardial infarction was clearly reaffirmed. In a National Heart, Lung, and Blood Institute workshop consensus report by Chandler et al,[7] it was emphasized that thrombotic occlusions exhibit consistent temporal and spatial relations to areas of acute transmural (Q wave) myocardial infarction.

In this chapter we examine the nature of coronary atherosclerosis, its distribution within the coronary arteries, its relation to the severity of atherosclerosis in other arterial sites and the striking inflammatory cellular infiltrates associated with lesions. We also provide a brief overview of the mechanisms involved in pathogenesis. Additionally, we describe and review the role of occlusive thrombosis in differing types of infarction, the contributions that thrombi might make to atherogenesis, and the factors influencing thrombogenesis and clinical events.

Important Features of Coronary Atherosclerosis

Coronary atherosclerosis, like lesions in other arterial sites, is a complex disease affecting all three layers of the arterial wall. Intimal thickening is a dominant feature in which extensive fibrosis, smooth muscle cells, macrophage-derived foam cells, lymphocytes, proteoglycans, and a central necrotic lipid core are most prominent. It is important to recognize that the relative contributions of each of these features may vary considerably from lesion to lesion, and even within lesions. Medial thinning, which is associated with smooth muscle loss, is almost invariably associated with advanced lesions. Within the adventitia, a triad of changes are typically seen, particularly with severe lesions, namely a lymphocytic infiltrate, fibrosis, and neovascularization.

These changes are thought to represent an underlying autoimmune inflammatory response that occurs during the later stages of plaque evolution.[8] Table 1 summarizes the prevalence and degrees of adventitial lymphocytic infiltration relative to coronary artery plaque severity. Simply stated, coronary arteries microscopically free of disease exhibit no adventitial lymphocytic infiltrates. With some disease present, ie, fatty streaks or early transitional lesions, adventitial lymphocytes are observed in 18% of sites, while in sites with histologically severe or advanced lesions, lymphocytic infiltrates are present in 75% of the blocks examined, of which 23% are of a marked degree.

Several additional features of this adventitial lymphocytic infiltration deserve comment. Overall, and with but few minor inconsistencies, it is not arterial site-, age-, or gender-specific. Furthermore, it exhibits the same prevalence and relation to plaque severity in patients with myocardial infarction as in individuals from an unselected necropsy sample.[8] However, as shown in Table 2, there is a complex relation between coronary artery adventitial cellularity and thrombosis. Here, the relation between plaque severity and the grade of adventitial cellular infiltration in men with myocardial infarction is subdivided according to the presence

TABLE 1

Prevalence and Degree of Coronary Artery Adventitial Lymphocytic Infiltration

Microscopic Coronary Plaque		Percentage of Histologic Blocks Examined (%) Grade of Cellularity	
Severity	Absent	Slight	Marked
Free n=223	100	0	0
Present n=149	82	15	3
Severe n=75	25	52	23

n = number of histologic blocks examined. Adapted from Reference 1.

TABLE 2

Prevalence (%) and Degree of Coronary Adventitial Lymphocytic Infiltration According to Plaque Severity and the Presence and Nature of Occluding Thrombi

Grade of Adventital Cellularity

Microscopic Coronary Plaque Severity	Blocks without Thrombi n=348			Blocks with Recent Thrombi n=56			Blocks with Recanalizing Thrombi n=66		
Severity	Absent	Slight	Marked	Absent	Slight	Marked	Absent	Slight	Marked
Free n=101	100	0	0	—	—	—	—	—	—
Present n=142	77	19	4	31	50	19	—	—	—
Severe n=227	35	41	24	5	65	30	30	48	22

Adapted from Reference 1.

n = number of histologic blocks examined

and histologic nature of occluding thrombi. In arteries with no histologic evidence of thrombosis, the relation between plaque severity and the degree of adventitial cellularity is similar to that in the unselected necropsy samples. However, in those arteries with recent but not recanalizing thrombi, the prevalence of adventitial lymphocytic infiltration is significantly greater for comparable degrees of plaque severity. Whether these findings reflect a thrombogenic influence of the underlying inflammatory process or an arterial response to the thrombosis is an important question requiring clarification.

Coronary Atherosclerosis: Distribution of Stenotic Lesions and Their Severity in Myocardial Infarction

Atherosclerosis does not affect the various branches of the coronary arteries in a uniform manner. In fact, all branches of the left coronary artery show a significantly greater prevalence of severe stenosis than their right coronary counterparts. The highest prevalence of severe stenosis is seen in the left anterior descending artery and its two main branches. These striking differences in prevalence of stenosis between the branches of the right and left coronary arteries, coupled with the predominance of lesions in the left anterior descending system, very likely reflect anatomically determined differences in fluid-mechanical stresses, together with arterial mechanical stresses differentially exerted on different arterial segments during the cardiac cycle. Furthermore, both age and gender influence the severity of coronary artery stenosis. Severe narrowing shows an increase in prevalence with age in both men and women, peaking in men in the age group 65 to 74 years, with an apparent decline thereafter. Men are more severely affected than women in all age groups up to 75 years and over, when the gender differences is much less distinct.[1]

When considering men and women with myocardial infarction, it is clear that as a group, they have more severe coronary artery stenosis than their age-matched counterparts from an unselected necropsy samples. However, it is important to note that there is substantial overlap between the groups, with many patients from unselected necropsy samples having considerably more coronary artery stenosis than patients with myocardial infarction. It is interesting that while men from an unselected necropsy sample under the age of 75 years have more coronary stenosis than their female counterparts, this gender difference is largely abolished or even reversed in women with myocardial infarction.[1] Additionally, a significant subset of patients with myocardial infarction have surprisingly low coronary stenosis grades. These observations suggest that it is not merely the degree nor extent of coronary stenosis alone that is a determinant of infarction, but rather the propensity to develop thrombotic occlusion. Thus, the emerging concept and potential significance of plaque stabilization and thromboresistance assume a new level of clinical relevance.

Coronary Atherosclerosis: A Manifestation of a Systemic Disorder

We have stated that coronary atherosclerosis does not occur uniformly within the branches of the coronary arteries, but exhibits a predictably consistent focal topography. Similarly, atherosclerotic lesions in other arterial sites including the carotid, iliac, and vertebral arteries, as well as the aorta do not occur at random, but develop in relation to areas of arterial branching, curvature, or flow dividers. Hemodynamically, lesions appear to develop preferentially in areas of low shear stress associated with domains of reversing blood flow.[9,10] In spite of the predictably focal nature of atherosclerosis, it is paradoxically a systemic process. In an unselected necropsy population, there is a clear and strong correlation between the degree of both carotid and iliac artery stenosis and the severity of coronary artery stenosis; this correlation between coronary, carotid, and iliac artery stenosis in enhanced even further in patients with myocardial infarction, in whom the prevalence and degree of carotid and iliac artery stenosis are significantly greater. Similarly, the aortic area affected by atherosclerotic lesions in patients with myocardial infarction is greater than in comparable individuals comprising an unselected necropsy sample.[1]

Both carotid artery and iliac artery plaque ulceration are clearly age-dependent phenomena, the frequency of plaque ulceration increasing with age in men and women. Plaque ulceration is also markedly gender dependent, with a lower prevalence in women than in men. In Table 3, the percentage prevalence of carotid and iliac artery plaque ulceration is greater in patients with myocardial infarction than in an unselected necropsy population of comparable age and gender. It is clear then, that patients with myocardial infarction, and a greater prevalence and degree of coronary artery stenosis, differ qualitatively as well as quantitatively in terms of disease in their carotid and iliac arterial systems. This observation is consistent with the greater aortic surface area affected

TABLE 3

Percentage Prevalence of Plaque Ulceration
According to Site in an Unselected Necropsy
Population and Patients with Myocardial Infarction

		Site Prevalence of Ulceration by Systems(%)		
	Neither	Carotid	Iliac	Both Carotid and Iliac
Unselected	79	4.4	14.3	2.3
Myocardial Infarction	65	6.1	21.5	7.4

Adapted from Reference 1.

by complicated plaques of which ulceration is a component. In summary, using cardiac infarction as an index, it is feasible to define a population that is more atherosclerotic quantitatively and qualitatively than a comparable population without infarction. These studies are consistent with the weight of clinical opinion that concludes that clinically overt occlusive arterial disease in any one site is but a manifestation of a widespread or systemic disorder.

Coronary Thrombosis in Myocardial Infarction

The consensus report by Chandler et al[7] concluded that occlusive coronary thrombi play a causal role in the development of acute transmural myocardial infarction. In the resolution of this problem, two issues were of particular importance. The first was the recognition that so-called subendocardial infarction is a different entity from transmural or Q wave infarction and is typically associated with a low frequency of occlusive thrombi.[11–14] In the preceding studies, the frequency of occlusive thrombi ranged from 10% to 27%. The second was the realization that only 30% to 40% of cases of sudden unexpected cardiac death are associated with myocardial infarction, thus providing an explanation for the low frequency (25% to 30%) of occlusive coronary thrombi found in these cases. It is important to add that the frequency of thrombotic occlusion is related to infarct age. In particular, infarcts having a histologic age of over 4 months exhibit an occlusion frequency of only 67%[1] (Table 4),

TABLE 4

Frequency and Nature of Occlusive Lesions in Patients with Myocardial
Infarction According to the Age of the Infarct or of the Youngest Infarct if More Than One is Present

Infarct Age (Histologic)	Number of Patients n	Distribution of Lesions, %		Nature of Occlusions (% Distribution)		
		Occlusions*	Stenosis Only	Thrombus	Recanalizing Thrombus	Plaque
<2 days	16	100	0	66.6	13.9 (n=35)**	19.5
2–13 days	24	96	4	69.2	17.3 (n=52)	13.5
2–4 weeks	7	100	0	25.0	56.3 (n=16)	18.7
1–4 months	11	100	0	4.0	64.0 (n=25)	32.0
Over 4 months	21	67	33	0.0	80.0 (n=30)	20.0

*This category includes lesions in which a minute channel or fleck of injection dye was observed.
**n = the number of occlusions seen in each infarct-age category.
Adapted from Reference 1.

whereas in more recent infarcts the occlusion frequency exceeds 95%. With increasing infarct age, the nature of the occluding lesions undergoes a transition from recent thrombus to recanalizing thrombus to atherosclerotic plaque (Table 4). Occlusive lesions are also frequently multiple.

Not surprisingly, coronary artery occlusions are predominantly located in the branches of the left coronary artery (69%) relative to all branches of the right coronary artery (31%) (Table 5). It is also interesting that 50% of all the occlusive lesions found are located in the left anterior descending artery and its two main branches (Table 5).

As indicated earlier, although patients with myocardial infarction have, as a group, a more severe grade of coronary artery stenosis than a comparable control population, cases of thrombotic occlusion are frequently found in association with relatively small lipid-rich plaques containing an extracellular lipid core and a thin collagenous cap. Plaque fissuring in such fragile or vulnerable lipid-rich lesions exposes their thrombogenic constituents,[15–17] and is in all likelihood a prelude to the initiation of occlusive thrombosis leading to the initiation of myocardial infarction or unstable angina. Ulceration, however, is not always associated with significant thrombosis.[18] Plaque fissures occur preferentially at the plaque shoulders, and particularly at sites where the macrophage density is greatest.[19–21] This important topic is reviewed by Davies[22] and by Richardson,[23] who have critically examined the mechanics of the processes involved. The subject is addressed further in Chapter 6 of this book by Falk. It remains unknown, however, if endothelial dysfunction associated with defective thromboresistance can facilitate

---

TABLE 5

Anatomic Distribution of Coronary Artery Occlusions Expressed as a Percentage of all Occlusions

Left Coronary System	%				Right Coronary System	%	
Left anterior descending	23						
Left anterior descending	1	17	17	51			
Left anterior descending	2	11	11				
Left circumflex	12				Right circumflex	14	
Left marginal	4				Right marginal	3	
Left posterior descending	2				Right posterior descending	3	3
All branches of left coronary system	69				All branches of right coronary system	31	

Adapted from Reference 1.

arterial thrombogenesis in the absence of endothelial denudation, ulceration, or plaque fissuring.

The Pathogenesis of Coronary Atherosclerosis

It is probable that the pathogenesis of coronary atherosclerosis is similar to that in different arterial beds. To simplify this subject, lesion pathogenesis has been divided into three stages that have been reviewed elsewhere.[10,24]

Initial Events in Pathogenesis: Stage I

In Table 6 we summarize the early events of atherogenesis that occur predictably and preferentially in lesion-prone sites, which are considered to be areas of low hemodynamic shear stress associated with domains of reversing blood flow. Many of the early events of stage I are strikingly amplified by hypercholesterolemia and its associated dyslipoproteinemias. The end result of this cascade of initial events is the so-called fatty streak, in which macrophage- derived foam cells are dominant, and the lipid is predominantly intracellular. There is considerable evidence that fatty streaks are reversible lesions. They are clearly regarded as precursors of the more advanced fibrous plaques, although it is by no means certain that all fatty streaks necessarily progress to become fibrous plaques. In other words, the mechanisms for their initiation and subsequent progression may differ. Key initial events are an enhanced focal intimal influx and accumulation of plasma proteins and lipoproteins, an increased net intimal oxidative stress, with a resulting oxidative modification of lipoprotein components, en-

---

TABLE 6

Stage I: Initial Events in Atherogenesis

The focal hemodynamic environment: low shear, reversing flow
Increased intimal influx and accumulation of plasma proteins and lipoproteins:
    LDL, LDL-B, Lp(a)
A net intimal oxidative stress status
Oxidative modification of intimal lipoproteins
Focal blood monocyte recruitment to the intima: endothelial activation,
    endothelium-leukocyte adhesion
Monocyte-macrophage activation
Intimal foam cell formation: macrophage scavenger receptors
The Fatty Streak

TABLE 7

Protean Biological Consequences of Lipoprotein Oxidation

Cytotoxicity: necrosis, apoptosis?

Recognition by the scavenger receptor pathways
Augmented gene expression and synthesis of MCP-1, IL-1B, MCSF, etc

Inactivation of the L-arginine-nitric oxide pathway
Endothelial activation: procoagulant activity
Immunogenicity
Altered platelet function
Augmented endothelin synthesis

dothelial activation, and a focally augmented recruitment of blood monocytes to the arterial intima. Because of the chemical and conformational changes that accompany oxidative modification of lipoproteins, they are avidly recognized and internalized via the nondownregulating macrophage scavenger pathways.[25] The result is the formation of the cholesterol- and cholesteryl ester-rich macrophage-derived foam cell, which is a dominant feature of the early and evolving atherosclerotic lesion. As outlined in Table 6, these interactive cascades ultimately give rise to the foam cell-rich lesion we know as the fatty streak. Before describing the mechanisms leading to the transition of the fatty streak to the fibrous plaque, it is appropriate to emphasize the protean nature of the biological consequences of low-density lipoprotein oxidation, which include influences on monocyte recruitment, vasomotor regulation, and possibly hemostasis/thrombosis. Some of the salient biological consequences of lipoprotein oxidation are listed in Table 7; these consequences underscore the potential importance of this phenomenon in vascular pathobiology.

Progression of the Fatty Streak to the Fibrous Plaque: Stage II

The formation of fibrous plaques has an explosive growth in the second and third decades of life. This transitional progression is of considerable importance as it represents the metamorphosis of the relatively reversible fatty streak to the less reversible fibrous plaque. As indicated above, not all fatty streaks necessarily undergo this transition. In Table 8 the key mechanisms leading to this progression sequence are listed. Progression of the fatty streak to the fibrous plaque is dependent not only on the persistence of the initial events

---

TABLE 8

Process Pivotal to Transition of the Fatty Streak to the Fibrous Plaque: Stage II

Persistence of mechanisms leading to lesion initiation
Inadequacy of processes facilitating lesion regression/reversal
Foam cell death: formation of an extracellular lipid core
Smooth muscle cell migration to or proliferation in the intima
Connective tissue synthesis: collagens, elastins, proteoglycans

---

leading to the development of the fatty streak (Table 6), but also on inadequacies in the mechanisms facilitating reversal or regression, together with the superimposition of several processes that are pivotal in the transitional process. The latter include foam cell death leading to the formation of an extracellular necrotic lipid core; smooth muscle cell migration to and proliferation in the intima; and the excessive synthesis of fibrillary and nonfibrillary connective tissue elements (collagens, elastins, proteoglycans). Possibly resulting from the cytotoxic influences of oxidatively modified low-density lipoproteins, foam cell death is likely a major contributor to the extracellular plaque core lipid. A plasma contribution is also feasible. This extracellular lipid core is important for at least two reasons. First, because it is interstitial, it constitutes an essentially metabolically inert lipid pool not readily accessible to biological clearance mechanisms. Second, in all likelihood it contributes to overall plaque fragility and vulnerability to plaque fissuring.

Smooth muscle cells are an important component of the evolving and established fibrous plaque. Teleologically they may reflect a reparative or healing process. Their migration to and proliferation in the arterial intima are another key transitional event that may be regulated by at least three families of proteins, including the fibroblast growth factors, platelet-derived growth factors, and thrombin, together with the proto-oncogenes c-*fos* and c-*myc*.[26–30] To date, the factors influencing connective tissue synthesis by intimal smooth muscle cells either qualitatively or quantitatively remain uncertain, but they appear likely to include both fluid mechanical as well as cyclical stretching forces.

Maturation of the Fibrous Plaque: Stage III

Features of the advanced or complex fibrous plaque are summarized in Table 9. Typically, these lesions exhibit a considerable

TABLE 9
Plaque Maturation: The Advanced or Complex Fibrous Plaque: Stage III

Surface ulceration or denudation
Plaque fissure or fracture
Thrombosis: mural or occlusive
Intramural hemorrhage
Calcification
Plaque neovascularization
Plaque granulomata
Adventitial lymphocytic inflammation: autoimmune

degree of medial thinning, and in 80% of lesions there is evidence of chronic inflammation as reflected by the adventitial lymphocytic infiltration. Other inflammatory components include the presence of granulomatous foci, usually surrounding the lipid core, and the presence of scattered lymphocytes within the plaque itself. Advanced lesions may exhibit areas of surface ulceration, mural thrombosis, or intramural plaque hemorrhage. The latter often occurs at the plaque shoulders, a site where plaque neovascularization is usually prominent. It is at these sites where hemosiderin deposits, presumably footprints of past hemorrhage, are usually seen. The plaque shoulders are also, as already discussed, the preferred location for the development of plaque fissures. Frequently, mural thrombi in varying stages of organization are observed. The important contribution thrombi make to the later stages of plaque development is discussed below. Calcification in advanced lesions is both common and frequently extensive. Under certain conditions, calcium deposits may alter arterial compliance and enhance the likelihood of plaque fissuring. Whether the presence of calcification detected by imaging technique can be used to identify coronary artery atherosclerotic lesions during life still needs further clinical evaluation.

The Role of Thrombosis in the Development of Coronary Atherosclerosis

No overview of the pathological background of coronary artery disease would be complete without a brief discussion of the important role thrombosis plays in the development and progression of atherosclerotic lesions. This topic has been the subject of a number of reviews.[31-33] Historically, the celebrated pathologist Carl von Rokitansky[34] is credited with the original proposal that thrombosis might contribute significantly to plaque pathogenesis. This thrombogenic or encrustation hypothesis had sporadic champions, but it was only after the landmark and incisive observations of Duguid in 1946[35] that this concept received wide acceptance. An extensive literature derived from pathological studies in man indicates that plaque growth is to a significant degree dependent upon the organization of mural thrombi by smooth muscle cells and their incorporation by endothelial overgrowth.[1,36-40] One study of particular interest is that of Woolf and Carstairs[40] in which the frequency and topographic distribution of fluorescein-labeled antiplatelet and antifibrin antibodies in fatty streaks, small lipid plaques and advanced fibrous plaques were determined. Significant banded patterns of both fibrin-fibrinogen and platelet antigens were detected in advanced fibrofatty (fibrous) plaques but not in fatty streaks. There is also an abundance of experimental data indicating that thrombi may undergo a variety of organizational changes leading to lesions with many of the essential features of the atherosclerotic plaque.[32] It is not surprising, therefore, that in the revised list of risk factors for clinical coronary disease we must now add potential determinants of abnormal hemostasis and thrombosis, including hyperfibrinogenemia, factor VII, and plasminogen activator- inhibitor-1 (PA1-I).[41]

Acknowledgement

Thanks to our secretaries, Ms. Anna Juiel and Mrs. Marie Hiller, for manuscript preparation. We also gratefully acknowledge the many colleagues who have participated in studies reported here.

References

1. Mitchell JRA, Schwartz CJ. *Arterial Disease.* Oxford: Blackwell Scientific Publications; 1965:235–240.
2. Heberden W. *Commentaries on the History and Cure of Diseases.* Boston: Wells and Lilly; 1818:292.
3. East T. *The Story of Heart Disease.* London: Dawson; 1957:103.
4. Lewis T. Pain in muscular ischaemia. *Arch Intern Med* 1932;49:713–727.
5. Brunton TL. On the use of nitrite of amyl in angina pectoris. *Lancet* 1867;ii:97–98.
6. Weigert C. Uber die Pathologischen Geriunungsvorgange. *Virchows Arch Path Anat* 1880;79:87.
7. Chandler AB, Chapman I, Erhardt LR, et al. Coronary thrombosis in

myocardial infarction. Report of a workshop on the role of coronary thrombosis in the pathogenesis of acute myocardial infarction. *Am J Cardiol* 1974;34:823–833.

8. Schwartz CJ, Mitchell JRA. Cellular infiltration of the human arterial adventitia associated with atheromatous plaques. *Circulation* 1962;26: 73–78.

9. Schwartz CJ, Sprague EA. Vascular endothelium and hemodynamic stress. *Nutr Metab Cardiovasc Dis* 1992;2:99–100.

10. Schwartz CJ, Valente AJ, Hildebrandt EF. The pathogenesis of atherosclerosis and coronary heart disease: An evolving consensus. In: Born GVR, Schwartz CJ, eds: *New Horizons in Coronary Heart Disease.* London: Current Science; 1993:1.1–1.10.

11. Miller RD, Burchell HB, Edwards JE. Myocardial infarction with and without acute coronary occlusion. A pathologic study. *Arch Intern Med* 1951;88:597–604.

12. Ehrlich JC, Shinohara Y. Low incidence of coronary thrombosis in myocardial infarction. A restudy by serial block technique. *Arch Pathol Lab Med* 1964;78:432–445.

13. Davies MJ, Woolf N, Robertson WB. Pathology of acute myocardial infarction with particular reference to occlusive coronary thrombi. *Br Heart J* 1976;38:659–664.

14. Silver MD, Baroldi G, Mariani P. The relationship between acute occlusive coronary thrombi and myocardial infarction studied in 100 consecutive patients. *Circulation* 1980;61:219–227.

15. Barstad RM, Hamers M, Kierulf P, et al. Procoagulant human monocytes mediate tissue factor/factor VIIa-dependent platelet-thrombus formation when exposed to flowing nonanticoagulated human blood. *Arterioscler Thromb Vasc Biol* 1995;15:11–16.

16. Fernandez-Ortiz A, Badimon JJ, Falk E, et al. Characterization of the relative thrombogenicity of atherosclerotic plaque components: Implications for consequences of plaque rupture. *J Am Coll Cardiol* 1994;23:1562–1569.

17. Wilcox JN, Smith KM, Schwartz SM, et al. Localization of tissue factor in the normal vessel wall and in the atherosclerotic plaque. *Proc Natl Acad Sci USA* 1989;86:2839–2843.

18. Frink RJ, Ostrach LH, Rooney PA, et al. Coronary thrombosis, ulcerated atherosclerotic plaques and platelet/fibrin microemboli in patients dying with acute coronary disease. A large autopsy study. *J Inv Cardiol* 1990;2:199–210.

19. Falk E. Why do plaques rupture? *Circulation* 1992;86(suppl III):III-30–III-42.

20. Lendon CL, Davies MJ, Born GVR, et al. Atherosclerotic plaque caps are locally weakened when macrophage is increased. *Atherosclerosis* 1991;87:87–90.

21. Davies MJ, Richardson P, Woolf N et al. Risk of thrombosis in human atherosclerotic plaques: Role of extracellular lipid, macrophage and smooth muscle content. *Br Heart J* 1993;69:377–381.

22. Davies MJ. The progression of atherosclerosis—Role of plaque fissuring and thrombosis I. In: Born GVR, Schwartz CJ, eds: *New Horizons in Coronary Heart Disease*. London: Current Science; 1993:10a.1–10a.8.

23. Richardson PD. The progression of atherosclerosis—Role of plaque fissuring and thrombosis II. In: Born GVR, Schwartz CJ, eds: *New Horizons in Coronary Heart Disease*. London: Current Science; 1993:10b.1–10b.5.

24. Schwartz CJ, Valente AJ, Hildebrandt EF. Prevention of Atherosclerosis and end-organ damage: A basis for antihypertensive interventional strategies. *J Hypertension* 1994;12(suppl 5):S3–S11.
25. Goldstein JL, Ho YK, Basu SK, et al. Binding site on macrophages that mediates uptake and degradation of acetylated low density lipoprotein, producing massive cholesterol deposition. *Proc Natl Acad Sci USA* 1979;76:333–337.
26. Maciag T, Zhan X. The role of fibroblast growth factor-1 as a regulator of restenosis. In: Born GVR, Schwartz CJ, eds. *New Horizons in Coronary Heart Disease*. London: Current Science; 1993:15.1–15.8.
27. Jawien A, Bowen-Pope DF, Lindner V, et al. Platelet-derived growth factor promotes smooth-muscle migration and intimal thickening in a rat model of balloon angioplasty. *J Clin Invest* 1992;89:507–511.
28. Reidy MA, Fingerle J, Lindner V. Factors controlling the development of arterial lesions after injury. *Circulation* 1992;86(suppl III):III-43–III-46.
29. McNamara CA, Sarembock IJ, Gimple IW, et al. Thrombin stimulates proliferation of cultured rat aortic smooth muscle cells by a proteolytically activated receptor. *J Clin Invest* 1993;91:94–98.
30. Bauters C, Degroote P, Adamantidis M, et al. Proto-oncogene expression in rabbit aorta after wall injury. First marker of the cellular process leading to restenosis after angioplasty? *Eur Heart J* 1992;13:556–559.
31. Schwartz CJ, Chandler AB, Gerrity RG, et al. Clinical and pathological aspects of arterial thrombosis and thromboembolism. In: Chandler AB, Eurenius K, McMillan GC, et al, eds. *The Thrombotic Process in Atherogenesis*. New York/London: Plenum Press; 1978:111–126.
32. Schwartz CJ, Valente AJ, Kelley JL et al. Thrombosis and the development of atherosclerosis. Rokitansky revisited. *Semin Thromb Hemostasis* 1988;14:189–195.
33. Chandler AB. An overview of thrombosis and platelet involvement in the development of the human atherosclerotic plaque. In: Glagov S, Newman WP III, Schaffer SA, eds. *Pathology of the Human Atherosclerotic Plaque*. New York: Springer-Verlag; 1990:359–377.
34. von Rokitansky C. *A Manual of Pathological Anatomy*. London: Sydenham Society; 1852.
35. Duguid JB. Thrombosis as a factor in the pathogenesis of coronary atherosclerosis. *J Pathol Bacteriol* 1946;58:207–212.
36. Crawford T. Thrombotic occlusion and the plaque. In: Jones RJ, ed: *Evolution of the Atherosclerotic Plaque*. Chicago: University of Chicago Press; 1963:279–290.
37. Haust MD, Movat HZ, Moore RH. The role of fibrin thrombi in the genesis of the common white plaque in arteriosclerosis. *Circulation* 1956;14:483.
38. Heard BE. Mural thrombosis in the renal artery and its relation to atherosclerosis. *J Pathol Bacterol* 1949;61:635–637.
39. Morgan AD. *The Pathogenesis of Coronary Occlusion*. Oxford: Blackwell Scientific Publications; 1956:171.
40. Woolf N, Carstairs KC. Infiltration and thrombosis in atherogenesis. A study using immunofluorescent techniques. *Am J Pathol* 1967;51:373–386.
41. Meade TW. Epidemiology of atheroma, thrombosis and coronary heart disease. In: Born GVR, Schwartz CJ, eds: *New Horizons in Coronary Heart Disease*. London: Current Science; 1993:2.1–2.6.

Chapter 3

Clinical Correlation of Atherosclerosis:
Aortic Disease

Christopher K. Zarins, MD,
Chengpei Xu, MD, and Seymour Glagov, MD

Introduction

The aorta is a common site of atherosclerotic plaque formation. The infrarenal abdominal aortic segment is particularly vulnerable, whereas the thoracic aorta is relatively spared. Differences in susceptibility may be due to differences in the structure, composition, and nutrition of the aortic wall as well as differences in flow conditions and mechanical stresses which have been shown to be associated with a predisposition to atherosclerosis. Plaque depo-sition is associated with localized dilation in relation to erosion, atrophy, and thinning of the media, which predisposes the atherosclerosis-prone abdominal aorta to aneurysm formation with eventual fibrosis and calcification of the aortic wall. Circulating levels of elastase have been proposed as etiologic factors, but aneurysm formation in this location is regularly associated with atherosclerosis. Life-threatening rupture of an aortic aneurysm may be quite sudden. Progressive enlargement and transverse dimensions >4.0 cm increase the probability of rupture. The role of aneurysm configuration, wall erosion, and atrophy as well as the presence of florid atherosclerosis are probable major factors in the tendency to disruption. Mural thrombus formation tends to restore normal lumen caliber and stable flow, but the contribution of mural thrombosis to the tensile strength of the wall is not clear. Plaque deposition and

Supported by NIH Grant HL 15062 (SCOR-Atherosclerosis).

From: Fuster V, (ed.) *Syndromes of Atherosclerosis: Correlations of Clinical Imaging and Pathology.* Armonk, NY: Futura Publishing Company, Inc.: © 1996.

thrombosis may also occur without associated medial thinning or dilation and result in the development of lumen stenosis, obstruction to flow, and/or embolization to the lower extremities. The clinical risk factors and individual tissue reactions that may determine these differences in response remain to be defined.

Aortic atherosclerosis is characterized by the formation of intimal plaques with the usual morphological features of atherosclerosis including cellular proliferation, lipid accumulation, inflammation, necrosis, fibrosis, and dystrophic calcification. Plaque ulceration may result in embolization of plaque elements or thrombus formation. Plaque deposition is accompanied by arterial wall changes that result in artery enlargement. Erosion, atrophy, and associated weakening of the aortic wall may eventually result in aneurysm formation. In medium-sized muscular arteries with relatively small diameters, such as the coronary arteries, vessel enlargement may play an important role in maintaining lumen patency. In the large-sized aorta, atherosclerosis-associated enlargement is more likely to predispose to aneurysm formation. In the aorta, plaque deposition does not occur uniformly. The abdominal aorta is particularly susceptible to both plaque formation and aneurysmal enlargement, whereas the thoracic aorta is relatively resistant to both of these processes. In this chapter we examine the differences between the thoracic aorta and abdominal aorta, which may account for these segmental differences in vulnerability. We also consider the features of the atherosclerotic process and the associated artery wall changes that may underlie the pathogenesis of aneurysmal degeneration.

Contrasting Susceptibility of the Thoracic and Abdominal Aortic Segments

Although both the thoracic and abdominal aortic segments are prone to plaque formation, thoracic aortic plaques are usually less abundant, more discrete, less complicated, and less calcific than those in the abdominal aorta of the same individual.[1] Thoracic aortic plaques tend to develop predominantly in relation to intercostal branch ostia, but occlusive or obstructive atherosclerosis is rarely seen. Infrarenal abdominal aortic plaques and thrombosis may obstruct blood flow leading to intermittent claudication and other manifestations of distal ischemia. The thoracic aorta is also less prone to developing aneurysmal disease, whereas the infrarenal abdominal aorta often becomes aneurysmal, particularly in elderly men. The different susceptibilities of the thoracic and abdominal aorta may be related to local differences in aortic flow conditions and mechanical stresses as well as to differences in aortic wall structure, composition, and nutrition.

Structural Differences

The major physical differences between thoracic and abdominal segments are shown in Figure 1. Thoracic aortic diameter is greater than that of the abdominal aorta, and accordingly, has a greater number of transmedial lamellar units.[2] The thoracic aorta also contains relatively more elastin and less collagen than the abdominal aorta, allowing greater distensibility and pulse propagation.[3] The abdominal aorta, which contains proportionately more collagen, is stiffer and less compliant than the thoracic segment. Each abdominal aortic lamellar unit supports approximately 3000 dynes/cm circumferential tension, whereas each thoracic lamellar unit supports about 2000 dynes/cm. The outer two thirds of the human thoracic aortic wall is supplied with intramural medial vasa vasorum,[4] whereas the abdominal aorta is largely devoid of medial vasa vasorum. Because intramural vasa vasorum are largely absent from the abdominal aorta, nutrition is presumably dependent primarily on diffusion from the lumen. Thus, even early

COMPARISON OF HUMAN THORACIC AND ABDOMINAL AORTA

	DIAMETER (MM)	WALL THICKNESS (CM)	LAMELLAR UNITS (LU)		TENSION		
			NUMBER	THICKNESS (MM)	TOTAL (DYNES/CM)	PER LU (DYNES/CM)	STRESS (DYNES/CM²)
THORACIC	17	9.5×10^{-2}	56	0.017	117,000	2,095	122×10^4
MEDIAL VASA IN OUTER 50%							
ABDOMINAL	13	7.3×10^{-2}	28	0.026	89,000	3,180	122×10^4
NO MEDIAL VASA							

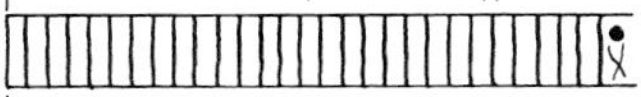

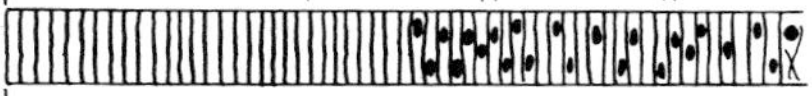

INTIMA

FIGURE 1. *Comparison of human thoracic and abdominal aortic segments. The thickness of the media of the abdominal aorta is appropriate for its diameter, but the number of its medial lamellar units is relatively low for the diameter compared with the thoracic aorta. Media total tension of the abdominal aorta is appropriate for its diameter, but tension per lamellar unit is higher than in the thoracic portion. Furthermore, the abdominal aortic media, only 29 lamellar units thick, is avascular. None of the the avascular aortic medias or avascular zones of vascular aortic medias of mammals studied are as thick as the abdominal aorta of humans. Other mammals aortas that have comparably elevated tensions per lamellar unit have more than 29 lammellae and vasa vasorum. LU indicates lamellar unit.*

intimal plaque deposition may augment the barrier to diffusion, rendering the abdominal aortic media vulnerable to ischemic degeneration and atrophy. Intimal plaque formation would also be expected to increase the diffusion distance across the wall, predisposing to processes that may promote inflammatory cell infiltration, lipid accumulation, and further plaque formation. Extension into the plaque of reactive vasa vasorum may help to clear lipid from the intimal lesion, but this may also induce further proliferation and plaque enlargement. Conversely, failure of vasa vasorum ingrowth may result in arterial wall atrophy and promote aneurysm formation. Thus, differences in structure and nutrition would appear to be associated with the differing vulnerabilities of the thoracic and abdominal aorta.

Flow Conditions

Hemodynamic factors are important in plaque localization, particularly at branch points, bends, and bifurcations. Detailed quantitative correlative studies of the carotid bifurcation reveal that plaques tend to form in regions of reduced wall shear stress and flow separation[5] and where wall shear stress oscillates in direction in the course of the cardiac cycle.[6] The thoracic aorta is exposed to relatively high flow rates, with outflow through the cerebral, upper extremity, and visceral artery branches. The renal arteries alone account for approximately 25% of the cardiac output. In contrast, the infrarenal abdominal aorta supplies mainly the lower extremities, where flow is quite variable depending on exercise conditions. In our increasingly sedentary society, walking and lower extremity exercise is diminished and the abdominal aorta is likely exposed to relatively low flow rates and oscillating wall shear stress over prolonged periods of time. In addition, flow reverses direction during the cardiac cycle in the abdominal aorta, as it is in vulnerable regions at the carotid bifurcation. Therefore, the abdominal aorta would be subjected to the adverse hemodynamic effects associated with low wall shear stress and oscillation of shear stress direction, which favor plaque formation.[7] In contrast, the thoracic aorta is not subjected to these flow-related predisposing hemodynamic risk factors. Experimental model flow studies of the abdominal aorta reveal, however, that the adverse hemodynamic conditions can be eliminated or minimized by simulating the high flow conditions that prevail during exercise.[8]

Atherosclerotic Arterial Enlargement

Arterial enlargement during atherogenesis may compensate for increasing plaque size and prevent or retard the development of lumen stenosis. This process may occur as a result of local increases in flow associated with periodic temporary narrowing of the lumen produced by an encroaching intimal plaque. The increase in wall shear stress may be expected to stimulate endothelial release of nitric oxide and/or other factors resulting in smooth muscle relaxation in the media and artery dilation.[9] Ongoing increases in radius would be expected to cease when baseline wall shear stress is restored, which has been noted in arteries proximal to arteriovenous fistulas.[10] Alternatively, the plaque may induce direct proteolytic or involutional changes in the media underlying the plaque with resulting dilation. Thinning of the media is commonly seen beneath atherosclerotic plaques regardless of location, with associated eccentric outward bulging of the underlying artery wall.[11] Compensatory enlargement has been demonstrated in human coronary arteries,[12,13] carotid arteries at the bifurcation,[14] and in the superficial femoral arteries[15] as well as in experimental atherosclerosis in primates in coronary,[16,17] carotid,[18] and superficial femoral artery sites.[19] Enlargement accompanied by increasing atherosclerotic plaque formation has also been demonstrated in our own recent studies of the human thoracic and abdominal aorta. We have found that abdominal aortic enlargement is closely related to the degree of atherosclerotic plaque deposition, whereas thoracic aorta enlargement is more closely linked to increasing age.

Atherosclerotic Medial Thinning

Thinning of the media with loss of normal structure and composition is a common feature in atherosclerosis and is a constant feature in abdominal aortic aneurysm formation. Human aortic aneurysms are characterized by extensive atrophy of the media with almost total loss of normal lamellar architecture (Figure 2). The media is usually almost totally devoid of the usual elastin layers and is converted into a narrow and calcific fibrous band. In nonaneurysmal aortas, recent morphological studies show that the abdominal aorta is much more prone to media atrophy beneath atherosclerotic lesions than is the thoracic aorta. The microanatomic features of abdominal aortic structure and the susceptibility of this region to atherosclerosis and to the resulting

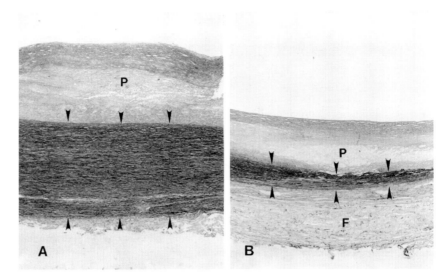

FIGURE 2. *Representative transverse sections of the thoracic and abdominal aorta. The thoracic aorta* **(A)** *has a well-developed plaque (P), but little or no thinning of the media. The lamellar micro-architecture of the aortic wall is largely preserved. The abdominal aorta* **(B)** *has a large plaque (P) with substantial atrophy and thinning of the underlying media (indicated by arrows) as well as associated fibrosis of the adventitia (F). (Magnification ×50).*

erosive effects on the media are the main features that correspond to the special susceptibility of this aortic segment to aneurysm formation. Experimental studies confirm the importance of the destruction of the medial lamellar architecture in the pathogenesis of aneurysms[20] and reveal that diet-induced atherosclerosis may result in the thinning of the media and aneurysm formation.[21] A controlled trial of cholesterol-lowering therapy in monkeys revealed plaque regression, thinning of the media, and aneurysmal dilation of the abdominal aorta.[21] These observations suggest that aneurysm formation is mainly a manifestation of atherosclerotic artery wall degeneration. Thus, observations of the atherosclerotic process in humans and experimental animals suggest possible mechanisms for aneurysm formation related directly to erosion of the artery wall by plaque components.

Although intimal plaque deposition is accompanied by compensatory arterial enlargement and is often associated with atrophy of the underlying media, stable early atherosclerotic plaques may actually lend structural tensile support to the artery wall, particu-

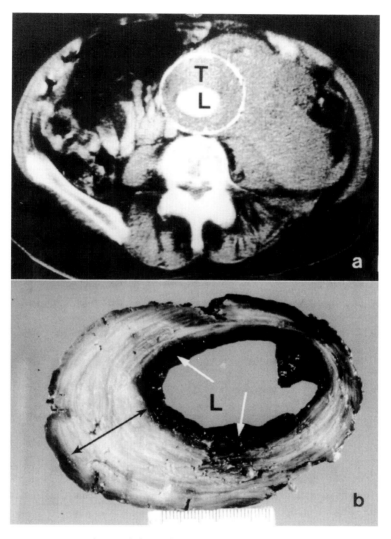

FIGURE 3. *A typical mural thrombus in an abdominal aortic aneurysm. (**a**) A computerized tomography scan shows the aneurysm containing the thrombus (T) and a lumen (L) of almost normal caliber. (**b**) The thrombus consists of layers of compressed fibrin (double arrow) and a superficial layer of fresh thrombus (white arrows). There is no evidence of fibrous cap formation or endothelium at the lumen side of such thrombi.*

larly when fibrogenesis is a principle feature of plaque formation.[14] During progression of the disease process, however, or during plaque regression, proteolytic enzymes such as matrix metallopro-teinases are released, and aortic wall thickness and plaque compo-sition are altered, resulting in insufficient tensile and structural support of the aortic wall.[22,23] Progressive aneurysmal enlargement would then be expected to occur, accounting for the localized and selective nature of aneurysm formation in the most atherosclerosis-prone segment of the human aorta. During the dilational reaction, the enlarged lumen tends to be partially filled by mural thrombus. The residual lumen is usually maintained at nearly normal caliber, and the thrombus is often compact and stable, tending to prevent distal embolization (Figure 3).[24] Presumably, flow rate at the thrombus surface associated with the persistence of near-normal lumen caliber prevents further platelet adhesion and thrombus ac-cretion, thus avoiding the progression to occlusion. The role of mural thrombus in providing tensile support to the thinned wall is not yet clear.

Conclusion

Aneurysms appear at a relatively late phase of plaque evolution when plaque and media atrophy predominate, rather than at ear-lier phases when cell proliferation, fibrogenesis, and lipid accumu-lation characterize plaque progression. The major late complication of abdominal aortic aneurysm formation is sudden life-threatening rupture. Rapid progression in aneurysm diameter and diameters exceeding 4.0 cm have been found to increase the probability of disruption and have been considered as indications for preventive surgical intervention. Macrophages involved with repair processes and resorption or alteration of lipids during evolution and regres-sion of atherosclerotic lesions are likely to be important sources of the proteolytic enzymes, which appear to be involved in aneurys-mal enlargement. Although circulating proteolytic enzymes such as elastase may play some role in abdominal aortic aneurysm forma-tion,[25] morphologically, abdominal aortic aneurysms are closely associated with atherosclerosis and the clinical risk factors associ-ated with atherosclerosis. Aneurysms rarely occur at this site in the absence of atherosclerosis and there is abundant evidence to indi-cate that the underlying changes in the aortic wall are associated with the metalloproteinases that are demonstrable in atheromatous plaques.

References

1. Glagov S. Hemodynamic risk factors: Mechanical stress, mural architecture, medial nutrition and the vulnerability of arteries to atherosclerosis. In: Wissler RW, Geer JC, eds. *The Pathogenesis of Atherosclerosis.* Baltimore: Williams and Wilkins; 1972:164–199.
2. Wolinsky H, Glagov S. Comparison of abdominal and thoracic aortic medial structure in mammals. Deviation from the usual pattern in man. *Circ Res* 1969;25:677–686.
3. Clark JM, Glagov S. Structural integration of the arterial wall: I. Relationships and attachments of medial smooth muscle cells in normally distended and hyperdistended aortas. *Lab Invest* 1979;40:587–602.
4. Wolinsky H, Glagov S. Nature of species differences in the medial distribution of aortic vasa vasorum in mammals. *Circ Res* 1973;20:409–421.
5. Zarins CK, Giddens DP, Bharadvaj BK, et al. Carotid bifurcation atherosclerosis. Quantitative correlation of plaque localization with flow velocity profiles and wall shear stress. *Circ Res* 1983;53:502–514.
6. Ku DN, Zarins CK, Giddens DP, et al. Pulsatile flow and atherosclerosis in the human carotid bifurcation: Positive correlation between plaque localization and low and oscillating shear stress. *Arteriosclerosis* 1985;5:292–302.
7. Zarins CK, Glagov S, Giddens DP, et al. Hemodynamic factors and atherosclerotic change in the aorta. In: Bergan JJ, Yao JST, eds. *Aortic Surgery.* Philadelphia: WB Saunders; 1988:17–25.
8. Ku DN, Glagov S, Moore JE, et al. Flow patterns in the abdominal aorta under simulated postprandial and exercise conditions: An experimental study. *J Vasc Surg* 1989;9:309–316.
9. Zarins CK. Adaptive responses of arteries. *J Vasc Surg* 1989;9:382.
10. Zarins CK, Zatina MA, Giddens DP, et al. Shear stress regulation of artery lumen diameter in experimental atherogenesis. *J Vasc Surg* 1987;5:413–420.
11. Glagov S, Zarins CK, Giddens DP, et al. Hemodynamics and atherosclerosis: Insights and perspectives gained from studies of human arteries. *Arch Path Lab Med* 1988;112:1018–1031.
12. Glagov S, Weisenberg E, Zarins CK, et al. Compensatory enlargement of human atherosclerotic coronary arteries. *N Engl J Med* 1987;316:1371–1375.
13. Zarins CK, Weisenberg E, Kolettis G, et al. Differential enlargement of artery segments in response to enlarging atherosclerotic plaques. *J Vasc Surg* 1988;7:386–394.
14. Massawa N, Glagov S, Zarins CK. Quantitative morphologic study of intimal thickening at the human carotid bifurcation. II. The compensatory enlargement response and the role of the intima in tensile support. *Atherosclerosis* 1994;107:147–155.
15. Blair JM, Glagov S, Zarins CK. Mechanism of superficial femoral artery adductor canal stenosis. *Surg Forum* 1990;41:359–360.
16. Bond MG, Adams MR, Bullock BC. Complicating factors in evaluating coronary artery atherosclerosis. *Artery* 1982;9:21–25.
17. Beere PA, Glagov S, Zarins CK. Retarding effect of lowered heart rate on conorary atherosclerosis. *Science* 1984;226:180–182.
18. Beere PA, Glagov S, Zarins CK. Experimental atherosclerosis at the carotid bifurcation of the cynomolgus monkey: Localization, compen-

satory enlargement and the sparing effect of lowered heart rate. *Arterioscler Thromb* 1992;12:1245–1253.

19. Armstrong ML, Heistad DD, Marcus ML, et al. Structural and hemodynamic responses of peripheral arteries of macague monkeys to atherogenic diet. *Arteriosclerosi*s 1985;5:336–346.

20. Zatina MA, Zarins CK, Gewertz BL, et al. Role of medial lamellar architecture in the pathogenesis of aortic aneurysms. *J Vasc Surg* 1984;1:442–448.

21. Zarins CK, Xu C-P, Glagov S. Aneurysmal enlargement of the aorta during regression of experimental atherosclerosis. *J Surg Res* 1992;15: 90–101.

22. McMillan WD, Patterson BK, Keen RR, et al. In situ localization and quantification of mRNA for 92-kD type IV collagenase and its inhibitor in aneurysmal, occlusive and normal aorta. *Arterioscler Thromb Vasc Biol* 1995;15:1139–1144.

23. Freestone T, Turner RJ, Coady A, et al. Inflammation and matrix metalloproteinases in the enlarging abdominal aortic aneurysm. *Arterioscler Thromb Vasc Biol* 1995;15:1145–1151.

24. Glagov S, Bassiouny HS, Giddens DP, et al. Intimal thickening: Morphogenesis, functional significance and detection. *J Vasc Invest* 1995;1:2–14.

25. Tilson MD, Newman KM. Proteolytic mechanisms in the pathogenesis of aortic aneurysms. In: Yao JST, Pearce WH, eds. *Aneurysms: New Findings and Treatments*. Norwalk; Appleton and Lange; 1994;3–10.

Chapter 4

Compositions of Atherosclerotic Lesions in Human Coronary Arteries and a Histologic Classification of Atherosclerosis

Herbert C. Stary, MD

Introduction

This chapter describes the compositions of atherosclerotic lesions in coronary arteries and provides a histologic classification of the lesions. Descriptions and classification are from a recent autopsy study of the coronary arteries and aortas of 1286 human subjects aged birth to 39 years who died as a result of accidents or violence in the New Orleans area.[1,2] Studies that were performed on the aortas of these cases are summarized in a companion chapter in this volume. The classification of the lesions is given in this chapter because although it was mainly derived from the studies of the coronary arteries, it also applies to the lesions in the aorta. Descriptions of lesions from other vascular beds by other authors indicate that the classification can also be used for lesions in other arteries. Our most detailed studies were in 691 cases in which the coronary arteries were restored to near in vivo dimensions and configurations by perfusing them with a fixative (glutaraldehyde) under pressure before removal from the heart. These 691 cases were selected from among the 1286 total cases for special handling and detailed histologic study because the interval between death and autopsy was relatively short (mean 9.5 hours) compared with the remaining cases, and we expected that the tissues would be well preserved. Sequential rather than single cross sections, each only 1μm thick, were evaluated, and the three-dimensional structure

From: Fuster V, (ed.) *Syndromes of Atherosclerosis: Correlations of Clinical Imaging and Pathology.* Armonk, NY: Futura Publishing Company, Inc.: © 1996.

TABLE 1

Terms Used to Designate Variants in Normal Intimal Histology

Terms for Thicker but Histologically Normal Intimal Segments Present in All Human Subjects From Birth	Other Terms Used in the Literature for Identical (and Probably Identical) Intimal Structures
Adaptive intimal thickening	
Eccentric type (eccentric intimal thickening)	Intimal cushion, intimal pad, spindle cell cushion, smooth muscle mass, mucoid fibromuscular plaque, focal intimal hyperplasia
Diffuse type (diffuse intimal thickening)	Musculoelastic intimal thickening, intimal hyperplasia

and composition of the coronary artery and of each lesion type were reconstructed. The best preserved cases were also studied by electron microscopy.

The natural history, ie, the sequence of lesions, was deduced by characterizing the intima and lesions in precisely defined locations of the coronary arteries in infants and children and then by studying the same locations in adolescents and young and middle-aged adults. The locations chosen for this study were known for their predisposition for developing pathologically advanced and clinically symptom-producing lesions. The locations are also known as advanced lesion-prone locations. When the advanced lesion-prone locations were examined in infants and older children,[3] the intima was found to be thicker than in adjacent locations in which advanced lesions in adults are not often found, or not found as early. To prevent possible misinterpretation of the normally thicker intima segments as lesions, their histology is described later in this chapter. Table 1 gives the nomenclature of the normally thicker intima segments.

Histologic Classification of Lesions

Eight characteristic types of lesion histology can be distinguished.[4,5] The contiguous nature of the histologies and the time of life at which each one emerges or predominates provide strong evidence that each represents a gradation or stage in a temporal sequence from the initial minimal change to changes associated with clinical manifestations.

The characteristic histologies were therefore arranged as a numbered sequence of lesion types. Table 2 gives an overview of the histologic nomenclature and compares it with nomenclature that is used when lesions are evaluated with the unaided eye. Lesion types I to IV are formed primarily through the accumulation of lipid in the intima. In types I and II, accumulation is mainly intracellular, in macrophages and smooth muscle cells. Type III lesions contain, in addition, at least as much lipid extracellularly. Type IV is the stage at which so much extracellular lipid has accumulated at the core of the intima that the intimal smooth muscle cells of that location are atrophic or dead. Clumps of mineral are microscopically visible in the dead cells and among the extracellular lipid particles.

Up to and including type IV, the lesions increase in size mainly because lipid accumulates in the intima at a relatively slow and predictable rate in the average susceptible individual. Lesion types V and VI are not just more advanced stages of lipid accumulation, but include components that formed through additional pathogenetic mechanisms. A main additional mechanism involves the accumulation of collagen. Presumably, intimal smooth muscle cells synthesize increased collagen after intimal structure is disorganized by the accumulated lipid. We designate a lesion as type V when substantial collagen has formed on top of a type IV lesion.

Other components that may increase lesion size are the thrombus and hematoma that may develop on or within a type IV or type V lesion. The result is the type VI morphology. Unless the episode is fatal, the thrombotic deposit and/or the hematoma are converted to extracellular matrix, particularly collagen. Thus a type VI morphology returns to the type V morphology, but the lesion is thicker and more obstructive than it was before the episode of thrombosis.

A type VII lesion is one that is largely calcified. The mineral replaces earlier accumulations of lipid and dead cells. Type VIII lesions consist mainly of layers of collagen, but lack lipid. Such lesions could be the consequence of lipid regression or of a thrombus that had formed in a part of the artery lacking a lipid accumulation.

By histologic criteria, lesion types IV, V, VI, VII, and VIII are considered advanced because they involve disorganization of the structure of the intima and changes in the contour of the arterial segment. Some lesions that are advanced histologically (especially type IV) may narrow the arterial lumen only minimally, and may not be visible by angiography. However, type IV lesions can quickly become clinically overt by developing a fissure at their surface, a hematoma, and a thrombus. Figure 1 gives an indication of the frequency of coronary artery lesions in the first four decades of life.

The effect of therapeutic lipid lowering on the histology of the various types of human lesions is not known. Clinical angiographic

TABLE 2

Terms Used to Designate Different Types of Human Atherosclerotic Lesions in Pathology

Terms for Atherosclerotic Lesions in the Histologic Classification		Other Terms for the Same Lesions Often Based on Appearance With the Unaided Eye	
Type I lesion	Initial lesion		
Type II lesion	Progression-prone (type IIa) Progression-resistant (type IIb)	Fatty streak	Early lesions
Type III lesion	Preatheroma	Intermediate lesion, transitional lesion	
Type IV lesion	Atheroma	Fibrolipid plaque, fibrous plaque, plaque	
Type V lesion	Fibroatheroma		Advanced lesions, raised lesions
Type VI lesion	Lesion with surface disruption, and/or hematoma-hemorrhage, and/or thrombotic deposit	Complicated lesion	
Type VII lesion	Calcific lesion	Calcified plaque	
Type VIII lesion	Fibrotic lesion	Fibrous plaque, plaque	

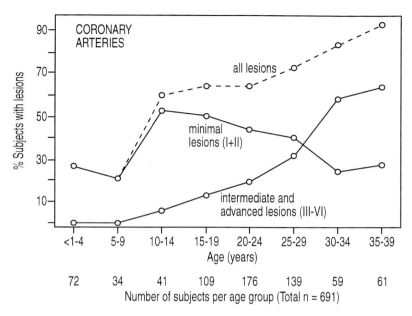

FIGURE 1. *The graph shows the percentages of all subjects with minimal lesions only or with intermediate (preatheroma) and advanced lesions plotted for successive 5-year age groups. The data were obtained by microscopy of 1-μm thick sections from the left coronary artery. Note that by the end of puberty, 61% of the population has some type of coronary artery lesion; by the end of the fourth decade, 95% of the population has some type of coronary artery lesion. The years after puberty are marked by a rise in preatheroma and advanced lesions that, as our microscopic data indicate, result from the progression of type IIa lesions. The progression of type IIa to preatheroma and advanced lesions is also the reason for the observed decline in the frequency of minimal lesions. Type VII and type VIII lesions were not found in the coronary arteries of this sample of the relatively young population. Reprinted with permission from Reference 2.*

studies that indicate the possibility of lesion regression in the coronary arteries of human subjects have not yet been clarified by histologic studies of these lesions. We have, however, investigated the histology of lesion regression in monkeys (unpublished observations), and some extrapolations to humans are possible. When the risk factors for atherosclerosis are drastically reduced, lesions of types I to III may disappear completely; the size of type IV may be reduced substantially; and types V and VI might be reduced somewhat. In some cases, type IV, V, and VI lesions might assume the compositions of type VII or type VIII lesions.

In addition to clarifying the natural history of atherosclerotic lesions, the present classification provides a framework of standard histologic morphologies with which images of lesions obtained with all types of clinical techniques can be compared. Matching the clinical image to the corresponding histologic lesion type could explain the clinical manifestations and allow individualization of treatment.

To provide a perspective for the histologic classification, earlier classifications are reviewed in the next section of this chapter. Subsequent sections describe intima in locations in which lesions tend to become advanced and also describe the eight types of atherosclerotic lesions.

A Brief History of Classifications of Atherosclerosis Used in Pathology

At least from the beginning of this century, fatty streaks and fibroatheromatous lesions (fibrous plaques) were suspected as two stages of atherosclerosis. Some observers, however, strongly disagreed that fibroatheromatous lesions were the consequence of fatty streak progression. Aschoff[6–8] recognized two components of atherosclerosis. One was lipid, which was deposited in the intima beginning in infancy. Aschoff designated this stage as atherosis (or atheromatosis). The other component was fibrosis (sclerosis, collagen formation), which was added to some of the lipid deposits in adults. Aschoff subdivided preadult atherosis into infant and pubertal phases. Atherosis in infants was described as yellow dots, visible at the root of the aorta with the unaided eye. Atherosis at puberty consisted of more extensive yellow streaks in many parts of the aorta and in coronary arteries. Microscopically, the dots and streaks consisted of mainly intracellular and some extracellular lipid in the intima. Both differed from adult lesions in the absence of fibrosis. In adults, atherosis and fibrosis (now called atherosclerosis) formed fibroatheromatous lesions.

After Aschoff, classifications were developed for the purpose of estimating the prevalence of individual lesion types in epidemiologic studies of risk factors. In these studies, lesions seen on the intimal surface of arteries that had been opened longitudinally, flattened, fixed in formalin, and stained for lipid were examined with the unaided eye. The terms for lesions used in these studies were close to the terms used by Aschoff. A classification described by several groups of investigators at about the same time[9–12] consists of the sequence *fatty streak, fibrous plaque,* and *complicated lesion.* The last term was used for fibroatheromatous lesions that developed a hematoma or had ulcerated or developed a thrombotic deposit. In addition to these three terms, the classification by the World Health Organization (WHO)[11] includes the term *atheroma* to distinguish advanced lesions with a predominantly lipid component (atheroma) from those with a predominantly collagenous one (fibrous plaque).

Whereas the terms *fibrous plaque* or *atheroma* are used in the above classifications, other authors substitute *fibroatheroma, atheromatous plaque, fibrolipid plaque,* or *fibrofatty plaque* (Table 2). In some studies the range of grossly visible lesion types was reduced to two: fatty streaks and raised lesions. The term atheroma as used in the WHO classification for a lesion type has sometimes been used to designate the entire disease process,[13] analogous to the term atherosclerosis. The classification consisting of the terms fatty streak, fibrous plaque, and complicated lesion was also used in histologic studies, but it became apparent that the histologic spectrum of lesion types was broader than that indicated by the gross terminology.

The Nature of the Intima in Locations in Which Advanced Lesions Tend to Develop in Coronary Arteries

Before describing individual lesion types in detail, it is necessary to define the undiseased intima of locations in which symptom-producing lesions are generally found. Human coronary arteries have both thin and thick intima segments normally. Differences in thickness are present in everyone from infancy, may develop in the fetus, and are the consequence of physiological variations in shear and tensile forces along the length of the arteries. The thicker intima segments are found at or near branches. These are the locations at which advanced lesions emerge in young adults and at which symptom-producing lesions are found. Without superimposed atherosclerosis, such adaptive thickening is self-limited in growth and does not obstruct blood flow at any age.[14]

In cross sections of a properly distended coronary artery, an adaptive thickening is an eccentric, crescent-shaped increase in the thickness of the outer wall of a bifurcation (Figure 2). The thickest part of the crescent may be up to twice the thickness of the media from infancy, although considerable individual variation in degree

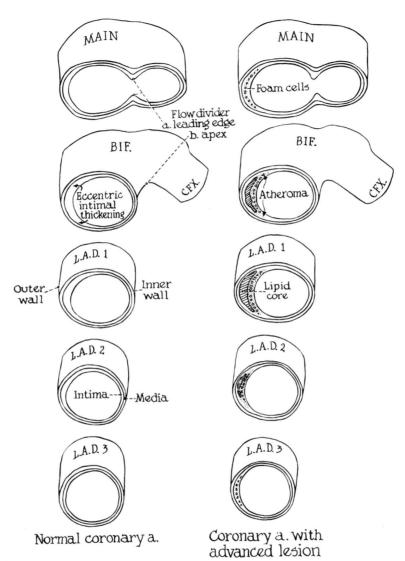

FIGURE 2. *Drawing of three-dimensional reconstructions of the proximal part of two coronary arteries. A normal coronary artery (**left**) shows the usual location, extent, and form of adaptive (eccentric) intimal thickening. The location, extent, and form of a type IV (atheroma) lesion is shown in the coronary artery to the right. Atheroma evolves in adaptive (eccentric) intimal thickening through several earlier lesion types or stages (see text). BIF. indicates bifuration; CFX., Circumflex; and L.A.D., left anterior descending. (Reprinted with permission from Reference 1.)*

has been found.[3] In an adult, it measures about 15 mm in length, is tapered at its proximal and distal ends, and is thickest at about the level of the apex of the flow divider or just beyond.

Adaptive intimal thickening is composed of two layers. To distinguish between the layers and discern their composition, 1-μm-thick sections must be used with light microscopy, or electron microscopy must be used. The inner layer is known as the proteoglycan-rich layer because it consists of a connective tissue matrix that is finely reticulated and interpreted as proteoglycan by electron microscopy. Smooth muscle cells are both rough endoplasmic reticulum -rich (synthetic) and myofilament-rich (contractile) types, and occur as widely spaced single cells. The part of the proteoglycan layer near the endothelium contains isolated macrophages. The usually much thicker, underlying layer is known as the musculoelastic layer because of the abundance of myofilament-rich smooth muscle cells and elastic fibers.

Adaptive thickening of the intima is often mistaken for an advanced lesion because the circumscribed extent, tapered periphery, and eccentric location are identical to the extent, outline, and location of an atheroma (Figures 2 and 3). The topographic correspondence between adaptive thickening and atheroma is explained by the fluid mechanical forces in these locations. The closely bounded low shear stress that elicits adaptive thickening also increases the time of interaction (the residence time) between blood-borne particles like low-density lipoprotein (LDL) and the lumen surface, consequently also increasing transendothelial diffusion.[15] Therefore, when atherogenic plasma lipoproteins and blood pressure exceed certain threshold levels in an individual, more LDL accumulates in these than in other locations. There is also evidence that components of the intima in the thicker segments retain LDL.[16] The frequent presence of even minimal accumulated lipid (such as would be called a fatty streak in locations with a thin intima) within or between the cells of an adaptive thickening has convinced many investigators that the entire thickening is atherosclerotic disease.

As a result of vascular collapse at death and recoil when in situ attachments are severed at autopsy, some localized adaptive thickenings may protrude above the remaining intimal surface. When coronary arteries are not redistended to in vivo dimensions before sections for microscopy are taken, the protrusions may appear as obstructions of the lumen. Unfortunately, at autopsy, collapsed rather than redistended coronary arteries are mostly examined, often with only the unaided eye, and distinguishing normal from atherosclerotic thickening may not be possible.

If adaptive thickening is accepted as a self-limited physiologi-

Coronary artery at
lesion-prone location

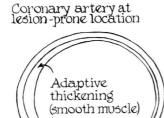

Type II lesion

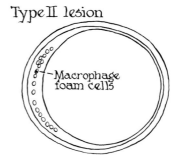

Type III (preatheroma)

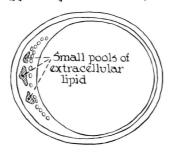

Type IV (atheroma)

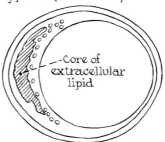

Type V (fibroatheroma)

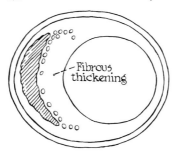

Type VI (complicated lesion)

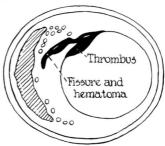

cal adjustment to normal differences in fluid mechanical forces along the length of arteries, then atherosclerotic disease constitutes only the superimposed changes. Thus adaptive intimal thickening is not a cause, prerequisite, or consequence of the lipid accumulation that occurs in the same location in hyperlipidemia. This topic is also discussed in the section on the type II lesion.

Type I Lesions

Type I lesions are the very initial and most minimal changes that do not thicken the arterial wall beyond what is normal for a location. They consist of only microscopically and chemically detectable lipid deposits in the intima and associated macrophage reactions. Type I lesions are frequent in infants and children and can also be found in some adults, particularly in those with little atherosclerosis or in locations of arteries that are lesion-resistant. Because of the limited technology available earlier in this century when many autopsy studies were performed, little was known about the initial histologic changes.

The histologic changes in the coronary artery intima consist of small, isolated groups of macrophages and macrophages that contain lipid droplets (macrophage foam cells).[1,3] These cells have been found to preferentially accumulate in regions of the intima with adaptive intimal thickening.

The accumulation of macrophages and macrophage foam cells in the arterial intima is also the initial cellular change in laboratory animals made hypercholesterolemic. Intimal foam cell accumulation is associated or preceded by an increased adherence of monocytes to the endothelium, particularly over atherosclerosis-prone regions of the intima.[17,18] Chemical and immunochemical data from laboratory animals indicate that the intimal macrophage increase and the formation of foam cells are a sequel to, and a cellular marker of pathological accumulations of LDL in the same locations.[19,20] The same lipoproteins are always present in the in-

---

FIGURE 3. *Drawing of cross sections taken from the identical, most proximal part of six left anterior descending coronary arteries. The morphology of the intima in this location ranges from adaptive intimal thickening that is always present in this lesion-prone location to a type VI lesion in a case with advanced atherosclerotic disease. The other cross sections show other atherosclerotic lesion types. Identical morphologies may be found in other lesion prone parts of the coronary and many other arteries. Reprinted with permissiom from Reference 5.*

tima but at lower concentrations. The threshold concentration that induces their accumulation and an increase in macrophages and the development of foam cells is not known.

Type II Lesions

Type II lesions include all those lesions that are known as fatty streaks. To the unaided eye, fatty streaks are visible on the inner surfaces of arteries as relatively flat, yellow-colored streaks or patches. They stain red with a Sudan dye and some become visible only at that time. The terms sudanophilic lesion or sudanophilia are sometimes used to refer to fatty streaks. However, the determining factor of a type II lesion is its histologic composition and not that it is often visible as a fatty streak. The nature of the arterial intima with which a type II lesion is colocalized determines in part whether and how it is seen on the intimal surface. When colocalized with an adaptive intimal thickening, macrophage foam cells accumulate some distance below the endothelial surface and may not be visible from the surface as a fatty streak even when stained with a Sudan dye. Type II lesions increase the thickness of the intima by less than a millimeter and do not obstruct arterial blood flow to any degree.

Type II lesions are more distinctly defined as lesions by light and electron microscopy than type I lesions and primarily consist of macrophage foam cells stratified in adjacent layers rather than being present as only isolated groups of a few cells. In addition to macrophages, intimal smooth muscle cells also contain lipid droplets. Macrophages without lipid droplets are more numerous than in type I lesions. T lymphocytes have been identified in type II lesions, but they are less numerous than macrophages.[21,22] The number of mast cells is greater than in the normal intima, but only isolated mast cells are found and their number is also much smaller than that of macrophages.[2] In laboratory animals the turnover of macrophage foam cells, endothelial cells, and smooth muscle cells is increased in experimentally produced fatty streaks.

Most of the lipid of type II lesions is in cells. The proportion of macrophages and smooth muscle cells containing lipid droplets varies, but in the coronary arteries most lipid is in macrophage foam cells. The extracellular space may contain lipid droplets that are smaller than in the cells and small vesicular particles. The derivation of this type of extracellular lipid is discussed in the section on the type IV lesion. Chemically, the lipid of type II lesions consists primarily of cholesterol esters, cholesterol, and phospholipids.

The main cholesterol ester fatty acids are cholesteryl oleate and cholesteryl linoleate.[23–26]

The locations in the arterial tree in which type II lesions can be found are relatively constant. Of the many type II lesions generally present in persons at risk, the subgroup that is colocalized with adaptive thickening tends to contain more lipid (more foam cells) and will be first to proceed to type III and then to atheroma (Figure 3). This subgroup has been called progression-prone, advanced lesion-prone, or the type IIa lesion. The larger subgroup of type II lesions that either do not progress, or progress only slowly, or only in persons with very high plasma levels of atherogenic lipoproteins, are found in segments with relatively thin intima and may be called progression-resistant or advanced lesion resistant, or type IIb. Whether a type II lesion develops at all and whether it is type IIa or type IIb is determined in large part by the mechanical forces that act on a particular part of the vessel wall. The influence of fluid mechanical forces on intima thickness and on the development of lesions was discussed in the section on the nature of the intima.

Type III Lesions

The *term type III* lesion applies to the stage of development that is histologically the bridge between minimal lesions and atheroma. The type III lesion is also known as preatheroma[1–3] and as intermediate lesion.[27] Type III lesions thicken the intima only slightly more than type II and do not obstruct blood flow. Compared with type II, extracellular lipid droplets and vesicular particles are increased to the extent that multiple separate but not sharply defined pools of this material are found among the layers of smooth muscle cells of adaptive intimal thickenings with which type III are usually colocalized (Figure 3). The extracellular droplets and particles are identical to those found only very thinly dispersed in type II lesions and that in much larger amounts constitute the cores of advanced lesions. This extracellular lipid accumulates below the layers of macrophage foam cells, replaces the proteoglycans and fibers that are normally present, and by increasing the extracellular matrix drives smooth muscle cells apart. By this definition, collections of extracellular lipid that disturb the coherence of some structural intimal smooth muscle cells in a circumscribed region of the intima constitute progression beyond a type II lesion. At this stage an extensive, well-delineated accumulation of extracellular lipid (a lipid core) has not developed. Studies of many cases indicate that the lipid core, the characteristic component of most advanced lesions, forms by the increase and confluence of the smaller, separate pools that characterize type III lesions.

The significance of type III lesions lies in the fact that they probably signal future clinical disease. They also provide the evidence that atheroma begins as a minimal lipid deposit. In the past, the belief that clinically significant atherosclerotic lesions develop from some type II (ie, some fatty streak) lesions encountered considerable skepticism. Because fatty streaks had been traditionally regarded as minimal lipid in thin intima, they were considered morphologically too different from atheroma to be its precursor. Nevertheless, some authors were convinced that advanced lesions originated in the minimal intimal lipid accumulations of fatty streaks or of a subgroup of fatty streaks.[28,29]

The bridge between the morphologies of the fatty streak and atheroma was found in the progression-prone regions of arteries (ie, the locations with adaptive intimal thickening). Early in life, progression-prone locations shelter minimal lipid accumulations (type IIa lesions). Later, in young adults, type III lesions and atheroma are found in the same locations. Because of the many layers of smooth muscle cells that are normal for these locations, minimal lipid accumulations in progression-prone locations are morphologically closer to atheroma than the minimal lipid accumulations in regions of the intima that are thin and consist of few smooth muscle cells (type IIb lesions).

Type IV Lesions

In type IV lesions, an extensive accumulation of extracellular lipid occupies the intima. The accumulation is known as the lipid core. The type IV lesion is known as atheroma. Type IV is the first lesion type to be considered as advanced in this histologic classification because of the dissolution of arterial structure caused by the large accumulation of extracellular lipid. All the features of type II (IIa) lesions are also present but increased collagen, disruption of the lesion surface, and thrombosis are not features at this stage of lesion development.

Type IV lesions are crescent-shaped increases in the thickness of an artery. The greatest thickness of a crescent is generally opposite the flow divider of a bifurcation or just beyond (Figure 2). Location and shape parallel those of the adaptive intimal thickening that is always present in this location and that contributes to the overall thickness of the arterial wall at that point, but not to any reduction of the lumen that the superimposed lesion may cause. The lesion may not narrow the arterial lumen much except in persons with very high plasma cholesterol levels. Thus, in many people, a type IV lesion may not be visible by angiography. Disruption of the coherence of structural smooth muscle cells by the accumulated lipid may allow an increase in the outer perimeter of the arterial segment involved. Although type IV lesions are generally clinically silent, their recognition with intravascular ultrasound or other techniques would be desirable because they have the potential to develop fissures, hematoma, and thrombus (see type VI lesion).

The characteristic core develops from an increase and the consequent confluence of the isolated pools of extracellular lipid that characterize the type III lesion. The increase in lipid results from continued insudation from the plasma. The mechanism and pathway whereby the particles of extracellular lipid form is unclear. The view that a large part is derived from lipid-laden cells is supported by the observation of partly disintegrated foam cells at the margins of lipid cores, by the extrusion of the residuals of intracytoplasmic lipid droplets from cells, and by the similarity between the extracellular and the intracellular lipid particles.[2,30,31] There is also evidence that some extracellular particles may be derived directly from the coalescence of smaller lipoprotein particles derived from the plasma and not previously taken up by cells.[32,33]

In the core, clumps of mineral are almost always visible by microscopy within the cytoplasm of smooth muscle cells that apparently have damaged organelles or are dead altogether, or associated with extracellular particles of lipid and cell debris. The size and amount of the mineral particles is extremely variable between lesions that are otherwise comparable. Mineral particles may be too small in many type IV lesions and even in more advanced lesion types to be visible by clinical imaging.

The lipid core is in the musculoelastic (the deep) part of the intima, and smooth muscle cells still surviving in the core are dispersed within the entire region of the core including its margins. Dispersed cells have attenuated and elongated cell bodies and may have unusually thick basement membranes. The intima that is between the lipid core and the lumen of the artery contains macrophages and smooth muscle cells with and without lipid droplet inclusions, lymphocytes,[34] and mast cells. Variable numbers of capillaries often border the lipid core, particularly at its lateral margins and at the aspect facing the lumen. The lateral margins are also the regions of greater density of macrophages, macrophage foam cells, and lymphocytes. The lipid core emerges before fibrous tissue that may subsequently additionally thicken the intimal lesion. This subsequent morphology, if it develops, is then designated as the type V lesion.

Type V Lesions

Type V lesions are defined as those in which a layer or layers of fibrous tissue (mainly collagen) are added to a type IV lesion (Figure 3). This morphology is also referred to as fibroatheroma. Generally, collagen is synthesized as a reaction to the cell and tissue disorganization and dissolution caused by a core of extracellular lipid. Thus, formation of a lipid core (type IV lesion) precedes collagen formation (type V lesion). Some thick layers of collagen represent the end stage of superimposed thrombi. Such lesions would be classified as type VI if evidence of a thrombus and its remnants had not been erased by the ingrowth of smooth muscle cells into the thrombus and by the formation of collagen. In spite of the layers of smooth muscle cells and newly formed extracellular matrix, type V lesions, like type IV, are susceptible to rupture (or re-rupture) and to formation (or re-formation) of mural thrombi. That is, they may periodically assume the morphology of a type VI lesion. The sequence is explained in the flow diagram in Figure 4. Multiple episodes may result in multilayered type V lesions.

Multilayered type V lesions consist of two or more lipid cores stacked irregularly one above the other and separated from each other by layers of fibrous tissue and cells. Presumably, multilayered type V lesions could also be the consequence of modifications in hemodynamic forces that follow the development of a vascular stenosis, thus modifying the site of lipid accumulation. Collagen often becomes the predominant feature of a lesion, accounting for more of the thickness than the underlying lipid accumulations. Increased collagen is associated with smooth muscle cells rich in rough-surfaced endoplasmic reticulum. Capillaries may be numer-

FIGURE 4. *The flow diagram in the center column indicates the pathways in the evolution, progression, and regression of human atherosclerotic lesions. The Roman numerals stand for the histologically characteristic types of lesion enumerated in Table 2 and defined in the column to the left of the flow diagram. The direction of the arrows indicates the sequence in which the characteristic morphologies may change. From type I to type IV, changes in lesion morphology occur primarily because of increasing accumulation of lipid. Once a type IV lesion has formed it may change and grow by mechanisms additional to lipid accumulation. The two loops between type IV and type VI illustrate how lesions advance when thrombotic deposits form on their surface. Thrombotic deposits may form many times in the same location and may constitute the principal mechanism for the gradual occlusion of medium-sized arteries. Reprinted with permission from Reference 5.*

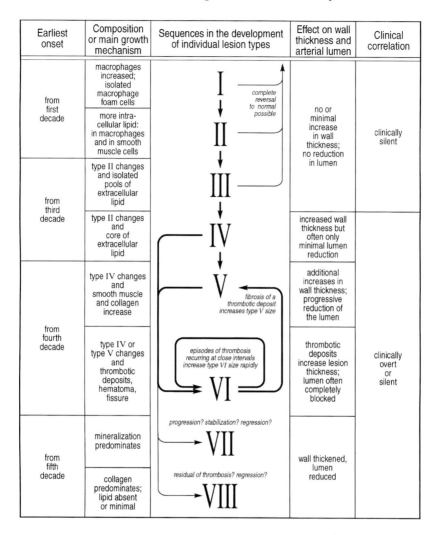

Earliest onset	Composition or main growth mechanism	Sequences in the development of individual lesion types	Effect on wall thickness and arterial lumen	Clinical correlation
from first decade	macrophages increased; isolated macrophage foam cells	I — complete reversal to normal possible	no or minimal increase in wall thickness; no reduction in lumen	clinically silent
	more intra-cellular lipid: in macrophages and in smooth muscle cells	II		
from third decade	type II changes and isolated pools of extracellular lipid	III		
	type II changes and core of extracellular lipid	IV	increased wall thickness but often only minimal lumen reduction	
from fourth decade	type IV changes and smooth muscle and collagen increase	V — fibrosis of a thrombotic deposit increases type V size	additional increases in wall thickness; progressive reduction of the lumen	
	type IV or type V changes and thrombotic deposits, hematoma, fissure	episodes of thrombosis recurring at close intervals increase type VI size rapidly — VI	thrombotic deposits increase lesion thickness; lumen often completely blocked	clinically overt or silent
from fifth decade	mineralization predominates	progression? stabilization? regression? — VII	wall thickened, lumen reduced	
	collagen predominates; lipid absent or minimal	residual of thrombosis? regression? — VIII		

ous and microhemorrhages may be present around the capillaries. Lipid may also accumulate in the adjacent media, and medial smooth muscle cells may be disarranged. The adjacent adventitia may contain focal and diffuse accumulations of lymphocytes, macrophages, and macrophage foam cells.

Type VI Lesions

The morbidity and mortality from coronary atherosclerosis derives largely from lesions classified as type VI and often referred to as complicated lesions. The type VI characteristics consist of disruptions of the lesion surface such as fissures, erosions or ulcerations, hematoma or hemorrhage, and thrombotic deposits (Figure 3). While most type VI lesions have the underlying morphology of type IV or type V lesions, fissure, hematoma, and thrombus are sometimes superimposed on lesser lesion types and even on intima without a perceptible lipid accumulation. The superimposed processes accelerate progression, at least temporarily, beyond the gradual rate. The histologic evidence indicates that the superimposed complicating episodes follow each other at variable and, so far, unpredictable intervals. Sometimes, complications appear to be interspersed by months or years without additional episodes. During that time fissures reseal and hematomas and thrombotic deposits are colonized by smooth muscle cells and converted to collagen. Conversion results in a return to a type V morphology, although to a type V lesion that is larger and more obstructive of the arterial lumen than before. In other instances, recurrent superimpositions of layers of thrombus follow in quick succession and an occlusion builds up within the coronary lumen within hours, days, or weeks (see Figure 4).

To date, there are no conclusive measures whereby the susceptibility of individual type IV and type V lesions to disruptions of the lesion surface can be measured clinically or histologically. Factors that could contribute to fissuring and other disruptions include structural weakness of the intimal lesion at the point of disruption,[35] modifications of the shear stress and tensile force to which a lesion is exposed,[15] spasm,[36] and the release of toxic substances and proteolytic enzymes from macrophages within the lesions.[29,37] While thrombotic deposits and their remnants are the consequence of disruptions of the lesion surface in many cases, thrombotic deposits may also form on lesions without an apparent surface defect, hematoma, or hemorrhage. Various systemic thrombogenic risk factors may contribute to the formation of thrombi.[38]

At autopsy, thrombotic deposits are frequently found superimposed on type IV or type V lesions in the coronary arteries and aortas in subjects in the fourth decade of life. Some data on the frequency of thrombosis are given in the companion chapter on the aorta.

Type VII and Type VIII Lesions

Some advanced atherosclerotic lesions, particularly after the fourth decade, are largely mineralized. The term calcific lesion (type VII) may be used here. Mineralization takes the form of calcium phosphate and apatite replacing the accumulated remnants of dead cells and extracellular lipid. Variable amounts of mineral are present in most advanced lesions. With refined microscopic methods, even the type IV lesions of young adults reveal aggregates of crystalline calcium phosphate among the lipid particles of lipid cores and within the cytoplasm of smooth muscle cells trapped and injured within lipid cores. Since most advanced lesions contain mineral deposits, the type VII classification is appropriate only when mineralization dominates the picture. However, it is understood that lesion components such as lipid deposits and increased fibrous tissue are generally also present.

Some atherosclerotic lesions may consist entirely or almost entirely of collagen, which is sometimes hyalinized. The lipidic component is minimal or absent. The term fibrotic lesion (type VIII) may be used here. Lipid may have been resorbed or may never have been present. A fibrotic lesion may be the consequence of a thrombotic extension of a lipidic lesion with the extension converted to collagen. Such lesions may severely obstruct the lumen of medium-sized arteries and may even be occlusive. Some lesions with the type VIII morphology could be in part or entirely the consequence of factors other than the established risk factors of atherosclerosis.

We did not encounter lesion types VII or VIII in the coronary arteries of the young population we studied. The descriptions of these lesion types are derived from parallel studies in older people that also included other vascular beds.

Acknowledgments

The content of this chapter is based for the most part on autopsy studies by the author that have been supported by the National Institutes of Health (grant HL-22739). The American Heart Association's Committee on Vascular Lesions recently reviewed and compiled data on the compositions of human atherosclerotic lesions and proposed a histologic classification.[14,27,39] The classification used in this chapter is in agreement with the conclusions of this committee.

References

1. Stary HC. Evoution and progression of atherosclerotic lesions in coronary arteries of children and young adults. *Arteriosclerosis* 1989;9(suppl I):I–19-I–32.

2. Stary HC. The sequence of cell and matrix changes in atherosclerotic lesions of coronary arteries in the first forty years of life. *Eur Heart J* 1990;11(suppl E):3–19.
3. Stary HC. Macrophages, macrophage foam cells, and eccentric intimal thickening in the coronary arteries of young children. *Atherosclerosis* 1987;64:91–108.
4. Stary HC. Composition and classification of human atherosclerotic lesions. *Virchows Archiv A (Pathol Anat)* 1992;421:277–290.
5. Stary HC. The histological classification of atherosclerotic lesions in human coronary arteries. In: Fuster V, Ross R, Topol E, eds. *Atherosclerosis and Coronary Artery Disease*. New York: Raven Press; 1995:000.
6. Aschoff L. *Lectures on Pathology*. Philadelphia: Lippincott-Raven Publishers; 1996:463–474.
7. Aschoff L. Die Arteriosklerose. *Mediz Klinik* 1930;(Suppl 1):1–20.
8. Aschoff L. Introduction. In: Cowdry EV, ed. *Arteriosclerosis. A Survey of the Problem*. New York: The Macmillan Company; 1933:1–18.
9. Gore I, Tejada C. The quantitative appraisal of atherosclerosis. *Am J Pathol* 1957;33:875–885.
10. Holman RL, McGill HC Jr, Strong JP, et al. Technics for studying atherosclerotic lesions. *Lab Invest* 1958;7:42–47.
11. World Health Organization. Classification of atherosclerotic lesions: Report of a study group. *WHO Techn Rep Ser* 1958;143:1–20.
12. Guzman MA, McMahan CA, McGill HC Jr, et al. Selected methodologic aspects of the international atherosclerosis project. *Lab Invest* 1968;18:479–497.
13. Davies MJ. *Color Atlas of Cardiovascular Pathology*. London: Harvey Miller; 1986.
14. Stary HC, Blankenhorn DH, Chandler AB, et al. A definition of the intima of human arteries and of its atherosclerosis-prone regions. *Circulation* 1992;85:391–405.
15. Glagov S, Zarins C, Giddens DP, et al. Hemodynamics and atherosclerosis: Insights and perspectives gained from studies of human arteries. *Arch Pathol Lab Med* 1988;112:1018–1031.
16. Williams KJ, Tabas I. The response-to-retention hypothesis of early atherogenesis. *Arterioscler Thromb Vasc Biol* 1995;15:551–561.
17. Gerrity RG. The role of the monocyte in atherogenesis. II. Migration of foam cells from atherosclerotic lesions. *Am J Pathol* 1981;103:191–200.
18. Lewis JC, Taylor RG, Jerome WG. Foam cell characteristics in coronary arteries and aortas of White Carneau pigeons with moderate hypercholesterolemia. *Ann NY Acad Sci* 1985;454:91–100.
19. Schwenke DC, Carew TE. Initiation of atherosclerotic lesions in cholesterol-fed rabbits I. Focal increases in arterial LDL concentration precede development of fatty streak lesions. *Arteriosclerosis* 1989;9:895–907.
20. Schwenke DC, Carew TE. Initiation of atherosclerotic lesions in cholesterol-fed rabbits. II. Selective retention of LDL vs. selective increases in LDL permeability in susceptible sites of arteries. *Arteriosclerosis* 1989;9:908–918.
21. Munro JM, Van der Walt JD, Munro CS, et al. An immunohistochemical analysis of human aortic fatty streaks. *Hum Pathol* 1987;18:375–380.
22. Katsuda S, Boyd HC, Fligner C, et al. Human atherosclerosis. III. Immunocytochemical analysis of the cell composition of lesions of young adults. *Am J Pathol* 1992;140:907–914.

23. Katz SS, Shipley GG, Small DM. Physical chemistry of the lipids of human atherosclerotic lesions: Demonstration of a lesion intermediate between fatty streaks and advanced plaques. *J Clin Invest* 1976;58:200–211.
24. Geer JC, Malcom GT. Cholesterol ester fatty acid composition of human aorta fatty streaks and normal intima. *Exp Mol Pathol* 1965;4:500–507.
25. Insull W, Bartsch GE. Cholesterol, triglyceride, and phospholipid content of intima, media, and atherosclerotic fatty streak in human thoracic aorta. *J Clin Invest* 1966;45:513–523.
26. Smith EB, Smith RH. Early changes in aortic intima. *Atherosclerosis Rev* 1976;1:119–236.
27. Stary HC, Chandler AB, Glagov S, et al. A definition of initial, fatty streak, and intermediate lesions of atherosclerosis. *Circulation* 1994; 89:2462–2478.
28. McGill HC. The lesion. In: Schettler G, Weizel A, eds. *Atherosclerosis III*. Berlin: Springer-Verlag; 1974:27–38.
29. Steinberg D, Witztum JL. Lipoproteins and atherogenesis. Current concepts. *JAMA* 1990;264:3047–3052.
30. Schmitz G, Muller G. Structure and function of lamellar bodies, lipid-protein complexes involved in storage and secretion of cellular lipids. *J Lipid Res* 1991;32:1539–1570.
31. Ball RY, Stowers EC, Burton JH, et al. Evidence that the death of macrophage foam cells contributes to the lipid core of atheroma. *Atherosclerosis* 1995;114:45–54.
32. Guyton JR, Klemp KF, Mims MP. Altered ultrastructural morphology of self-aggregated low density lipoproteins. Coalescence of lipid domains forming droplets and vesicles. *J Lipid Res* 1991;32:953–962.
33. Guyton JR, Klemp KF. Development of the atherosclerotic core region. *Arterioscler Thromb* 1994;14:1305–1314.
34. Jonasson L, Holm J, Skalli O, et al. Regional accumulations of T cells, macrophages, and smooth muscle cells in the human atherosclerotic plaque. *Arteriosclerosis* 1986;6:131–138.
35. Richardson PD, Davies MJ, Born GVR. Influence of plaque configuration and stress distribution on fissuring of coronary atherosclerotic plaques. *Lancet* 1989;2:941–944.
36. Nobuyoshi M, Tanaka M, Nosaka H, et al. Progression of coronary atherosclerosis: Is coronary spasm related to progression? *J Am Coll Cardiol* 1991;18:904–910.
37. Henney AM, Wakeley PR, Davies MJ, et al. Localization of stromelysin gene expression in atherosclerotic plaques by in situ hybridization. *Proc Natl Acad Sci USA* 1991;88:8154–8158.
38. Fuster V. Mechanisms leading to myocardial infarction: Insights from studies of vascular biology. *Circulation* 1994;90:2126–2146.
39. Stary HC, Chandler AB, Dinsmore RE, et al. A definition of advanced types of atherosclerotic lesions and a histological classification of atheroslerosis. *Arterioscler Thromb Vasc Biol* 1995;15:1512–1531.

Chapter 5

Early Evolution of Coronary Artery Lesions in Young People:
From Fatty Streak to Fibrous Plaque— Implications for Imaging

Robert W. Wissler, MD, PhD,
Laura Hiltscher, ASCP,
and Matthew Wahden

Introduction

This chapter uses observations and data from our Pathobiological Determinants of Atherosclerosis in Youth (PDAY) study, as well as our quantitative analysis of the coronary artery standard samples of the perfusion fixed left anterior descending (LAD) coronary arteries from almost 1000 cases. These PDAY forensic cases represent an autopsy population of young people, 15–34 years of age, who died suddenly and unexpectedly, usually from acute trauma.[1] They have recently been used extensively to demonstrate the usefulness of quantitative risk factor analysis data when related to the measurements of plaque extent and severity as well as the microscopically measured lesion components.[2] These cases have also been used to develop a new and useful classification of the microscopically highly variable raised lesions that are sometimes referred to as fatty plaques or intermediate lesions.[3–5]

In this chapter we present some recently obtained results from applying this classification system to a study of LAD standard samples. The chapter concentrates on type V lesions using the criteria

This work was partially supported by HL 33740 and HL 45715 from the NIH Heart, Lung and Blood Institute.

A listing of the PDAY Research Group is found at the end of this chapter.

From: Fuster V, (ed.) *Syndromes of Atherosclerosis: Correlations of Clinical Imaging and Pathology*. Armonk, NY: Futura Publishing Company, Inc.: © 1996.

from the recently published numerical system that represents a new modern comprehensive atherosclerotic lesion definition and classification as developed by the American Heart Association (AHA) Committee on Lesions.[6,7]

Activities and Unique Features of PDAY

The PDAY Steering Committee has had a constant and sustained involvement and is its most important personnel. (Its members and the principal investigators of the 14 centers involved in the multicenter study during its definitive period are listed at the end of this chapter.) All of the steering committee members are experienced investigators who have demonstrated their remarkable interest and ability to study atherosclerosis in novel and productive ways. This and a few of the other important aspects of the structure and function of PDAY that have augmented its value and the uniqueness of its contributions are as follows:

- Forensic cases allow elimination of many diseases that influence risk factors.

- First study of young people focusing on correlation of risk factors with development of lesions.

- Age, sex, and race factors are well represented and balanced.

- Macro- and microinterpretation and classification facilitated by standardized sampling strategy and en face color macrophotographs of core samples.

- Computer assisted mapping and both micro- and macro-morphometry.

- Excellent preservation of intima and wide variety of microscopic preparations available for quantitative evaluation of lesion components.

- Many special studies increase the new information gained about autoimmune and immune complex atheroarteritis, special effects of smoking, hypertension, mast cells, and vasoactive amines, etc.

One of the unexpected results of our work on classifications of intermediate lesions (Table 1) was the finding that in this series of nearly 1000 cases of young people ranging from 15 to 34 years of age, the proximal LAD had almost three times as many advanced (type V) fibrous plaques in the coronary samples as we had found

TABLE 1

Classification of Atherosclerotic Lesions Including a New Microscopic Subgrouping of the Intermediate Lesion

- No lesions.

- Fatty streak.
    Gross: Discolored, fuzzy borders, not raised.
    Microscopic: Preponderance of MØ foam cells.

- Fatty plaque (intermediate lesion).
    Gross: Raised, discrete borders, usually yellow.
    Microscopic subgroups:
    1. Mostly intracellular lipid, mainly in SMC, few if any MØ foam cells.
    2. Mostly extracellular lipid, relatively few SMC or MØ foam cells.
    3. Mostly intracellular lipid, with more than 20% MØ foam cells.
    4. Mostly intracellular lipid, with or without MØ foam cells, but with a large component of lymphocytes.

- Fibrous plaque.
    Gross: Raised, firm, discrete borders, often white and glistening.

- Complicated plaque.
    Gross: Plaque with fracture, ulceration, thrombosis, etc.

in the lower abdominal aorta. This is surprising because many studies have recorded advanced fibrous lesions appearing sooner in the lower abdominal aorta than in the proximal coronary arteries. In fact, some experienced observers have indicated that the lower abdominal aortic lesions tend to progress to raised lesions and type V fibrous plaques about a decade before they reach the same extent and severity in the proximal coronary arteries.

The study also revealed that the stages and types of microscopic intermediate lesions in the coronary arteries were similar in lesion components to the microscopic features of the stages and types in the aorta, and that the coronary lesions could be classified just as easily. Table 2 indicates the similarities and contrasts between proximal LAD coronary artery lesion types and aortic lesion types in this quantitative study of young people's lesions.[5] It is clear from this table that many more of the LAD coronary artery core samples had no appreciable lipid containing intimal lesions as compared with any of the aortic samples. Conversely, fatty streaks

TABLE 2

The Analysis of All Available Cases with Gross and Microscopic Lesion Classification Using the New Criteria for Intermediate Lesion Microscopic Types

Sample No.	No Micro Lesion	Micro Fatty Streaks	FATTY PLAQUES				
			Intracell Lipid Predom "1"	Extracell Lipid >50% "2"	MØ Foam Cell >20% "3"	Rich in Lymphocytes "4"	Fibrous Plaques
01	235	174	175	117	121	5	2
18	264	128	216	155	102	0	7
16	250	53	164	225	89	1	38
45	388	47	58	206	69	4	102

were much more prominent in the thoracic and upper abdominal aorta than in the lower abdominal or the LAD coronary artery core samples. In fact, in many respects, the distribution of intermediate fatty plaque lesion types was somewhat similar in the lower abdominal and LAD coronary artery core samples.

The Correlates of LAD Advanced Coronary Plaques with Age, Race, Sex, and Risk Factors

In an effort to obtain a better understanding of why we saw many more advanced coronary artery fibrous plaques than expected, we carried out a number of studies of the correlation of these advanced plaques with other observations that we made.

We found that these type V plaques are almost equally present in the black and white members of this large group of cases, which was almost exactly balanced between the races. As might be expected, type V lesions tended to be more frequent in the older age group because age is the most powerful risk factor in the PDAY study. There was a much greater frequency of advanced lesions in males than in females. This was substantially greater than the preponderance of males in this population group. In general, advanced coronary lesions in females tended to be smaller and thinner fibrous plaques, but with a higher proportion of fibrous cap predominance as compared with the males. Among the most interesting observed relationships with risk factors was the high direct correlation of advanced coronary artery atherosclerotic plaques with evidence of smoking (Table 3). Other relationships of advanced lesions with the risk factors that were routinely measured are also given in Table 3. It is clear that there is an association of fibrous plaques in the LAD coronary arteries with evidence of

TABLE 3

Coronary Artery Fibrous Plaques
% Positive for Selected Risk Factors

	% of cases*
Elevated cholesterol	46
Elevated thiocyanate	72
Combined elevated cholesterol and thiocyanate	45
Glycosylated Hbg	20
Evidence of high blood pressure	16

*Limited to those on which blood samples permitted analyses.

smoking. Elevated serum cholesterol is also associated with a substantial increase in percentage of cases with advanced proximal coronary artery plaques, as compared with either elevated glycosylated hemoglobin or evidence of hypertension. While each of these percentages is higher than the occurrence of these risk factors in the entire PDAY autopsy population, the increase associated with smoking is the most impressive, and certainly underscores the importance of this risk factor for progression to a fibrous plaque. Of interest is the fact that in terms of fibrous plaque incidence, the combination of hypercholesterolemia and positive serum thiocyanate levels does not seem to impose the added risk that it does for extent of aortic lesions as evaluated grossly.[8]

Correlates of the Severity and the Components of Fibrous Plaques with the Problems of Imaging

An analysis of the components of the fibrous plaques of the coronary arteries was performed. The goal was to assess the way that these simplified features of the advanced plaques might present problems as well as opportunities for developing data from the several modes of imaging that might be useful in evaluating the coronary lesions in the living patient. Table 4 shows the results of this analysis and separates the general distribution of components between fibrous cap and necrotic center in the slightly more than 100 coronary fibrous plaques that were analyzed. It shows the component balance as they relate to plaque size, which in this case refers to the relative amount of space occupied in the cross section

TABLE 4

Distribution of 102 Left Anterior Descending Coronary Artery Fibrous Plaques According to Size and According to % Predominance of Fibrous Caps and Lipid/Cholesterol Rich Cores

		% Predominance	
	Size	Fibrous Cap	Fat/Cholesterol Core
Most marked	9	33	11
Severe	31	35	23
Moderate	48	29	40
Mild	14	14	79

of the artery, not to stenosis. It is now widely recognized that most of the small- and medium-sized plaques displace the artery wall externally and do not appreciably narrow the lumen.[9]

The results clearly indicate that many of the smaller proximal LAD coronary artery plaques that are definitely advanced fibrous type V in relation to their well-developed necrotic core with a definite fibrous cap of varying thickness are present in this population. Furthermore, they call attention to the probability that some of these smaller plaques, while not perceptibly narrowing the lumen, probably should be classified as clinically dangerous because their necrotic core is very near the luminal surface, especially at the shoulder of the plaque.

Figures 1 and 2 illustrate the types of lesions that we have been classifying as fibrous plaques. They are arranged as composites and are arranged from the largest to the smallest and with fibrous cap predominance and fatty core predominance side by side.

It is evident that although there are very large variations in the size of fibrous plaque, the proportions of fibrous component to necrotic core component can be at remarkable extremes for each size of plaque. In some of the larger and more stenotic ones the fibrous cap is very thick (Figure 1A) and in some of these most severe lesions the fibrous component is quite thin (Figure 1B). These same contrasts are shown from two additional examples in this same figure (Figures 1C and 1D). Even the smaller fibrous plaques that almost certainly would not show on contrast media angiography have the same contrast in proportions of fibrous and fatty components as reflected in Figure 2A through 2D.

We and others believe[10–12] that many of these relatively small fibrous plaques with rather superficial cholesterol-rich core centers and thin fibrous caps (Figures 3A and 3B) pose a substantial threat that can be triggered by the pathogenesis of plaque rupture and/or fibrous cap fracture pathogenetically sequenced by collagenolytic and elastinolytic enzymes from macrophages and hemodynamic influences as developed by the evidence from recent studies by Lendon et al[13] and Davies et al.[14]

In support of these rupture of plaque pathogenetic proposals, we have also observed frequent accumulations of macrophage foam cells near the lumen at the shoulders of these fibrous caps of varying size (Figure 3B) in this relatively young autopsy population. Therefore, the fundamental premise, ie, that it is plaque components rather than size that determine clinical danger of thrombosis seems to be supported by study of these advanced coronary artery plaques in young people.

Obviously, much more work is needed, but thus far, the PDAY

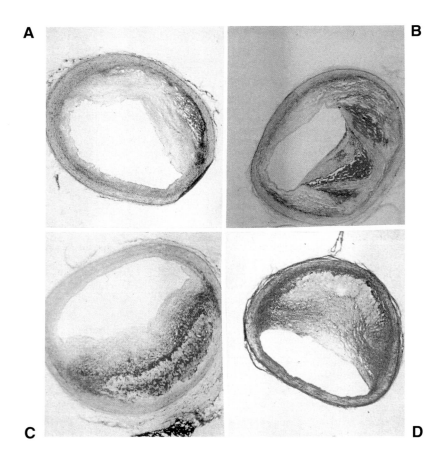

FIGURE 1. *A: This stenosing lesion, which is stained with oil red O and counterstained with hematoxylin, is from a 30-year-old white male. Note the rather thick, but relatively immature fibrous cap that is obviously made up primarily of smooth muscle cells with little or no stainable lipid and collagen. The lipid-rich core is rather irregular and also contains calcium, cholesterol clefts, and a few monocyte-derived foam cells, especially in the shoulder areas. **B:** This lesion was found in the proximal left anterior descending (LAD) coronary artery of a 32-year-old black male. The artery shows severe stenosis as a result of a very large and lipid-rich plaque with a poorly formed and irregular fibrous cap and a multiplicity of lipid-rich core areas, which are mostly acellular and some of which show deposits of calcium. It is easy to visualize a potential fracture of the fibrous cap in areas where the friable lipid-rich core is very near the arterial lumen. **C:** This advanced lesion is from a 27-year-old white male and shows approximately 50% stenosis of the lumen with a thick fibrous cap making up between one fourth and one third of the total cross-sectional plaque area. The largely acellular core area is very rich in lipid stained with oil red O and shows adjacent monocyte-derived macrophage foam cells, especially in the shoulder regions of the plaque. The adventitia has a prominent accumulation of lymphocytes and the lesion is reminiscent of the plaques that we have described as typical of those produced in rhesus monkeys fed a diet rich in coconut oil. **D:** This stenotic advanced atherosclerotic plaque is from a 22-year-old black male and has a thin, poorly formed fibrous cap that shows abundant oil red O positive lipid, particularly at the shoulder, and a large cell-free area much more lightly stained for lipid near the center.*

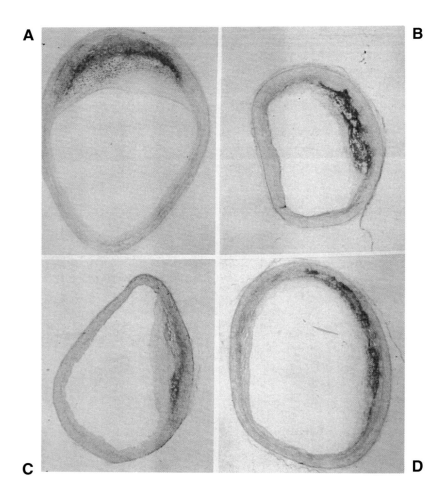

FIGURE 2. *This figure contains photomicrographs of lesions found in the standard samples of the left anterior descending (LAD) proximal coronary artery of four different individuals and demonstrates that even relatively small nonstenosing coronary arteries in individuals between 22 and 31 years of age can represent fibrous plaques as defined as lesions with fibrous caps and cell-free lipid-rich centers. **A:** This cross section is from a 31-year-old black female and demonstrates a fibrous plaque with a relatively thick fibrous cap. The more superficial part consists of smooth muscle cells with little or no stainable lipids; the deeper part consists of a mixture of smooth muscle cells and monocyte derived macrophage foam cells, both of which are positive for stainable cytoplasmic lipid. The lipid-rich acellular core is prominent, but makes up less than half of the total area of the lesion seen in this transverse section. **B:** This plaque, which probably would not be visualized by angiography, is from a 22-year-old black male and shows a thin fibrous cap and a relatively large acellular center that stains intensively for both lipid and calcium. **C:** This proximal coronary artery from a 27-year-old white male has a dominant fibrous cap and a relatively small lipid-rich acellular core that lies rather deep and away from the lumen. **D:** This section comes from the proximal LAD coronary artery of a 25-year-old white male and shows a relatively small, but advanced plaque with a thin fibrous cap and a relatively large and irregular oil red O positive acellular area. It is not difficult to visualize a situation in which some of the thrombogenic material from the lipid-rich core might be exposed to the bloodstream and induce thrombosis.*

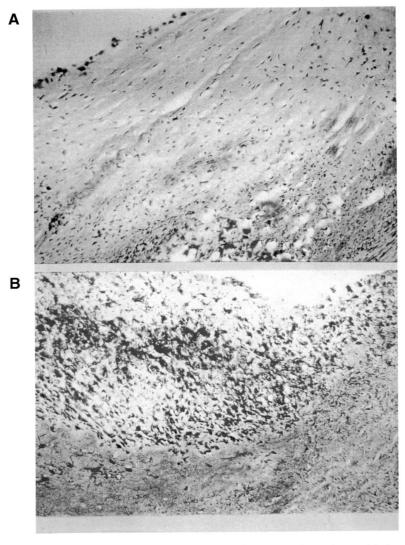

FIGURE 3. *These two high-power magnifications of portions of left anterior descending (LAD) proximal coronary artery plaques included in this study illustrate in greater detail a remarkable contrast in the areas near the shoulders.* **A:** *This figure is from a 31-year-old white male and demonstrates the shoulder region from a raised lesion that has a thick fibrous cap with a nest of macrophages located at some distance from the arterial lumen, but near the periphery of the cell-free oil red O rich core.* **B:** *This is the shoulder of a plaque where the rather "soft" fibrous cap is rich in macrophage foam cells that occupy much of the space between the lipid-rich acellular zone and the surface of the plaque near the lumen.*

studies and the observations we have made may offer a framework for arterial imaging professionals to further develop their hardware and methods. As was pointed out in a recent NATO conference,[15] this rapidly developing branch of medicine needs to be encouraged to increase the potential of its imaging approaches for recognizing and quantifying the components of the fibrous plaques, even the small ones, which are likely to lead to serious clinical events.

Summary

It is clear from this study of advanced type V fibrous plaques from young people that there are a number of findings that may be of great practical value. These findings include:

- The primary premise that artery stenosis and plaque severity are not related.
- The strong probability that clinical threat or danger is not very well correlated with degree of stenosis or plaque size, but rather with plaque composition.
- The need for quantitative imaging data during life regarding the relative thickness of the fibrous caps of each plaque, especially at the shoulders.
- The need for quantitative data on size and consistency of the lipid-rich core of the fibrous plaque.
- The need for greater sensitivity of imaging methods to detect and measure the components of small and rather thin fibrous plaques, especially those with relatively large lipid-rich centers.

The results of this study reveal some of the major challenges for the future for the further development of imaging approaches: a better precision for quantitation of the following plaque components including collagen, the cholesterol-rich core, the thickness of the plaque shoulders, ulcerations (size and location) as well as microthrombi (size and location). Arterial imaging professionals may want to consider some or all of the following questions as they work to increase the value of imaging procedures for atherosclerotic muscular arteries.

In what ways will quantitation of fibrous atherosclerotic plaque components be useful to prevent clinical events, ie, plaque rupture and thrombosis? Will it be possible to develop imaging technology that will make it possible to reproducibly quantify the major plaque components in coronary arteries and carotid arteries? What new and useful plaque component analytical technologies and approaches are feasible and likely? What is the potential for improving existing technology and methods for identifying and quantifying coronary artery lesion components, even when the lesions are relatively small?

The answers to these questions, when used with the findings described in this study may help establish the next era of imaging that will benefit all patients with vascular disease, especially those relatively young people with advanced plaques.

Acknowledgments

Special thanks and recognition are due to Gertrud Friedman, Blanche Berger, Taryn McFadden, Philip Tasca, and Ashish Mahajan.

Pathobiological Determinants of Atherosclerosis in Youth (PDAY Research Group)

Director/Program Director: R.W. Wissler, PhD, MD University of Chicago.

Associate Directors: A.L. Robertson, Jr, MD, PhD University of Illinois (1987–1992); J.P. Strong, MD Louisiana State University (1992–present).

Steering Committee: J.F. Cornhill, D.Phil Ohio State University; H.C. McGill, Jr, MD Southwest Foundation for Biomedical Research; C.A. McMahan, PhD University of Texas Health Science Center (San Antonio); A.L. Robertson, Jr, MD, PhD University of Illinois; J.P. Strong, MD Louisiana State University Medical Center; R.W. Wissler, PhD, MD University of Chicago.

Standard Operating Protocol and Manual of Procedures Committee Chairperson: M.C. Oalmann, DrPH Louisiana State University Medical Center.

Participating Centers:

University of A1labama (Birmingham), Department of Medicine—Principal Investigator (P.I.): S. Gay, MD. Coinvestigators: R.E. Gay, MD, G.-Q. Huang, MD (HL-33733); Department of Biochemistry—Principal Investigator: E.J. Miller, PhD; Coinvestigators: D.K. Furuto, PhD, M.S. Vail, A.J. Narkates (HL-33728).

Albany Medical College (Albany, NY)—Principal Investigator: A. Daoud, MD; Coinvestigators: A.S. Frank, PhD, M.A. Hyer, E.C. McGovern (HL-33765).

Baylor College of Medicine (Houston)—Principal Investigator: L.C. Smith, PhD; Coinvestigator: F.M. Strickland, PhD (HL-33750).

University of Chicago (Chicago)—Principal Investigator: R.W. Wissler, PhD, MD; Coinvestigators: D. Vesselinovitch, DVM, MS, A. Komatsu, MD, PhD, Y. Kusumi, MD, G.M. Culen, DPM, A. Chien, BA, A. Demopoulos, BA, G. Friedman, BA, R.T. Bridenstine, MS, R.J. Stein, MD, R.H. Kirschner, MD, M. Bekermeier, ASCP, B. Berger, ASCP, L. Hiltscher, ASCP (HL-33740).

University of Illinois (Chicago)—Principal Investigator: A.L. Robertson, Jr, MD, PhD; Coinvestigators: R.J. Stein, MD, E.R. Donoghue, MD, R.J.

Buschmann, PhD, Y. Katsura, MD, T. Lyong An, MD, E. Choi, MD, N. Jones, MD, M.S. Kalelkar, MD, Y. Konakci, MD, B. Lifschultz, MD, V.R. Gumidyala, MD, R.M. Harper, BS, F. Norris, HTL (ASCP) (HL-33758).

Louisiana State University Medical Center (New Orleans)—Principal Investigator: J.P. Strong, MD; Coinvestigators: G.T. Malcom, PhD, W.P. Newman III, MD, M.C. Oalmann, DrPH, P.S. Roheim, MD, A.K. Bhattacharyya, PhD, M.A. Guzman, PhD, A.A. Hatem, MD, C.A. Hornick, PhD, C.D. Restrepo, MD, R.E. Tracy, MD, PhD, C.C. Breaux, MS, S.E. Hubbard, C.S. Zsembik, D.G. Gibbs, D.A. Trosclair (HL-33746).

University of Maryland (Baltimore)—Principal Investigator: W. Mergner, MD, PhD; Coinvestigators: J.H. Resau, PhD, R.D. Vigorito, MS, P.A. Q.-C. Yu, MD, J. Smialek, MD (HL-33752).

Medical College of Georgia (Augusta)—Co-Principal Investigators: A.B. Chandler, MD, R.N. Rao, MD; Coinvestigators: D.G. Falls, MD, R.G. Gerrity, PhD, B.O. Spurlock, BA; Associate Investigators: K.B. Sharma, MD, J.S. Sexton, MD, Research Assistants: K.K. Smith, HT (ASCP), G.W. Forbes (HL-33772).

University of Nebraska Medical Center (Omaha)—Principal Investigator: B.M. McManus, MD, PhD; Coinvestigators: J.W. Jones, MD, T.J. Kendall, MS, J.A. Remmenga, BS, W.C. Rogler, BS (HL-33778).

Ohio State University (Columbus)—Principal Investigator: J.F. Cornhill, D.Phil; Coinvestigators: W.R. Adrion, MD, P.M. Fardel, MD, B. Gara, MS, E. Herderick, BS, J. Meimer, MS, L.R. Tate, MD (HL-33760).

Southwest Foundation for Biomedical Research (San Antonio)—Principal Investigators: J.E. Hixson, PhD, P.K. Powers (HL 39913).

University of Texas Health Science Center (San Antonio)—Principal Investigator: C.A. McMahan, PhD; Coinvestigators: H.C. McGill, Jr, MD, G.M. Barnwell, PhD, Y. Marinez, MA, T.J. Prihoda, PhD, H.S. Wigodsky, MD, PhD (HL-33749).

Vanderbilt University—Principal Investigator: R. Virmani, MD; Coinvestigators: J.B. Atkinson, MD, PhD, C.W. Harland, MD, L. Gleaves, RA, C. Gleaves, HT, P. Manik, RA (HL-33770).

West Virginia University—Principal Investigator: S.N. Jagannathan, PhD; Coinvestigators: B. Caterson, PhD, J.L. Frost, MD, K.M.K. Rao, MD, P. Johnson, N.F. Rodman, MD (HL-33748).

References

1. Wissler RW. USA multicenter study of the pathobiology of atherosclerosis in youth. *Ann NY Acad Sci* 1991;623:26–39.
2. Wissler RW, and PDAY collaborating investigators. New insights into the pathogenesis of atherosclerosis as revealed by PDAY. *Atherosclerosis* 1994:108(suppl S):S3–S20.
3. Wissler RW, Komatsu A, Curi E, et al. Classification of the intermediate atherosclerotic lesions in young people. Abstract, XI International Symposium on Drugs Affecting Lipid Metabolism. 1992.
4. Wissler RW, Hiltscher L, Gage A, et al. A useful classification of the intermediate atherosclerotic lesion in the aortas of young people (gross and microscopic lesions). Poster presented at the 26th Hugh Lofland Conference on Arterial Wall Metabolism, Bowman-Gray School of Medicine, Winston-Salem, North Carolina. May 1993.

5. Wissler RW, Hiltscher L, Oinuma T, et al. Pathogenesis of atherosclerosis—The lesions of atherosclerosis in the young: from fatty streaks to intermediate lesions. In: Fuster V, Ross R, Topol E, eds. *Atherosclerosis and Coronary Artery Disease.* New York: Lippincott-Raven Press; 1995:475–489.

6. Fuster V. Mechanisms leading to myocardial infarction: Insights from studies of vascular biology. Lewis A. Conner Memorial Lecture. Circulation 1994;90:2126–2146.

7. Stary HC, Chandler AB, Dinsmore RE, et al. Definitions of advanced types of atherosclerotic lesions and a histological classification of atherosclerosis. *Arterioscler Thromb Vasc Biol* 1995;15:1512–1531.

8. PDAY Research Group. Relationship of atherosclerosis in young men to serum lipoprotein cholesterol concentrations and smoking: A preliminary report from the Pathobiological Determinants of Atherosclerosis in Youth (PDAY) Research Group. *JAMA* 1990;264:3018–3024.

9. Zarins CK, Glagov S. Pathophysiology of human atherosclerosis. In: Veith FJ, Hobson RW, Williams RA, et al. eds. *Vascular Surgery Principles and Practice.* New York: McGraw-Hill; 1994:21–39.

10. Fuster V, Badimon L, Badimon JJ, et al. The pathogenesis of coronary artery disease and the acute coronary syndromes (first of two parts). *N Engl J Med* 1992;326:242–250.

11. Fuster V, Badimon L, Badimon JJ, et al. The pathogenesis of coronary artery disease and the acute coronary syndromes (second of two parts). *N Engl J Med* 1992;326:310–318.

12. Brown BG, Zhao X-Q, Socco DE, et al. Lipid lowering and plaque regression: New insights into prevention of plaque disruption and clinical events in coronary disease. *Circulation* 1993;87:1781–1791.

13. Lendon C, Briggs AD, Born GV, et al. Mechanical testing of connective tissue in the search for determinants of atherosclerotic plaque cap rupture. *Biochem Soc Trans* 1988;16:1032–1033.

14. Davies MJ, Woolf N, Katz DR. The role of endothelial denudation injury, plaque fissuring, and thrombosis in the progression of human atherosclerosis. In: Weber PC, Leaf A, eds. *Atherosclerosis Reviews 23.* New York: Raven Press; 1991:105–113.

15. Wissler RW, Bond MG, Mercuri M, et al, eds. *Atherosclerotic Plaques: Advances in Imaging for Sequential Quantitative Evaluation.* New York: Plenum Press; 1991.

Chapter 6

Advanced Lesions and Acute Coronary Syndromes:
A Pathologist's View

Erling Falk, MD, PhD

Introduction

Atherosclerosis and its complications are the result of a complex interaction between endothelial cells, monocytes/macrophages, T lymphocytes, smooth muscle cells (SMC), and thrombogenic factors involving several quite different pathological processes: <u>inflammation</u> with increased endothelial permeability,[1,2] endothelial activation,[3–8] and monocyte recruitment;[9–12] <u>growth</u> with SMC proliferation, migration, and matrix synthesis;[13] <u>degeneration</u> with cellular and extracellular lipid accumulation;[14–17] <u>calcification and/or ossification</u>;[18] <u>necrosis</u>, possibly due to cytotoxic effects of oxidized low-density lipoproteins (LDL);[17,19,20] and <u>thrombosis</u> involving platelet adherence, aggregation, and degranulation and coagulation with thrombin generation and fibrin formation.[21] Coronary atherosclerosis starts early in life, but takes decades to develop mature plaques responsible for ischemic heart disease (IHD).[22,23] Proliferation of SMC, matrix synthesis, and lipid accumulation may gradually narrow the arterial lumen and ultimately lead to myocardial ischemia and anginal pain, but the chance for survival is good as long as thrombotic complications do not supervene. If thrombosis is superimposed on mature plaques, it may turn an otherwise benign disease into a life-treatening condition that is mainly responsible for acute coronary syndromes of unstable angina, acute myocardial infarction, and sudden coronary death.[24] Therefore, the vital question is not why atherosclerosis develops, but

From: Fuster V, (ed.) *Syndromes of Atherosclerosis: Correlations of Clinical Imaging and Pathology.* Armonk, NY: Futura Publishing Company, Inc.: © 1996.

rather why some plaques remain thrombus-resistant and innocuous while other plaques, after years of indolent growth, become thrombus-prone and life-threatening. Therefore, the composition of plaque has emerged as a much more important factor than plaque size and stenosis severity. Plaques containing a core of soft lipid-rich atheromatous "gruel" are particularly dangerous because such plaques are unstable and vulnerable to rupture whereby highly thrombogenic plaque components are exposed to flowing blood.[25,26] Plaque disruption, or fissuring, with thrombosis superimposed is the most frequent cause of acute coronary syndromes.[24,27,28]

Mature Uncomplicated Plaques

In patients with IHD, the coronary arteries are diffusely involved with confluent "plaquing".[29] The composition, consistency, vulnerability and thrombogenicity of individual plaques vary greatly without any obvious relation to risk factors for clinical disease.[30–33] Most importantly, there is no simple relation among plaque type, plaque volume, or stenosis severity.

Atherosclerosis: Atherosis + Sclerosis

As the term atherosclerosis implies, mature plaques consist typically of two main components: atheromatous "gruel" that is lipid-rich and soft, and sclerotic tissue that is collagen-rich and hard (Figure 1). Although the sclerotic component usually is the most voluminous constituting >70% of an average stenotic coronary plaque,[34,35] it is a relatively benign component because collagen secreted by SMC probably stabilizes plaques, protecting them against disruption. In contrast, the atheromatous component is by far the most dangerous, because the soft atheromatous gruel destabilizes plaques, making them vulnerable to rupture with high risk of subsequent thrombus formation.[26] Accordingly, a significant atheromatous component is usually present in culprit lesions responsible for thrombus-mediated acute coronary syndromes.[28,36]

The atheromatous core within a plaque lacks supporting collagen;[36] it is rich in extracellular lipids, predominantly cholesterol and its esters;[37,38] it is avascular[39,40] and hypocellular (macrophage foam cells are, however, frequently present at the periphery of the core);[20,39,41,42] and it is usually soft. It is generally believed that foam cell necrosis, possibly due to cytotoxic effects of oxidized LDL

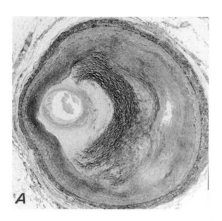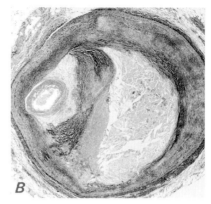

FIGURE 1. *Mature atherosclerotic plaques vary in composition, consisting typically of two main components: <u>atheromatous</u> "gruel" and <u>sclerotic</u> tissue.* **A.** *Stenotic plaque consisting predominantly of hard, collagen-rich sclerotic tissue.* **B.** *Stenotic plaque containing a soft, lipid-rich atheromatous core that is separated from the vascular lumen by a thick cap of fibrous tissue. Trichrome staining.*

taken up by macrophages via scavenger receptors, plays an important role in extracellular lipid accumulation and core formation,[17,19,20] which is why the atheromatous core and the processes leading to its formation are also called necrotic core and atheronecrosis, respectively.[19,37] Insudating lipoproteins trapped and retained within the extracellular space, without first being taken up and released by macrophages, may, however, also contribute to extracellular lipid accumulation, core formation and core enlargement.[43]

Vulnerable Plaques

A small subset of mature uncomplicated plaques is unstable and rupture-prone. There are three major determinants of a plaque's vulnerability to rupture: 1) the size and consistency of the atheromatous core; 2) the thickness of the fibrous cap covering the core; and 3) inflammation within the cap. Furthermore, long-term repetitive cyclic stresses may probably weaken the fibrous cap and increase its vulnerability, ultimately leading to sudden and unprovoked (ie, untriggered) mechanical failure due to fatigue.

Core Size and Consistency

The size of the atheromatous core is critical for the stability of individual plaques. Gertz and Roberts[40] reported the composition of plaques in 5-mm segments from 17 infarct-related arteries examined postmortem and found much larger atheromatous cores in the 39 segments with plaque rupture than in the 229 segments with intact surface (32% and 5% to 12% of plaque area, respectively). By studying aortic plaques, Davies et al[44] found a similar relation between core size and plaque rupture and identified a critical threshold; intact aortic plaques containing a core occupying more than 40% of the plaque area were considered particularly vulnerable and at high risk of rupture and thrombosis.

The consistency of the core, which probably is important for plaque stability, depends on temperature and lipid composition. The core gruel usually has a consistency similar to toothpaste at room temperature postmortem and it is even softer at body temperature in vivo.[37,38] Liquid cholesteryl esters soften gruel while crystalline cholesterol has the opposite effect.[37,38] Based on animal experiments,[37,45] lipid-lowering therapy in humans is expected to deplete plaque lipid with an overall reduction in liquid cholesteryl esters and a relative increase in crystalline cholesterol, theoretically resulting in a stiffer and more stable plaque.[46]

Cap Thickness

Thickness, cellularity, matrix, strength, and stiffness of fibrous caps vary widely. Cap thinning and reduced collagen content increase a plaque's vulnerability to rupture.[47] Caps of eccentric plaques are often thinnest and most heavily foam cell infiltrated at their shoulder regions where they most frequently rupture.[48] Collagen is important for the tensile strength of tissues, and ruptured aortic caps contain less collagen than intact caps.[49] For fibrous caps of same tensile strength, caps covering mildly or moderately stenotic plaques are probably more prone to rupture than caps covering stenotic plaques because the former have to bear a greater circumferential tension (according to Laplace's law).[47] Loss of cells and calcification in fibrous caps are associated with increased stiffness,[50] but the significance of cap stiffness for rupture-propensity is unknown.

Cap Inflammation

Disrupted fibrous caps usually are heavily infiltrated by macrophage foam cells,[39,51,52] and recent observations revealed that such rupture-related macrophages are activated, indicating ongoing inflammation at the site of plaque disruption.[53] For eccentric plaques, the shoulder regions are sites of predilection for both active inflammation (endothelial activation and macrophage infiltration) and disruption,[4,5,48] and mechanical testing of aortic fibrous caps indicate that foam cell infiltration indeed weakens caps locally, reducing their tensile strength.[54] van der Wal et al[53] identified superficial macrophage infiltration in plaques beneath all 20 coronary thrombi examined, whether the underlying plaque was disrupted or just eroded. Evaluated by immunohistochemical technique, the macrophages and adjacent T lymphocytes (SMCs were usually lacking at rupture sites) were activated, indicating ongoing disease activity. These postmortem studies of patients dying of coronary thrombosis have recently been expanded by an in vivo study of atherectomy specimens from culprit lesions responsible for stable angina, unstable rest angina or non-Q wave infarction.[55] Culprit lesions responsible for the acute coronary syndromes contained significantly more macrophages than did lesions responsible for stable angina pectoris (14% versus 3% of plaque tissue occupied by macrophages).[55] Macrophages are capable of degrading extracellular matrix by phagocytosis or by secreting proteolytic enzymes such as plasminogen activators and metalloproteinases, which may weaken the fibrous cap, predisposing it to rupture.[56] Collagen is the main component of caps responsible for their tensile strength, and human monocyte-derived macrophages grown in culture may express collagenase and degrade collagen of aortic fibrous caps during incubation.[57] Particularly lipid-filled macrophages (foam cells) seem to possess such matrix degrading potential.[58] Several studies have now identified matrix degrading proteinases in human plaques,[59–61] and macrophages could be critical in destabilizing plaques, predisposing them to rupture. Furthermore, activated monocytes/macrophages could also play a detrimental role after plaque disruption, promoting thrombin generation and luminal thrombosis.[62–64]

Activated mast cells in plaques may secrete powerful proteolytic enzymes, and mast cells are indeed present in shoulder regions of mature plaques, but at very low density (mast cell to macrophage ratio about 1:20).[65–67] Neutrophils are also capable of destroying tissue by secreting proteolytic enzymes,[68] but neutrophils are rarely found in intact plaques.[53,69] They may occasionally be found in disrupted plaques beneath coronary thrombi, probably entering these plaques shortly after disruption,[53] and neutrophils may also migrate into the arterial wall shortly after reperfusion of occluded arteries in response to ischemia/reperfusion.[70]

Plaque Composition and Risk Factors

Clinical observations indicate that endothelial dysfunction, even evaluated in vessels resistant to atherosclerosis, is an early and reliable marker for the presence of atherogenic risk factors.[71,72] It is unknown, however, how these various risk factors for clinical disease influence the development, composition, and vulnerability of coronary plaques. Age, male gender, hypercholesterolemia, hypertension, smoking, and diabetes correlate with the extent of coronary "plaquing" present postmortem (percentage of surface covered with mature plaques),[73–75] but possible differences in plaque composition have not been reported. On the contrary, fibrous tissue seems to constitute the most voluminous component of mature coronary plaques, irrespective of individual risk factors.[30–33] Preliminary data indicate, however, that smokers may have more extracellular lipids, particularly oxidized LDL, in their plaques than nonsmokers.[76]

Plaque Disruption

Disruption of vulnerable plaques occurs frequently. It is followed by variable amounts of luminal thrombosis and/or hemorrhage into the soft gruel (also called intraplaque thrombosis)[27] causing rapid growth of the lesion. Autopsy data indicate that 9% of "normal" healthy persons have disrupted plaques (without superimposed thrombosis) in their coronary arteries; the number increases to 22% in persons with diabetes or hypertension,[77] and one or more disrupted plaques, with or without superimposed thrombosis are usually present in coronary arteries of patients who died of IHD.[52,78] Disruption of the plaque surface occurs most often where the cap is thinnest and most heavily infiltrated by macrophages and therefore weakest, namely at the cap's shoulders.[26,48] The weak shoulder regions are, however, also points where biomechanical and hemodynamic forces acting on plaques often are concentrated.[48,79] Therefore, the risk of plaque disruption is related to both *intrinsic* plaque features (actual vulnerability) and *extrinsic* stresses imposed on plaque (rupture triggers). The former (discussed above) predispose a plaque to rupture, while the latter (to be discussed below) may precipitate it, if the plaque is vulnerable. As the presence of a vulnerable plaque is a prerequisite for plaque disruption, vulnerability is probably more important than triggers in determining the risk for a future heart attack. If no vulnerable plaques are present in the coronary arteries, there is no rupture-prone substrate for a potential trigger to work on.

Rupture Triggers

Coronary plaques are constantly stressed by a variety of bio-mechanical and hemodynamic forces that may precipitate or "trigger" disruption of vulnerable plaques.[26,80,81] Plaque disruption may occur from the lumen into the plaque due to an increase in luminal blood presssure, or the cap may rupture from the plaque into the lumen due to an increase in intraplaque pressure caused by, for example, vasospasm, bleeding from vasa vasorum, plaque edema, and/or collapse of compliant stenoses.

Blood Pressure

The luminal pressure induces both circumferential tension in and radial compression of the vessel wall. The circumferential wall tension (tensile stress) caused by the blood pressure is given by Laplace's law that relates luminal pressure and radius to wall tension: the higher the blood pressure and the larger the luminal diameter, the more tension develops in the wall.[81] If components within the wall (soft gruel, for example) are unable to bear the imposed load, the stress is redistributed to adjacent structures (fibrous cap over gruel, for example) where it may be critically concentrated.[47,48,79] As mentioned, the consistency of the gruel may be important for stress distribution within plaques; the stiffer the gruel, the more stress it can bear and correspondingly less is redistributed to the adjacent fibrous cap.[46] Importantly, the thickness of the fibrous cap is most critical for the peak circumferential stress: the thinner the fibrous cap, the higher stress develops in it.[47]

Pulse Pressure

The propagating pulse wave causes cyclic changes in lumen size and shape with deformation and bending of plaques, particularly the "soft" ones. Eccentric plaques typically bend at their edges, ie, at the junction between the stiff plaque and the more compliant plaque-free vessel wall.[80] Also, changes in vascular tone cause bending of eccentric plaques at their edges. Cyclic bending may in the long term weaken these points leading to unprovoked "spontaneous" fatigue disruption, while a sudden accentuated bending may "trigger" rupture of a weakened cap.

Heart Contraction

The coronary arteries tethered to the surface of the beating heart undergo cyclic longitudinal deformations by axial bending (flexion) and stretching, particularly the left anterior descending coronary artery.[82] Angiographically, the angle of flexion was recently found to correlate with subsequent lesion progression, but the coefficient of correlation was low.[82] Similar to circumferential bending, a sudden accentuated longitudinal flexion may "trigger" plaque disruption, while long-term cyclic flexion may "fatigue" and weaken the plaque.

Spasm

Plaque rupture and vasospasm do frequently coexist, but the former most likely causes the latter rather than vice versa.[83–85] Onset of myocardial infarction is uncommon during or shortly after drug-induced spasm of even severely diseased coronary arteries,[86,87] indicating that spasm infrequently precipitates plaque disruption and/or luminal thrombosis.

Capillary Plaque Bleeding

Bleeding and/or transudation (edema) into plaques from thin-walled new vessels originating from vasa vasorum and frequently found at the plaque base[78,88] could theoretically increase the intraplaque pressure with resultant cap rupture from the inside.[89] Although frequently found,[78] it is difficult to imagine how a small capillary bleeding at the base of an advanced plaque may disrupt a fibrous cap against the much higher luminal pressure.

Fluid Dynamic Stress

High blood velocity within stenotic lesions may shear the endothelium away, but whether high hemodynamic shear stress alone may disrupt a stenotic plaque is questionable.[40] Hemodynamic stresses are usually much smaller than mechanical stresses imposed by blood and pulse pressures.[80]

Triggering of Disease Onset

Onset of acute coronary syndromes does not occur randomly.[90] Myocardial infarction occurs at increased frequency in the morning, particularly within the first hour after awakening; on Mondays; during winter months and on colder days at other times of the year; and during emotional stress and vigorous exercise.[90–92] Although only about 5% of all myocardial infarctions seem to be related, or triggered, by heavy physical exertion such as shoveling snow[92] (thought to be a potent trigger activity), possible triggers of disease onset—also called acute risk factors[90]—have been reported by nearly 50% of patients with infarction.[93] The pathophysiologic mechanisms responsible for the nonrandom and apparently often triggered onset of myocardial infarction are unknown but probably related to[90]: 1) plaque disruption, likely caused by surges in sympathetic activity with a sudden increase in blood pressure, pulse rate, heart contraction, and coronary blood flow; 2) thrombosis, occurring on previously disrupted or intact plaques when the systemic thrombotic tendency is high because of platelet activation, hypercoagulability, and/or impaired fibrinolysis; and 3) vasoconstriction, occurring locally around a coronary plaque or generalized.

The beneficial effect of β-blockade in the secondary prevention after myocardial infarction provides strong evidence for the theory that plaque disruption may trigger disease onset. β-Blocker therapy reduces reinfarction by 25%[94] despite the lack of any obvious antiatherogenic, direct antithrombotic, fibrinolytic, or spasmolytic effects in humans. On the contrary, β-blockers may induce or potentiate atherogenic dyslipoproteinemia,[95] platelet aggregation,[96] and vasoconstriction.[97] β-blockade does, however, blunt the sympathetic surge in the morning and also blunts the morning peak in onset of infarction,[90] indicating that biomechanical and hemodynamic forces could be critical in triggering plaque disruption and disease onset. Furthermore, the beneficial effect of β-blockade on reinfarction has been related to the reduction in heart rate,[98] and a similar effect on reinfarction has been obtained by the heart rate reducing calcium antagonists verapamil and deltiazem[99,100]— in sharp contrast to the results obtained with the heart rate increasing nifedipine.[100] It should be emphasized, however, that activation of the sympathetic nervous system and hypercatecholaminemia associated with arousal, exercise, emotional stress, and smoking, for example, could trigger onset of infarction not only via β-adrenoceptors but also via α-receptors, promoting platelet aggregation and vasoconstriction. Sudden thrombus growth on previously disrupted or intact plaques due to changes in platelet function and other hemostatic factors are probably a common triggering mechanism of disease onset.[24]

Plaque Thrombosis

Coronary thrombosis is the result of a dynamic interplay between the arterial wall and the flowing blood. About 75% of thrombi responsible for acute coronary syndromes are precipitated by plaque disruption whereby thrombogenic material is exposed to the flowing blood (Figure 2).[25] Superficial plaque inflammation with intimal erosion but no frank disruption, ie, no deep injury, are found beneath the remaining fatal thrombi,[53] usually in combination with a severe atherosclerotic stenosis.

Determinants of Thrombosis

Most disrupted plaques are resealed by a small mural thrombus, and only sometimes does a major luminal thrombus evolve. There are three major determinants for the thrombotic response to plaque disruption/erosion: 1) character and extent of exposed thrombogenic plaque materials (thrombogenic substrates); 2) degree of stenosis and surface irregularities (local flow disturbances); and 3) thrombotic-thrombolytic equilibrium at the time of plaque disruption/erosion (systemic thrombotic tendency).

Thrombogenic Substrates

Limited and conflicting information is available on the thrombogenicity of individual plaque components and it remains unclear which components or factors within the plaque initiate the thrombotic response after plaque disruption and which pathway(s) is (are) involved. Two recent studies evaluated the thrombogenicity of human plaques by analyzing platelet deposition on specimens exposed to flowing blood in perfusion chambers.[101,102] One study tested gross plaque specimens obtained from human aortas and found significantly more platelet deposition on lipid-rich atheromatous "gruel" than on collagen-rich sclerotic matrix.[101] The other study examined microscopic cryostat sections of human coronary arteries and found just the opposite; plaque collagen (types I and/or III) appeared most reactive towards platelets in this experimental set-up.[102]

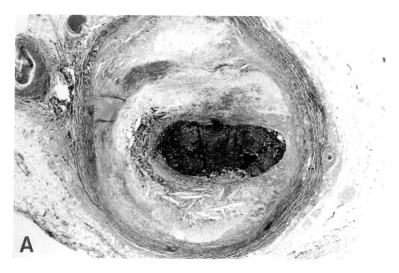

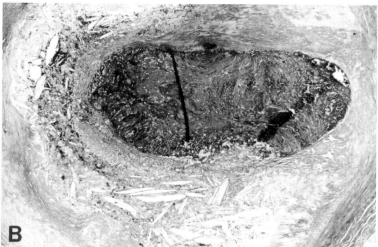

FIGURE 2. *Most coronary thrombi are precipitated by plaque disruption whereby thrombogenic plaque components are exposed to the flowing blood.* **A.** *Disrupted plaque with occlusive luminal thrombosis superimposed.* **B.** *Higher magnification of the plaque thrombus interface, revealing heavily foam cell infiltration in the disrupted cap beneath the thrombus. Some of the soft atheromatous gruel has been extruded through the disrupted surface into the lumen where it is buried within the thrombus, clearly indicating the temporal sequence of events: plaque disruption followed by luminal thrombosis.*

The lipid-rich atheromatous gruel and plaque macrophages are not only important for plaque stability and rupture risk, lipid and macrophages may also be critical in the thrombotic response to plaque disruption.[101] The soft gruel is derived from insudated and retained serum lipids, necrotic and disintegrated cells (preferentially macrophage foam cells), and degraded extracellular matrix. It contains free cholesterol (hard crystals), cholesteryl esters (soft droplets), lipoprotein(a), phospholipids, cellular debris, and collagen degradation products. The component(s) responsible for the high thrombogenicity is unknown, but tissue factor has been suggested as a possible[101] and even likely[103] candidate. Using immunohistochemical techniques, tissue factor protein has been identified in lipid-filled macrophages (foam cells) as well as extracellularly within the atheromatous core (derived from disintegrated macrophages?) of human carotid plaques,[62,103] but not in aortic plaques.[104] Tissue factor expressed by activated macrophages could also be critical for the thrombotic response associated with superficial intimal erosion without frank plaque disruption.

Coronary thrombi are rich in platelets, activated directly by exposed plaque components and shear forces or indirectly via thrombin generation. Thrombin may be generated via the intrinsic (contact activation) or extrinsic (tissue-factor dependent) coagulation pathway, and preliminary data indicate that the former rather than the latter is mainly responsible for thrombin generation in patients with acute coronary syndromes.[105,106] If it is true, the suggested critical role of tissue factor in initiating the thrombotic response after plaque disruption needs to be reconsidered.

Local Flow Disturbances

The severity of stenosis and surface irregularities at the site of plaque disruption influence the thrombotic response: the tighter the stenosis and the rougher the surface, the more platelets are activated and deposited.[52,101,107,108] A platelet thrombus may indeed form and grow within a severe stenosis where the blood velocity and shear forces are highest,[109] probably due to shear-induced platelet activation.[110]

Systemic Thrombotic Tendency

Thrombogenic factors such as platelet hyperaggregability, hypercoagulability, and impaired fibrinolysis are associated with increased risk of thrombus-mediated coronary events.[24] A transient or persistent hypercoagulable state, probably partly mediated by activated monocytes in the peripheral blood, can be identified in many patients with acute coronary syndromes.[64,111] The importance of the actual thrombotic-thrombolytic equilibrium at the time of plaque disruption is clearly documented by the protective effect of antiplatelet agents and anticoagulants against myocardial infarction and coronary death in patients with IHD.[24]

Dynamics of Thrombosis

The thrombotic response to plaque disruption is dynamic; thrombosis/rethrombosis and thrombolysis/embolization occur simultaneously in many patients with acute coronary syndromes, with or without concomitant vasospasm, causing intermittent flow obstructions.[25] The initial flow obstruction is usually due to platelet aggregation, but fibrin is important for subsequent stabilization of the early and fragile platelet thrombus. Therefore, both platelets and fibrin play a role in the evolution of a persisting coronary thrombus.

Secondary to the reduced flow caused by the white platelet-rich thrombus at the rupture site, a red erythrocyte/fibrin-rich venous-type thrombus may form and propagate up- and/or downstream, contributing to the overall thrombotic burden of occluded arteries.[25] This phenomenon tends to occur particularly in coronary vein grafts, which compared to native coronary arteries, lack side branches and are of larger caliber. Although the secondarily formed venous-type thrombus is probably more easily lysed than the primary platelet-rich thrombus at the rupture site, a "clot" several centimeters long may contribute significantly to the thrombotic burden.

Plaque Imaging

Evaluated angiographically, coronary atherosclerosis appears to be a focal disease, and it is so in the sense that it causes intimal plaques to develop that involve the coronary tree unevenly, longitudinally as well as circumferentially. However, in patients with IHD, the extent of "plaquing" is usually so widespread (diffuse) that virtually no vascular segment is left entirely unaffected.[29] Coronary arteries undergo compensatory enlargement during early plaque growth and may thus preserve a normal lumen despite rather severe vessel wall disease.[112,113] Therefore, angiography usually underestimates the extent of disease as well as the degree and length of stenoses, and vascular segments judged normal (because the lumen appears normal) are frequently severely diseased. Disrupted plaques with or without superimposed nonocclusive thrombosis may be identified angiographically due to irregular luminal borders and/or intraluminal lucencies—the "complex" angiographic morphology (Figure 3).[114–116]

Visualization of the arterial wall rather than the lumen is necessary to reveal the full extent of coronary artery disease and to identify early lesions and nonstenotic vulnerable plaques. Intravascular ultrasound[117,118] and angioscopy[119] may reveal important plaque and surface features not seen angiographically, and nuclear magnetic resonance imaging,[120,121] spectroscopy,[122,123] and scintigraphy[124–127] may in the near future improve the in vivo identification and characterization of coronary plaques further. Increased endothelial permeability with insudation of plasma constituents, lipoprotein accumulation, endothelial activation with expression of adhesion molecules recruiting monocytes, macrophage activation and retention in lesions, endothelial denudation with platelet adhesion, aggregation and degranulation, activation of coagulation (thrombin generation) and fibrinolysis (tissue-plasminogen acivator and plasminogen activator inhibitor-1 release) characterize active ongoing atherosclerosis and vulnerable high-risk plaques—features that may be visualized in living persons by appropriate imaging technique.

Clinical Manifestations

The occurrence and course of coronary atherosclerosis and IHD are unpredictable. For individuals with the same number and degree of stenoses evaluated angiographically, some may live for years without any symptoms while others are severely handicapped by angina pectoris, experience life-threatening heart attacks, or die suddenly. The composition of plaques (plaque type) is most important for clinical presentation and outcome in IHD.

Stable Angina

Davies et al[128] categorized the plaque type in 54 men with stable angina and found that 60% of the plaques were fibrous and 40% were lipid-rich. More interestingly, all the plaques were fibrous in 15% of the patients and not a single plaque with a large lipid pool was found in as many as one third of the patients. Apparently, many patients with stable angina lack the appropriate pathoanatomic substrate for plaque disruption, and may consequently be at low

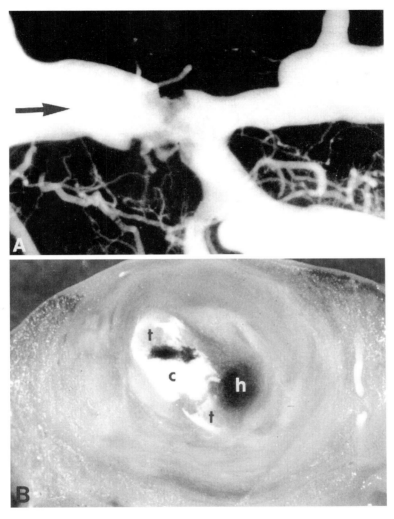

FIGURE 3. *A disrupted plaque, with or without superimposed nonocclusive thrombosis, may give rise to a "complex" angiographic morphology.* ***A.*** *Postmortem coronary angiogram showing a complex lesion in the circumflex branch with irregular borders and intraluminal lucencies.* ***B.*** *The corresponding cross section revealing plaque disruption with hemorrhage into the plaque (h) and nonoccluding thrombi (t) projecting into the narrowed lumen. Arrow in A indicates flow direction; c, contrast medium injected postmortem.*

risk of an acute coronary syndrome. It should be noted, however, that in the same patient individual plaques usually differ significantly, and the composition of one plaque does not predict the compsition of a nearby plaque in the same artery.

Silent Plaque Disruption

Plaque disruption itself is asymptomatic, and also the associated rapid plaque growth is usually clinically silent. It is probably the most important mechanism responsible for the unpredictable, sudden, and nonlinear progression of coronary lesions frequently observed angiographically.[129]

Acute Coronary Syndromes

After plaque disruption, hemorrhage into the plaque, luminal thrombosis, and/or vasospasm may cause sudden flow obstruction, either causing new symptoms to develop or existing symptoms to change. The culprit lesion is frequently dynamic causing intermittent flow obstruction, and the clinical presentation and the outcome depend on the severity and duration of myocardial ischemia. A nonocclusive or transiently occlusive thrombus most frequently underlie primary unstable angina with pain at rest and non-Q wave infarction (often but not always subendocardial) while a more stable and occlusive thrombus is most frequently seen in Q wave infarction (often but not always transmural)—overall modified by vascular tone and collateral flow.[24] The lesion responsible for out-of-hospital cardiac arrest or sudden death is often similar to that of unstable angina: a disrupted plaque with superimposed nonocclusive thrombosis.[24,78,130]

Conclusions

Atherosclerosis without thrombosis is in general a benign disease. However, acute thrombosis frequently complicates the course of coronary atherosclerosis, causing unstable angina, myocardial infarction and sudden death. The mechanism responsible for the sudden conversion of a stable disease to a life-threatening condition is usually plaque disruption with superimposed thrombosis. The risk of plaque disruption depends more on plaque type than on plaque size or stenosis severity. Major determinants of a plaque's vulnerability to rupture are: 1) size and consistency of the lipid-rich atheromatous core; 2) thickness of the fibrous cap covering the core; and 3) ongoing inflammation within the cap. Plaque disruption tends to occur at points where the plaque surface is weakest and most vulnerable, which coincide with points where stresses resulting from biomechanical and hemodynamic forces acting on plaques are concentrated. Therefore, both plaque vulnerability (intrinsic disease) and rupture triggers (extrinsic forces) are important for plaque disruption. The former predisposes the plaque to rupture while the latter may precipitate it. The resultant thrombotic response is important for the clinical presentation and outcome. The challenge is to identify and treat the dangerous vulnerable plaques responsible for infarction and death—to find and treat only angina-producing stenotic lesions is no longer enough. Culprit lesion-based interventions usually eliminate anginal pain, but do not substantially improve the long-term outcome; myocardial infarction and death depend more on coexisting non-symptomatic vulnerable plaques than on stenotic angina-producing lesions. For prevention and treatment, a systemic approach that addresses all coronary plaques will prove to be most rewarding.

References

1. Valenzuela R, Shainoff JR, DiBello PM, et al. Immunoelectrophoretic and immunohistochemical characterizations of fibrinogen derivatives in atherosclerotic aortic intimas and vascular prosthesis pseudointimas. *Am J Pathol* 1992;141:861–880.
2. Zhang Y, Cliff WJ, Schoefl GI, et al. Plasma protein insudation as an index of early coronary atherogenesis. *Am J Pathol* 1993;143:496–506.
3. van der Wal AC, Das PK, Tigges AJ, et al. Adhesion molecules on the endothelium and mononuclear cells in human atherosclerotic lesions. *Am JPathol* 1992;141:1427–1433.
4. Poston RN, Haskard DO, Coucher JR, et al. Expression of intercellular adhesion molecule-1 in atherosclerotic plaques. *Am J Pathol* 1992;140: 665–673.
5. Johnson-Tidey RR, McGregor JL, Taylor PR, et al. Increase in the adhesion molecule P-selectin in endothelium overlying atherosclerotic plaques. *Am J Pathol* 1994;144:952–961.
6. Davies MJ, Gordon JL, Gearing AJH, et al. The expression of the adhesion molecules ICAM-1, VCAM-1, PECAM, and E-selectin in human atherosclerosis. *J Pathol* 1993;171:223–229.
7. Wood KM, Cadogan MD, Ramshaw AL, et al. The distribution of adhesion molecules in human atherosclerosis. *Histopathology* 1993;22:437–444.
8. Bürrig K-F. The endothelium of advanced arteriosclerotic plaques in humans. *Arterioscler Thromb* 1991;11:1678–1689.
9. Ylä-Herttuala S, Lipton BA, Rosenfeld ME, et al. Expression of monocyte chemoattractant protein 1 in macrophage-rich areas of human and rabbit atherosclerotic lesions. *Proc Natl Acad Sci USA* 1991;88:5252–5256.

10. Nelken NA, Coughlin SR, Gordon D, et al. Monocyte chemoattractant protein-1 in human atheromatous plaques. *J Clin Invest* 1991;88:1121–1127.
11. Faruqi RM, DiCorleto PE. Mechanisms of monocyte recruitment and accumulation. *Br Heart J* 1993;69(suppl):S19–S29.
12. Hansson GK. Immune and inflammatory mechanisms in the development of atherosclerosis. *Br Heart J* 1993;69(suppl):S38–S41.
13. Ross R. The pathogenesis of atherosclerosis: A perspective for the 1990s. *Nature* 1993;362:801–809.
14. Ylä-Herttuala S, Rosenfeld ME, Parthasarathy S, et al. Gene expression in macrophage-rich human atherosclerotic lesions. 15-lipoxygenase and acetyl low density lipoprotein receptor messenger RNA colocalize with oxidation specific lipid-protein adducts. *J Clin Invest* 1991;87:1146–1152
15. Ylä-Herttuala S: Macrophages and oxidized low density lipoproteins in the pathogenesis of atherosclerosis. *Ann Med* 1991;23:561–567.
16. Guyton JR, Klemp KF, Black BL, et al. Extracellular lipid deposition in atherosclerosis. *Eur Heart J.* 1990;(suppl E);11:20–28.
17. Witztum JL. The oxidation hypothesis of atherosclerosis. *Lancet* 1994;344:793–795.
18. Demer LL, Watson KE, Boström K. Mechanism of calcification in atherosclerosis. *Trends Cardiovasc Med* 1994;4:45–49.
19. Schwartz CJ, Valente AJ, Sprague EA, et al. The pathogenesis of atherosclerosis: An overview. *Clin Cardiol* 1991;14(suppl I):1–16.
20. Mitchinson MJ. The new face of atherosclerosis. *BJCP* 1994;48:149–151.
21. Fuster V, Badimon L, Badimon J, et al. The pathogenesis of coronary artery disease and the acute coronary syndromes. *N Engl J Med* 1992;326:242–250 and 310–318.
22. Stary HC, Blankenhorn DH, Chandler AB, et al. A definition of the intima of human arteries and of its atherosclerosis-prone regions. A report from the Committee on Vascular Lesions of the Council on Arteriosclerosis, American Heart Association. *Circulation* 1992;85:391–405.
23. Stary HC, Chandler AB, Glagov S, et al. A definition of initial, fatty streak, and intermediate lesions of atherosclerosis. A report from the Committee on Vascular Lesions of the Council on Arteriosclerosis, American Heart Association. *Circulation* 1994;89:2462–2478.
24. Fuster V. Lewis A. Conner Memorial Lecture. Mechanisms leading to myocardial infarction: Insights from studies of vascular biology. *Circulation* 1994;90:2126–2146.
25. Falk E. Coronary thrombosis: Pathogenesis and clinical manifestations. *Am J Cardiol* 1991;68(suppl B):28B–35B.
26. Falk E. Why do plaques rupture? *Circulation* 1992;86(suppl III):III-30–III-42.
27. Davies MJ, Thomas AC. Plaque fissuring—the cause of acute myocardial infarction, sudden ischaemic death, and crescendo angina. *Br Heart J* 1985;53:363–373.
28. Falk E. Morphologic features of unstable atherothrombotic plaques underlying acute coronary syndromes. *Am J Cardiol* 1989;63(suppl E):114E–120E.
29. Roberts WC. Diffuse extent of coronary atherosclerosis in fatal coronary artery disease. *Am J Cardiol* 1990;65(suppl F):2F–6F.
30. Kragel AH, Roberts WC. Composition of atherosclerotic plaques in the

coronary arteries in homozygous familial hypercholesterolemia. *Am Heart J* 1991;121:210–211.

31. Gertz SD, Malekzadeh S, Dollar AL, et al. Composition of atherosclerotic plaques in the four major epicardial coronary arteries in patients ≥90 years of age. *Am J Cardiol* 1991;67:1228–1233.

32. Dollar AL, Kragel AH, Fernicola DJ, et al. Composition of Atherosclerotic Plaques in Coronary Arteries in Women <40 Years of Age with Fatal Coronary Artery Disease and Implications for Plaque Reversibility. *Am J Cardiol* 1991;67:1223–1227.

33. Mautner SL, Lin F, Roberts WC. Composition of atherosclerotic plaques in the epicardial coronary arteries in juvenile (type I) diabetes mellitus. *Am J Cardiol* 1992;70:1264–1268.

34. Kragel AH, Reddy SG, Wittes JT, et al. Morphometric analysis of the composition of atherosclerotic plaques in the four major epicardial coronary arteries in acute myocardial infarction and in sudden coronary death. *Circulation* 1989;80: 1747–1756.

35. Kragel AH, Reddy SG, Wittes JT, et al. Morphometric analysis of the composition of coronary arterial plaques in isolated unstable angina pectoris with pain at rest. *Am J Cardiol* 1990;66:562–567.

36. Davies MJ. A macro and micro view of coronary vascular insult in ischemic heart disease. *Circulation* 1990;82(suppl II):II-38–II-46.

37. Small DM. Progression and regression of atherosclerotic le sions. Insights from lipid physical biochemistry. *Arteriosclerosis* 1988;8:103–129.

38. Lundberg B. Chemical composition and physical state of lipid deposits in atherosclerosis. *Atherosclerosis* 1985;56:93–110.

39. Friedman M. The coronary thrombus: Its origin and fate. *Hum Pathol* 1971;2:81–128.

40. Gertz SD, Roberts WC. Hemodynamic shear force in rupture of coronary arterial atherosclerotic plaques. *Am J Cardiol* 1990;66:1368–1372.

41. Stary HC. Evolution and progression of atherosclerotic lesions in coronary arteries of children and young adults. *Arteriosclerosis* 1989;9 (suppl I):I-19–I-32.

42. Guyton JR, Klemp KF. The lipid-rich core region of human atherosclerotic fibrous plaques. Prevalence of small lipid droplets and vesicles by electron microscopy. *Am J Pathol* 1989;134:705–717.

43. Wight TN. Cell biology of arterial proteoglycans. *Arteriosclerosis* 1989;9:1–20.

44. Davies MJ, Richardson PD, Woolf N, et al. Risk of thrombosis in human atherosclerotic plaques: Role of extracel lular lipid, macrophage, and smooth muscle cell content. *Br Heart J* 1993;69:377–381.

45. Wagner WD, St. Clair RW, Clarkson TB, et al. A study of atherosclerosis regression in Macaca mulatta: III. Chemical changes in arteries from animals with atherosclerosis induced for 19 months and regressed for 48 months at plasma cholesterol concentrations of 300 or 200 mg/dl. *Am J Pathol* 1980;100:633–650.

46. Loree HM, Tobias BJ, Gibson LJ, et al. Mechanical properties of model atherosclerotic lesion lipid pools. *Arterioscler Thromb* 1994;14:230–234.

47. Loree HM, Kamm RD, Stringfellow RG, et al. Effects of fibrous cap thickness on peak cumferential stress in model at herosclerotic vessels. *Circ Res* 1992;71:850–858.

48. Richardson PD, Davies MJ, Born GVR. Influence of plaque configuration and stress distribution on fissuring of coronary atherosclerotic plaques. *Lancet* 1989;ii:941–944.

49. Burleigh MC, Briggs AD, Lendon CL, et al. Collagen types I and III, collagen content, GAGs and mechanical strength of human atherosclerotic plaque caps: Span-wise variations. *Atherosclerosis* 1992;96: 71–81.
50. Lee RT, Grodzinsky AJ, Frank EH, et al. Structure-dependent dynamic mechanical behavior of fibrous caps from human atherosclerotic plaques. *Circulation* 1991;83:1764–1770.
51. Constantinides P. Plaque fissures in human coronary thrombosis. *J Atheroscler Res* 1966;6:1–17.
52. Falk E. Plaque rupture with severe pre-existing stenosis precipitating coronary thrombosis. Characteristics of coronary atherosclerotic plaques underlying fatal occlusive thrombi. *Br Heart J* 1983;50:127–134.
53. van der Wal AC, Becker AE, van der Loos CM, et al. Site of intimal rupture or erosion of thrombosed coronary atherosclerotic plaques is characterized by an inflammatory process irrespective of the dominant plaque morphology. *Circulation* 1994;89:36–44.
54. Lendon CL, Davies MJ, Born GVR, et al. Atherosclerotic plaque caps are locally weakened when macrophages density is increased. *Atherosclerosis* 1991;87:87–90.
55. Moreno PR, Falk E, Palacios IF, et al. Macrophage infiltration in acute coronary syndromes: Implications for plaque rupture. *Circulation* 1994;90:775–778.
56. Matrisian, LM. The matrix degrading metalloproteinases. *Bioessays* 1992;14:455–463.
57. Shah PK, Falk E, Badimon JJ, et al. Human monocyte-derived macrophages express collagenase and induce collagen breakdown in atherosclerotic fibrous caps: Implications for plaque rupture. *Circulation* 1993;88(suppl I):I–254. Abstract.
58. Rennick RE, Ling KLE, Humphries SE, et al. Effect of acetyl-LDL on monocyte/macrophage expression of matrix metalloproteinases. *Atherosclerosis* 1994;109 (suppl):192. Abstract.
59. Henney AM, Wakeley PR, Davies MJ, et al. Localization of stromelysin gene expression in atherosclerotic plaques by in situ hybridization. *Proc Natl Acad Sci USA* 1991;88:8154–8158.
60. Galis ZS, Sukhova GK, Lark MW, et al. Increased expression of matrix-metalloproteinases and matrix degrading activity in vulnerable regions of human atherosclerotic plaques. *J Clin Invest* 1994;94:2493–2503.
61. Brown DL, Hibbs MS, Kearney M, et al. Expression and cellular localization of 92 kda gelatinase in coronary lesions of patients with unstable angina. *J Am Coll Cardiol* 1994;(suppl A):436A. Abstract.
62. Wilcox JN, Smith KM, Schwartz SM, et al. Localization of tissue factor in the normal vessel wall and in the atherosclerotic plaque. *Proc Natl Acad Sci USA* 1989;86:2839–2843.
63. Palabrica T, Lobb R, Furie BC, et al. Leukocyte accumulation promoting fibrin deposition is mediated in vivo by P-selectin on adherent platelets. *Nature* 1992;359:848–851.
64. Jude B, Agraou B, McFadden EP, et al. Evidence for time-dependent activation of monocytes in the systemic circulation in unstable angina but not in acute myocardial infarction or in stable angina. *Circulation* 1994;90:1662–1668.
65. Kaartinen M, Penttilä A, Kovanen PT. Mast cells of two types differing in neutral protease composition in the human aortic intima. Demonstration of tryptase- and tryptase/chymase-containing mast cells in

normal intimas, fatty streaks, and the shoulder region of atheromas. *Arterioscler Thromb* 1994;14:966–972.

66. Kaartinen M, Penttilä A, Kovanen PT. Accumulation of activated mast cells in the shoulder region of human coronary atheroma, the predilection site of atheromatous rupture. *Circulation* 1994;90:1669–1678.

67. Atkinson JB, Harlan CW, Harlan GC, et al. The role of mast cells in atherogenesis: A morphologic study of early atherosclerotic lesions in young people. *Human Pathol* In press.

68. Weiss SJ. Tissue destruction by neutrophils. *N Engl J Med* 1989;320:365–376.

69. Jonasson L, Holm J, Skalli O, et al. Regional accumulations of T cells, macrophages, and smooth muscle cells in the human atherosclerotic plaque. *Arteriosclerosis* 1986;6:131–138.

70. Kloner RA, Giacomelli F, Alker KJ, et al. Influx of neutrophils into the walls of large epicardial coronary arteries in response to ischemia/reperfusion. *Circulation* 1991;84:1758–1772.

71. Celermajer DS, Sorensen KE, Gooch VM, et al. Non-invasive detection of endothelial dysfunction in children and adults at risk of atherosclerosis. *Lancet* 1992;340:1111–1115.

72. Reddy KG, Nair RN, Sheehan HM, et al. Evidence that selective endothelial dysfunction may occur in the absence of angiographic or ultrasound atherosclerosis in patients with risk factors for atherosclerosis. *J Am Coll Cardiol* 1994;23:833–843.

73. Solberg LA, Strong JP. Risk factors and atherosclerotic lesions. A review of autopsy studies. *Arteriosclerosis* 1983;3:187–198.

74. Reed DM, Strong JP, Resch J, et al. Serum lipids and lipoproteins as predictors of atherosclerosis: An autopsy study. *Arteriosclerosis* 1989;9:560–564.

75. Pathobiological Determinants of Atherosclerosis in Youth (PDAY) Research Group. Natural history of aortic and coronary atherosclerotic lesions in youth. Findings from the PDAY study. *Arterioscler Thromb* 1993;13:1291–1298.

76. Wissler RW, the PDAY Collaborating Investigators. New insights into the pathogenesis of atherosclerosis as revealed by PDAY. *Atherosclerosis* 1994;108(suppl):S3–S20.

77. Davies MJ, Bland JM, Hangartner JRW, et al. Factors influencing the presence or absence of acute coronary artery thrombi in sudden ischaemic death. *Eur Heart J* 1989;10:203–208.

78. Davies MJ, Thomas A. Thrombosis and acute coronary-artery lesions in sudden cardiac ischemic death. *N Engl J Med* 1984;310:1137–1140.

79. Cheng GC, Loree HM, Kamm RD, et al. Distribution of circumferential stress in ruptured and stable atherosclerotic lesions. A structural analysis with histopathological correlation. *Circulation* 1993; 87:1179–1187.

80. MacIsaac AI, Thomas JD, Topol EJ. Toward the quiescent coronary plaque. *J Am Coll Cardiol* 1993;22:1228–1241. Review article.

81. Lee RT, Kamm RD. Vascular mechanics for the cardiologist. *J Am Coll Cardiol* 1994;23:1289–1295.

82. Stein PD, Hamid MS, Shivkumar K, et al. Effects of cyclic flexion of coronary arteries on progression of atherosclerosis. *Am J Cardiol* 1994; 73:431–437.

83. Etsuda H, Mizuno K, Arakawa K, et al. Angioscopy in variant angina: Coronary artery spasm and intimal injury. *Lancet* 1993;342:1322–1324.

84. Bogaty P, Hackett D, Davies G, et al. Vasoreactivity of the culprit lesion in unstable angina. *Circulation* 1994;90:5–11.
85. Zeiher AM, Schächinger V, Weitzel SH, et al. Intracoronary thrombus formation causes focal vasoconstriction of epicardial arteries in patients with coronary artery disease. *Circulation* 1991;83:1519–1525.
86. Bertrand ME, LaBlanche JM, Tilmant PY, et al. Frequency of provoked coronary arterial spasm in 1089 consecutive patients undergoing coronary arteriography. *Circulation* 1982;65:1299–1306.
87. Kaski JC, Tousoulis D, McFadden E, et al. Variant angina pectoris. Role of coronary spasm in the development of fixed coronary obstructions. *Circulation* 1992;85:619–626.
88. Zhang Y, Cliff WJ, Schoefl GI, et al. Immunohistochemical study of intimal microvessels in coronary atherosclerosis. *Am J Pathol* 1993;143: 164–172.
89. Barger AC, Beeuwkes R. Rupture of coronary vasa vasorum as a trigger of acute myocardial infarction. *Am J Cardiol* 1990;66(suppl G):41G–43G.
90. Muller JE, Abela GS, Nesto RW, et al. Triggers, acute risk factors and vulnerable plaques: The lexicon of a new frontier. *J Am Coll Cardiol* 1994;23:809–813.
91. Willich SN, Löwel H, Lewis M, et al. Weekly variation of acute myocardial infarction. Increased Monday risk in the working population. *Circulation* 1994;90:87–93.
92. Curfman GD. Is exercise beneficial—or hazardous—to your heart? *N Engl J Med* 1993;329:1730–1731. Editorial.
93. Tofler GH, Stone PH, Maclure M, et al. Analysis of possible triggers of acute myocardial infarction (The MILIS Study). *Am J Cardiol* 1990;66:22–27.
94. Yusuf S, Peto J, Lewis J, et al. Beta blockade during and after myocardial infarction: An overview of the randomized trials. *Prog Cardiovasc Dis* 1985;27:335–371.
95. Leren P. Ischaemic heart disease: How well are the risk profiles modulated by current beta blockers? *Cardiology* 1993;82(suppl 3):8–12.
96. Hjemdahl P, Larsson PT, Wallen NH. Effects of stress and beta-blockade on platelet function. *Circulation* 1991;84(suppl VI):VI44–VI61.
97. Heintzen MP, Strauer BE. Peripheral vascular effects of beta-blockers. *Eur Heart J* 1994;15(suppl C):2–7.
98. Kjekshus JK. Importance of heart rate in determining beta-blocker efficacy in acute and long-term acute myocardial infarction intervention trials. *Am J Cardiol* 1986;57(suppl F):43F–49F.
99. The Danish Study Group on Verapamil in Myocardial Infarction. The effect of verapamil on mortality and major events after myocardial infarction. The Danish Verapamil Infarction Trial II (DAVIT II). *Am J Cardiol* 1990;66:779–785.
100. Held PH, Yusuf S. Calcium antagonists in the treatment of ischemic heart disease: Myocardial infarction. *Coronary Artery Dis* 1994;5:21–26.
101. Fernandez-Ortiz A, Badimon JJ, Falk E, et al. Characterization of the relative thrombogenicity of atherosclerotic plaque components: Implications for consequen ces of plaque rupture. *J Am Coll Cardiol* 1994;23:1562–1569.
102. van Zanten GH, de Graaf S, Slootweg PJ, et al. Increased platelet deposition on atherosclerotic coronary arteries. *J Clin Invest* 1994;93: 615–632.

103. Wilcox JN, Harker LA. Molecular and cellular mechanisms of atherogenesis: Studies of human lesions linked with animal modelling. In: Bloom AL, Forbes CD, Thomas DP, Tuddenham EGD, eds. *Haemostasis and Thrombosis*. London: Churchill Livingstone; 1994:1139–1152.
104. Sueishi K, Yasunaga C, Murata T, et al. Endothelial function in thrombosis and thrombolysis. *Jpn Circ J* 1992;56:192–198.
105. Merlini PA, Spinola A, Ardissino D, et al. Activated factor VII and increased thrombin activity in acute coronary syndromes. *Circulation* 1994;90(suppl I):I–179.
106. Hoffmeister HM, Jur M, Ruf M, et al. Activation of the contact phase of the coagulation in patients with unstable angina pectoris. *Circulation* 1995; 91:2520–2527.
107. de Cesare NB, Ellis SG, Williamson PR, et al. Early reocclusion after successful thrombolysis is related to lesion length and roughness. *Coronary Artery Dis* 1993;4:159–166.
108. Folts J. An in vivo model of experimental arterial steno sis, intimal damage, and periodic thrombosis. *Circulation* 1991;83(suppl IV):IV-3–IV-14.
109. Badimon L, Badimon JJ. Mechanism of arterial thrombosis in nonparallel streamlines: Platelet thrombi grow on the apex of stenotic severely injured vessel wall. *J Clin Invest* 1989;84:1134–1144.
110. Ruggeri ZM. Mechanisms of shear-induced platelet adhesion and aggregation. *Thromb Haemostas* 1993;70:119–123.
111. Merlini PA, Bauer KA, Oltrona L, et al. Persistent activation of coagulation mechanism in unstable angina and myocardial infarction. *Circulation* 1994;90:61–68.
112. Glagov S, Weisenberg E, Christopher BA, et al. Compensatory enlargement of human atherosclerotic coronary arteries. *N Engl J Med* 1987;316:1371–1375.
113. Stiel GM, Stiel LSG, Schofer J, et al: Impact of compensatory enlargement of atherosclerotic coronary arteries on angiographic assessment of coronary artery disease. *Circulation* 1989;80:1603.
114. Levin D, Fallon JT: Significance of the angiographic morphology of localized coronary stenoses: Histopathologic correlations. *Circulation* 1982; 66:316–320.
115. Ambrose JA, Winters SL, Stern A, et al. Angiographic morphology and the pathogenesis of unstable angina pectoris. *J Am Coll Cardiol* 1985;5:609–614.
116. Haft JI, Al-Zarka AM. The origin and fate of complex coronary lesions. *Am Heart J* 1991;121:1050–1061.
117. Nissen SE, Gurley JC, Grines CL, et al. Intravascular ultrasound assessment of lumen size and wall morphology in normal subjects and patients with coronary artery disease. *Circulation* 1991;84:1087–1099.
118. Roelandt JRTC, di Mario C, Pandian NG, et al. Three-dimensional reconstruction of intracoronary ultrasound images. Rationale, approaches, problems, and directions. *Circulation* 1994;90:1044–1055.
119. den Heijer P, Foley DP, Hillege HL, et al. The "Ermenonville" classification of observations at coronary angioscopy—Evaluation of intra- and inter-observer agreement. *Eur Heart J* 1994;15:815–822.
120. Merickel MB, Berr S, Spetz K, et al. Noninvasive quantitative evaluation of atherosclerosis using MRI and image analysis. *Arterioscler Thromb* 1993;13:1180–1186.
121. Toussaint J-F, Southern JF, Falk E, et al. Atherosclerotic plaque com-

ponents imaged by nuclear magnetic resonance. *Arterioscler Thromb* In press.

122. Toussaint J-F, Southern JF, Fuster V, et al. ^{13}C-NMR spectroscopy of human atherosclerotic lesions: Relation between fatty acid saturation, cholesteryl ester content and luminal obstruction. *Arterioscler Thromb* In press.

123. Baraga JJ, Feld MS, Rava RP. In situ optical histochemistry of human artery using near infrared Fourier transform Raman spectroscopy. *Proc Natl Acad Sci USA* 1992;89:3473–3477.

124. Vallabhajosula S, Paidi M, Badimon JJ, et al. Radiotracers for low density lipoprotein biodistribution studies in vivo: Technetium-99m low density lipoprotein versus radioiodinated low density lipoprotein preparations. *J Nucl Med* 1988;29:1237–1245.

125. Lupattelli G, Fedeli L, Fiacconi M, et al. Scintigraphic detection of atherosclerosis by means of radiolabelled lipoproteins. *Thromb Haemorrh Disorders* 1991;3/2:61–65.

126. Lees RS, Lees AM. Radiopharmaceutical imaging of active atherosclerosis. *Atherosclerosis* 1994;109(suppl):352. Abstract.

127. Miller DD, Rivera FJ, Garcia OJ, et al. Imaging of vascular injury with ^{99m}Tc-labeled monoclonal antiplatelet antibody S12. Preliminary experience in human percutaneous transluminal angioplasty. *Circulation* 1992;85:1354–1363.

128. Hangartner JRW, Charleston AJ, Davies MJ, et al. Morphological characteristics of clinically significant coronary artery stenosis in stable angina. *Br Heart J* 1986;56:501–508.

129. Bruschke AVG, Kramer JR, Bal ET, et al. The dynamics of progression of coronary atherosclerosis studied in 168 medically treated patients who underwent coronary arteriography three times. *Am Heart J* 1989;117:296–305.

130. Lo Y-SA, Cutler JE, Blake K, et al. Angiographic coronary morphology in survivors of cardiac arrest. *Am Heart J* 1988;115:781–785.

Chapter 7

Angiographic Correlations of Advanced Coronary Lesions in Acute Coronary Syndromes

John A. Ambrose, MD

Introduction

The pathophysiology of acute coronary syndromes has been a source of controversy throughout this century. Recently, a large body of evidence has suggested that a common pathogenetic mechanism related to the occurrence of minor or major plaque fissuring complicated by intraintimal and/or intraluminal thrombosis may explain these syndromes.[1-5] These acute syndromes appear as a continuum—the clinical presentation being the end result of multiple factors including the severity and acuteness of obstruction, the presence and/or duration of total coronary occlusion, the ability to acutely recruit collaterals, and perhaps to a lesser extent, myocardial oxygen demands.[6-8] This chapter reviews the angiographic findings of these advanced or complex lesions.

Pathophysiology of Acute Coronary Syndromes

In unstable angina, plaque fissuring or disruption leads to an abrupt increase in luminal obstruction. A mural thrombus largely composed of platelets forms initially within the intima, which in itself may increase luminal obstruction. Thrombus may extend into the lumen and transiently decrease myocardial blood flow. Episodic embolization may also occur. Total coronary occlusion is

From: Fuster V, (ed.) *Syndromes of Atherosclerosis: Correlations of Clinical Imaging and Pathology.* Armonk, NY: Futura Publishing Company, Inc.: © 1996.

infrequent, but has been described in 10% to 20% of patients.[9] However, total occlusion followed by spontaneous opening of the artery is a possible mechanism of ischemia/necrosis in unstable angina as well as in non-Q wave infarction.[10] Ischemia at rest in unstable angina may be related to either transient decreases in myocardial oxygen supply related to vasoconstriction or enhanced vasomotion at or distal to the site of coronary narrowing as well as to changes in the thrombus.[11] As a new lesion has formed in the coronary artery causing a new imbalance between myocardial supply and demand, ischemic rest pain may also be precipitated by transient increases in myocardial oxygen demand.[12]

The syndrome of non-Q wave myocardial infarction occupies an intermediate position in the continuum of the acute coronary syndromes between unstable angina and Q wave infarction. A severely stenotic but patent infarct-related artery is found in 60% to 80% of cases. In the remaining 20% to 40%, total coronary occlusion is demonstrated angiographically.[9,13] In many cases of non-Q wave infarction where total occlusion is not found, it has been postulated that spontaneous reperfusion occurs. This has been suggested by the frequent finding of ST segment elevation on the electrocardiogram (ECG) during infarction and an early peak of creatine kinase after infarction.

In patients who present with Q wave myocardial infarction there is total coronary occlusion in 80% to 90% of cases as determined by angiography performed within 6 hours of the onset of acute myocardial infarction.[14,15] A thrombus rich in fibrin and red cells extends from the intima obstructing the lumen of the artery. In a majority of cases of Q wave infarction, a deep tear into the intima of a lipid-rich plaque can be demonstrated.[16] The amount of thrombus that forms after plaque disruption is a complex phenomenon and depends at least in part on the degree of plaque disruption as well as the hypercoagulability of the blood and hemodynamic factors that may potentiate vasospasm after plaque disruption. The latter may lead to the formation of a fibrin-rich, stasis thrombus.[17,18]

Recent data also suggest a potential role for inflammation in the pathogenesis of unstable angina.[19,20] Increased expression of granulocyte and monocyte adhesion receptors can be demonstrated in the coronary sinus of patients with unstable angina. Activated monocytes capable of expressing a tissue factor-like procoagulant activity have also been demonstrated in unstable but not stable syndromes. It is likely that inflammatory cell infiltrates in the fibrous cap are a trigger for plaque disruption.[21] Epicardial "streaks" on the surface of the heart containing inflammatory cells have also been seen at autopsy in patients who died after an episode of unstable angina.[22] Whether the presence of these inflammatory mediators indicates an additional pathophysiologic mechanism for inflammation in unstable angina and acute myocardial infarction is unknown at present. However, thrombosis and inflammation are not incompatable and neutrophil-platelet interactions, as well as the release of inflammatory mediators occur commonly at sites of thrombosis. Prolonged ischemia may also lead to inflammatory infiltrates in the microcirculation.[23,24]

Pathological-Angiographic Correlations in Acute Coronary Syndromes

The angiographic features of such disrupted or complex plaques were first described by Levin and Fallon[25] who examined the heart and coronary arteries and performed post-mortem angiography on patients who died after acute myocardial infarction or after coronary bypass surgery. They found a strong relationship between complicated stenoses as determined angiographically and histologic features of plaque rupture, plaque hemorrhage, superimposed partially occluding thrombi, or recannalized thrombi. These pathological features corresponded to a distinctive angiographic appearance characterized by eccentric, irregular, and shaggy borders with intraluminal haziness. Among 35 lesions with none of these angiographic features and only stenoses with smooth borders, 11.4% were complicated histologically. Among stenoses manifesting one or more of these complex angiographic morphologies, 79% were complicated histologically. Postmortem angiography had a sensitivity of 88% and a specificity of 79% for detecting a complicated stenosis on the basis of these angiographic findings. In a more recent study, Onodera et al[26] re-examined the relationship between postmortem coronary angiographic morphology and coronary histology in patients who died after intracoronary thrombolysis. This study reaffirmed the correlation between atheromatous plaque rupture and hemorrhage with the angiographic features of irregular stenosis borders and filling defects. Eighty percent of such irregular lesions manifested these histologic characteristics. More recently, angiographic-histologic correlations have been made at the time of directional atherectomy.[27–29] These studies show a strong association between the presence of complex lesion on angiography and the presence of an intracoronary thrombus on pathological examination.

Angiographic Correlations in Unstable Angina

Early studies on the angiographic findings in unstable angina found no significant difference in the number of diseased vessels, the stenosis severity, or left ventricular function when compared with patients with stable angina.[30,31] It was only when certain morphological characteristics of lesions were compared between syndromes that significant differences were noted between coronary syndromes.[4,32–36] Angiographic morphology refers to the assessment of lesion shape rather than the severity of stenosis. In general, two lesion characteristics are identified that are usually easy to ascertain. These characteristics are lesion symmetry and the regularity or irregularity of lesion borders. The assessment of morphology requires high-resolution image intensifiers or digital subtraction. This analysis could not have been performed in the early days of angiography when resolution on cine film was suboptimal.

Concerning the qualitative assessment of coronary morphology one must realize that it is subjective. There are multiple shapes and forms of atherosclerotic lesions as demonstrated by angiography. Yet, with careful attention to detail this analysis of symmetry and irregularity can be very reproducible. We can consistently obtain an inter- and intraobserver reproducibility above 90% for the detection of complex lesions. To qualitatively assess coronary morphology one must view the lesion in multiple projections without foreshortening or overlap of vessels. This analysis is performed best both in stop frame and in motion because the eye appears to integrate images better while in motion. It is also helpful to magnify the images by projecting the cine film on a white wall with magnification of about four times normal. It is not sufficient to view lesions in a single projection. Orthogonal views are often necessary because in one view a lesion may look rather smooth while complex features are only seen in the other projection.

In general, lesions that are <100% occluded can be divided qualitatively into simple and complex (Figure 1). There are four aspects to defining a lesion as complex. These include overhanging edges or irregular borders, ulcerations, abrupt faces (≤90%), or filling defects proximal or distal to a stenosis (Figures 2–4). A lesion with one or more of these features is designated as complex. These angiographic analyses of coronary morphology are purely qualitative. Some investigators have attempted to quantitize morphology by measuring the amount of plaque ulceration or the irregularity of lesion borders by complex computer-based analyses.[37,38] While

C.M. OF DISCRETE LESIONS
Simple

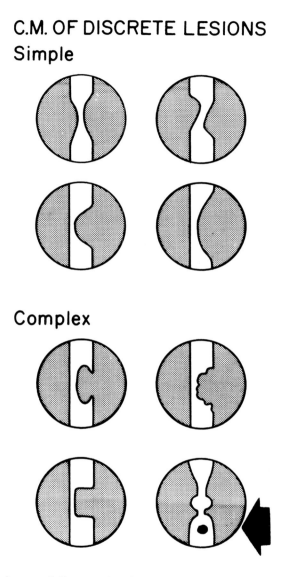

Complex

FIGURE 1. *Schema of discrete simple versus complex lesions showing the most frequent lesion geometries noted. The arrow points to a filling defect (FD), which can be seen proximal or distal to any lesion, and if present in a lesion with simple morphology automatically changes the classification to complex. Modified with permission from Ambrose JA, Israel D. Am J Cardiol 1991;68:78B–84B.*

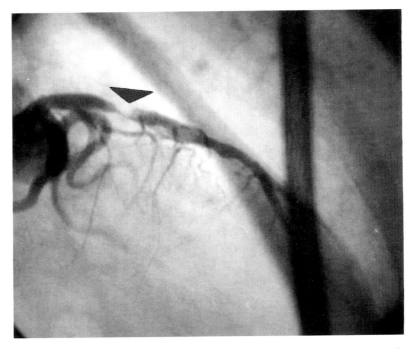

FIGURE 2. *Complex lesion (arrow) in proximal left anterior descending artery, right anterior oblique projection. The lesion has an abrupt distal face with a distal filling defect. This patient presented with pain at rest.*

these techniques may have some advantages over purely qualitative approaches, they have not gained wide acceptance. However, qualitative approaches to assess coronary morphology are widely used.

In our initial study of coronary morphology in unstable angina we evaluated the morphological features of 110 patients with either stable or unstable angina.[4] Unstable angina was defined as pain at rest or crescendo angina. In all cases there was an abrupt change or onset of symptoms. This definition would include most, but not all patients with a diagnosis of unstable angina. In these patients, the presence of an asymmetric or eccentric stenosis with a narrow neck and/or irregular borders was seen in 54% of vessels as opposed to 7% with stable angina. When the lesion responsible for symptoms could be identified by clinical, electrocardiographic, and ventriculographic criteria, this specific type II morphology was identifiable in 71% of "culprit" lesions with unstable angina but in only 16% of lesions were stable angina. Our initial nomenclature classified these lesions as type II eccentric to distinguish them from

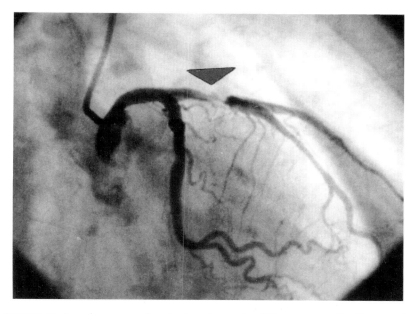

FIGURE 3. *Another complex lesion (arrow) of the proximal left anterior descending artery in the right anterior oblique projection showing an ulceration at the proximal end of the stenosis.*

eccentric or concentric stenoses with smooth borders. As mentioned, we now tend to classify these type II lesions as complex or complicated lesions. As lesion complexity may also be associated with concentric as opposed to eccentric stenosis this newer designation seemed appropriate.

These qualitative observations have been collaborated by other investigators who have characterized similiar appearing lesions as "T" lesions, intracoronary thrombi, or complex plaques.[32–36] In several studies, these angiographic features were found in a majority of patients with unstable angina while in only a minority of patients with stable angina (Table 1). It should be noted that the term complex lesion has also been used to characterize lesions at risk for adverse ischemic events during coronary intervention. Here, the complexity refers to certain anatomic characteristics like lesion tortuosity, calcification, etc. that decrease success and/or increase complications.[39] It is necessary to distinguish between these two designations of complex.

In patients with recent non-Q wave infarction or with a Q wave myocardial infarction and a patent infarct-related artery these angiograhpic features are also commonly seen with an incidence si-

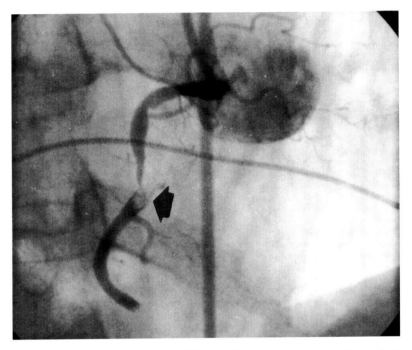

FIGURE 4. *The arrow points to a flling defect distal to a significant lesion of the right coronary artery in the right anterior oblique projection. The patient had a recent myocardial infarction. The distal flow in the coronary artery was decreased (TIMI II flow).*

miliar to that found in unstable angina. However, while 80% to 90% of culprit lesions are <100% occluded in patients with unstable angina this percentage is significantly less in patients who present with myocardial infarction. Within the first 6 hours of myocardial infarction total coronary occlusion is found in about 90% of patients with Q wave myocardial infarction. The incidence of total coronary occlusion in non-Q wave infarction varies between 20% and 40%. Angiographic signs of acute thrombotic coronary occlusion include either dye staining of the occlusion, convex borders to the occlusion, or multiple filling defects without distal filling or when distal filling of the artery is markedly delayed and incomplete (TIMI 0 or 1 flow).[40]

The incidence of complex lesions on angiography is similiar in patients with unstable angina and myocardial infarction with a patent vessel, but there are differences between the appearance of lesions in these syndromes. It has been our experience that multiple filling defects or distal filling defects are seen more frequently

TABLE 1

Complex Lesions or Intracoronary Thrombi in Unstable Angina

	Number	Unstable Angina Complex Lesions/ICT	Stable Angina Complex Lesions/ICT
Ambrose et al[4]	41U 29S	71%	16%
Capone et al[36]	119U	52% -last pain<1 day	0%
	35S	28% -last pain 1–14 days	
Bresnahan et al[35]	67U 201S	35%	2.5%
Haft et al[32]	73U 36S	73%	47%
Williams et al[33]	93U	62%	—
Rehr et al[34]	50U 42S	70%	21%

U indicates unstable angina; S: stable angina; Complex Lesions/ICT: complex lesion morphology or the presence of intracoronary thrombus.

after myocardial infarction than unstable angina. Other investigators have reported similiar findings. Patients presenting with non-Q wave infarction are more likely to exhibit thrombotic features on angiography than patients with unstable angina.[41] Furthermore, serial angiographic studies after myocardial infarction often reveal a gradual decrease in the degree of complexity on subsequent angiography suggesting ongoing thrombolysis.[42,43] In one of these studies, nearly half of the lesions that were classified as complex early after successful thrombolysis changed to smooth lesions in the subsequent 3-month period.[42] These progressive changes in morphology on serial angiography appear less frequent in unstable angina possibly due to a lesser amount of fibrin thrombus in lesions in unstable angina than in myocardial infarction. In fact, in one study 57% of complex lesions detected angiographically remained complex on follow-up.[44] This progressive decrease in the degree of lesion complexity after myocardial infarction has not been observed by all investigators. Nakagawa et al[45] showed that once there was dissolution of overlying mural thrombus, one may see features of plaque disruption (ulceration, overhanging edges, etc.) on subsequent angiography after myocardial infarction.

While lesion complexity and severity may decrease after myocardial infarction, the opposite may be seen after unstable angina. In a preliminary investigation assessing progression of ischemia-related stenosis in unstable angina, Chen et al[46] noted differences between the progression of culprit and nonculprit lesions in unstable angina. After medical stabilization, 25% of culprit lesions were found to have progressed by >20% or to total occlusion in comparison with only 7% of nonculprit lesions ($P=0.001$). In addition, 18 of 53 culprit lesions with complex morphology progressed compared with only 3 of 31 smooth lesions (34% vs. 10% $P=0.02$).

Thus, a majority of lesions in unstable angina show these angiographic characteristics suggesting a complex plaque; however, why do approximately 20% to 30% of lesions in culprit vessels not exhibit an angiographic morphology suggesting a complex lesion? There are several possibilities. First, angiography may be performed long enough after the episode of unstable angina for the lesion to have undergone some remodeling and healing. As mentioned before, this is more likely to occur after myocardial infarction than unstable angina. This remodeling is likely related to organization of mural thrombus. In the experimental model, the surfaces of mural thrombi become endothelialized as fibrin and platelets are replaced by smooth muscle cells, fibroblasts and connective tissue.[47] The original thrombus is no longer recognized as such histologically and the complex features are correspondingly obscured angiographically. The incidence of complex features on angiography are seen more frequently when angiography is performed soon after an episode of unstable angina than when performed days or weeks later.[48] Perhaps the most important reason for this relative insensitivity of angiography to pick up complex plaques is related to the limitations of angiography itself. Angiography only visualizes the lumen of the artery. The details of the intima cannot be seen by even the most high resolution of systems. It has been clearly shown that angioscopy is a more sensitive technique than angiography for assessing the presence of thrombus.[49,50] Therefore, many patients with unstable angina may have a smooth appearing angiographic culprit lesion yet angioscopy will detect intracoronary thrombus or other features of a complex plaque. Of course, it is also possible that clinical instability may occur without plaque disruption and thrombus formation and be related to other processes including vasospasm, increased myocardial oxygen demand, or secondary factors related to conditions like anemia or congestive heart failure.[7,12]

Conversely, why are complex lesions and thrombi that were detected angiographically seen in 7% to 21% of patients with stable angina? This finding supports the hypothesis of intermittency of acute plaque disruption and thrombus formation as an important mechanism of plaque progression. Particularly in patients with new onset of stable angina, these angiographic features of complex lesions may be commonly seen. However, its exact incidence in this group of patients has not been adequately assessed.

Intracoronary Thrombus

The angiographic detection of intracoronary thrombus is extremely variable in studies on unstable angina being reported in between 1% and 85% of cases.[32-36,51-54] This dramatic variation depends on numerous factors including the definition of angiographic thrombus, the timing of angiography in relationship to the last episode of pain, and the medical therapy prior to angiography. The most important factor, in our opinion, relates to the definition of intracoronary thrombus. There is no standardized angiographic definition of intracoronary thrombus in a nonoccluded vessel. Thrombus is often defined in angiographic studies as a filling defect surrounded by contrast on at least three sides. Other definitions used to define thrombus have been identical to criteria used to define complex or type II eccentric lesions. Lesion translucency has also been used to define thrombus. Therefore, there is considerable overlap in angiographic definitions of thrombus vs. complex lesions that clouds the distinction between complex lesions and intracoronary thrombi. This distinction is, in part, semantics, because most complex lesions undoubtedly contain some thrombus as shown in pathological studies and by angioscopy. The thrombotic component in the lesion may consist of platelet-rich intimal thrombi only, but often includes laminar mural thrombus anchored to the intimal component or a free intraluminal fibrin-rich tail anchored to the site of intimal disruption. It is likely that this latter feature is what is detected when filling defects are clearly visualized angiographically proximal or distal to a significant stenosis (Figure 4). The study by Nakagawa et al[45] provides strong evidence for the co-existence of mural thrombus within complex lesions and demonstrates the difficulties in making an angiographic diagnosis of mural thrombus overlying a complex lesion. In spite of these difficulties and lack of a clear distinction between a complex lesion and an intraluminal thrombus, we have tried to standardize the definition of intracoronary thrombus. We define an intracoronary thrombus as a clear-cut filling defect located proximal or distal to a significant narrowing in a coronary artery. Translucency or a filling defect at the site of a lesion are considered in the definition of a complex plaque.

A second important factor in the detection of intracoronary thrombus is the timing of angiography in relationship to the onset of unstable angina or last ischemic episode.[48] When patients are studied late after the onset of unstable angina, the thrombus may undergo endogenous lysis or may organize and become incorporated into the plaque. In either case this might lead to failure to detect a prior thrombus by angiographic techniques. In recent studies where patients were studied within hours or days of the onset of unstable angina the angiographic appreciation of thrombus was made in 40% to 50% of the cases.[35,36]

Angiographic Evolution of Coronary Lesion in Acute Coronary Syndromes

Several angiographic studies in which more than one angiogram was performed on a patient who subsequently developed an acute syndrome have shown that a majority of these syndromes develop from atherosclerotic plaques that did not cause severe obstruction on the initial angiogram.[55-59] In a majority of patients who developed unstable angina or acute myocardial infarction, the culprit lesion was <70% narrowed on the initial angiogram. In retrospective studies of acute myocardial infarction 78% to 97% of lesions were <70% or 75% obstructed on the initial angiogram while only 3% to 23% were >70% or 75% narrowed initially. Less than 50% narrowing was found in 48% of myocardial infarcitons by Ambrose et al[56] and in 66% by Little et al.[57] In a more recent prospective study of the effects of lipid lowering therapy on progression of coronary atherosclerosis, Brown et al[60] found that in 69% of patients the lesion subsequently responsible for either unstable angina, myocardial infarction or death was <70% narrowed on the first angiogram. Although all of these studies have selected out a population of patients in whom serial angiography was performed, these results differ significantly from patients who had been restudied and found to have had a new total coronary occlusion, but without an intervening infarction. In this latter group, a severe lesion with >70% narrowing was found on the first angiogram in the majority.[56,61]

In addition to the above, angiographic studies after successful thrombolysis often show only moderate coronary stenoses in the infarct-related artery. Of 32 patients studied by Brown et al[62] after successful thrombolysis, in 32% the underlying stenoses was <50% obstructive, and in 66% the lumen was narrowed by <60%. Other angiograhpic studies post-thrombolysis indicate that moderate stenoses causing a 50% to 70% diameter reduction are the rule rather than the exception in the infarct-related artery.[63,64] Furthermore, particularly in patients with acute myocardial infarction in whom thrombolysis was given, there is remodeling of the infarct-related lesion in the first week to 10 days after myocardial infarction.[42] This remodeling is associated with an increase in minimal lumen diameter and a decrease in the degree of irregularity of the lesion. Undoubtedly, this is related to endogenous thrombolysis which continues to dissolve residual thrombus even after thrombolytic therapy has opened an occluded artery. This observation of continued thrombolysis of the culprit lesion has been reconfirmed in the APRICOT trial and reported recently in a preliminary publication.[43] A progressive decrease in lesion irregularity and severity of stenoses was found at 3 months following myocardial infarction and this effect was potentiated by the use of antithrombotic and anticoagulant therapy after infarction. While these angiographic observations are extremely interesting and potentially important, we must realize that angiography often underestimates the degree of atherosclerosis. From studies of intravascular ultrasound and pathologic studies in pressure-fixed arteries, angiography will consistently under estimate the amount of atherosclerotic narrowing since it does not visualize the arterial wall.[65,66] Therefore, in all of these angiographic studies which assessed the degree of luminal narrowing prior to an acute syndrome even with the most sophisticated of quantitative coronary angiographic techniques the amount of narrowing of the artery may be unpredictably underestimated in some cases.

Furthermore, not all angiographic data support the notion that acute syndromes develop from less than severe lesions.[67,68] These studies suggest that in about one third of cases, infarction developed from a lesion that was severe (>70% obstructed) on the first angiogram. However, even in these studies, the data are not completely consistent with the concept that a severe lesion is a sensitive and specific indicator of subsequent infarction. Moise et al found new coronary occlusion in 31% of 313 patients restudied after medical therapy for coronary disease.[67] A new occlusion was strongly associated with an interim infarction. The best predictor of infarction on initial study was the presence of at least an 80% narrowing of an artery supplying a non akinetic left ventricular segment. However, in 54% of arteries the site of occlusion appeared to be distal to or at a different segment of the same artery remote from the 80%

narrowing. Similiar observations have been reported by Neill et al[68] who found a new total occlusion in 30% of severely stenotic lesions on follow-up angiography. This finding was associated in a large percentage with an interim infarction. However, six additional patients with progression of coronary disease to a new total occlusion did not develop a Q wave infarction after occlusion. In these patients, as in the other angiographic studies where a severe narrowing was present on the initial angiogram, new total occlusion did not result in infarction probably because the acute recruitment of collaterals prevented or limited the amount of the damage.

References

1. Ross R. The pathogenesis of atherosclerosis. In: Braunwald E, ed. *Heart Disease.* Philadelphia: WB Saunders; 1992:1106–1124.
2. Fuster V, Badimon L, Badimon JJ, et al. Coronary artery disease. Progression and acute coronary syndromes. Parts 1 and 2. *N Engl J Med* 1992;326:242–250 and 310–318.
3. Falk E. Unstable angina with fatal outcome. Dynamic coronary thrombosis leading to infarction and/or sudden death. *Circulation* 1985;71:699–708.
4. Ambrose JA, Winter SL, Stern A, et al. Angiographic morphology and the pathogenesis of unstable angina pectoris. *J Am Coll Cardiol* 1985;5:609–616.
5. Davies MJ, Thomas AC. Plaque fissuring: The cause of acute myocardial infarction, sudden ischaemic death, and crescendo angina. *Br Heart J* 1985;53:363–373.
6. Ambrose JA. Coronary angiographic findings in the acute coronary syndromes in unstable angina. In: Bleifeld W, Braunwald WE, Hamm C, eds. *Unstable Angina.* Berlin/Heidelbert: Springer-Verlag; 1990:112–128.
7. Ambrose JA, Monsen C. Arteriographic anatomy and mechanisms of myocardial ischemia in unstable angina. *J Am Coll Cardiol* 1987;9:1397–1402. Editorial.
8. Gorlin R, Fuster V, Ambrose JA. Anatomic-physiological links between the acute coronary syndromes. *Circulation* 1986;74:6–9.
9. Ambrose JA, Monsen C, Borrico S, et al. Angiographic demonstration of a common link between unstable angina pectoris and non-Q wave acute myocardial infarction. *Am J Cardiol* 1988;61:244–247.
10. Huey Bl, Gheorghiade M, Crampton RS, et al. Acute non-Q wave myocardial infarction associated with early ST segment elevation for spontaneous coronary reperfusion and implications for thrombolytic trials. *J Am Coll Cardiol* 1987;9:18–25.
11. Willerson JT, Hills LD, Winniford M, et al. Speculation regarding mechanisms responsible for acute ischemic heart disease syndromes. *J Am Coll Cardiol* 1986;8:245–250.
12. Langer A, Freeman MR, Armstrong PW. ST segment shift in unstable angina. Pathophysiology and association with coronary anatomy and hospital outcome. *J Am Coll Cardiol* 1989;13:1495–1502.

13. DeWood MA, Stifler WF, Simpson CS, et al. Coronary arteriographic findings soon after non-Q wave myocardial infarction. *N Engl J Med* 1986;315:417–423.
14. DeWood MA, Spores J, Notske RN, et al. Prevalence of total coronary occlusion during the early hours of transmural myocardial infarction. *N Engl J Med* 1980;303:897–902.
15. Rentrop KP, Feit F, Blanke H, et al. Effects of intracoronary streptokinase and intracoronary nitroglycerin infusion on coronary angiographic patterns and mortality in patients with acute myocardial infarction. *N Engl J Med* 1984;311:1456–1463.
16. Richardson PD, Davies MJ, Born GVR. Influence of plaque configuration and stress distribution on fissuring of coronary atherosclerotic plaques. *Lancet* 1989;2:941–944.
17. Ambrose JA. Plaque disruption and the acute coronary syndromes of unstable angina and myocardial infarction: If the substrate is similar, why is the clinical presentation different? *J Am Coll Cardiol* 1992;19:1653–1658.
18. Mizuno K, Satomuro K, Miyamato A, et al. Angioscopic evaluation of the character of coronary thrombi in acute coronary syndromes. *N Engl J Med* 1992;326:287–291.
19. Mazzone A, DeServi S, Ricevuti G, et al. Increased expression of neutrophil and monocyte adhesion molecules in unstable coronary artery disease. *Circulation* 1993;88:358–363.
20. Neri Serneri GG, Albate R, Gori AM, et al. Transient intermittent lymphocyte activation is responsible for the instability of angina. *Circulation* 1992;86:790–797.
21. Van der Wal A, Becker AE, Van der Loos CM, et al. Site of intimal rupture or erosion of thrombosed coronary atherosclerotic plaques is characterized by an inflammatory process irrespective of the dominant dominant plaque morphology. *Circulation* 1994;89:36–44.
22. Kohchi K, Takebayashi S, Hiroki T, et al. Significance of adventitial inflammation of the coronary artery in patients with unstable angina: Results at autopsy. *Circulation* 1985;71:709–716.
23. Entman ML, Ballantyne CM. Inflammation in acute coronary syndromes. *Circulation* 1993;88:800–803.
24. Bazzoni G, Dejana E, Del Maschio A. Platelet-neutrophil interactions: Possible relevance in the pathogenesis of thrombosis and inflammation. *Haematologica* 1991;76:491–499.
25. Levin DC, Fallon JT. Significance of the angiographic morphology of localized coronary stenoses: Histopathologic correlations. *Circulation* 1982;66:316–320.
26. Onodera T, Fujiwara H, Tanaka M, et al. Cineangiographic and pathological features of the infarct related vessel in successfull and unsuccessfull thrombolysis. *Br Heart J* 1989;61:385–389.
27. Sharma SK, Israel DH, Fyfe B, et al. Coronary thrombus: Clinical and angiographic correlates in 185 lesions undergoing directional coronary atherectomy. *Circulation* 1993;88:I–208. Abstract.
28. Christou CP, Haft JI, Goldstein JE, et al. Correlation of ischemic coronary syndromes with angiographic morphology and lesion histology. *J Am Coll Cardiol* 1992;19:375A.
29. Isner JM, Brinker JA, Gottlieb RS, et al. Coronary thrombus: Clinical features and angiographic diagnosis in 370 patients studied by directional atherectomy. *Circulation* 1992;86:I–649. Abstract.

30. Alison HW, Russell RO Jr, Mantle JA, et al. Coronary anatomy and arteriography in patients with unstable angina pectoris. *Am J Cardiol* 1978;41:204–209.
31. Fuster V, Frye RL, Connolly DC, et al. Arteriographic patterns early in the onset of the coronary syndromes. *Br Heart J* 1975;37:1250–1255.
32. Haft JI, Goldstein JE, Niemiera ML. Coronary arteriographic lesion of unstable angina. *Chest* 1987;92:609–612.
33. Williams AE, Freeman MR, Chisholm RJ, et al. Angiographic morphology in unstable angina pectoris. *Am J Cardiol* 1988;62:1024–1027.
34. Rehr R, DiSciascio G, Vetrovec G, et al. Angiographic morphology of coronary artery stenosis in prolonged rest angina. Evidence of intracoronary thrombosis. *J Am Coll Cardiol* 1989;14:1429–1437.
35. Bresnahan DR, Davis DR, Holmes DR Jr, et al. Angiographic occurence and clinical correlates of intraluminal coronary artery thrombus: Role of unstable angina. *J Am Coll Cardiol* 1985;6:285–289.
36. Capone G, Wolf NM, Meyer B, et al. Frequency of intracoronary filling defects by angiography in angina pectoris at rest. *Am J Cardiol* 1985;56:403–406.
37. Wilson FR, Holida MD, White CW. Quantitative angiographic morphology of coronary stenoses leading to myocardial infarction or unstable angina. *Circulation* 1986;73:286–293.
38. Kalbfleisch SJ, McGillen MJ, Simon SB, et al. Automated quantitation of indexes of coronary lesion complexity: Comparison between patients with stable and unstable angina. *Circulation* 1990;82:439–447.
39. Ellis SG, Vandormael MG, Cowley MJ, et al. Coronary morphology & clinical determinants of procedural outcome with angioplasty for multivessel coronary disease. Implications for patient selection. *Circulation* 1990;82:1193–1202.
40. The TIMI Study Group. Comparison of invasive and conservative strategies following intravenous tissue plasminogen activator in acute myocardial infarction: Results of the thrombolysis in myocardial infarction (TIMI) II trial. *N Engl J Med* 1989;320:618–628.
41. Rivera W, Sharaf BL, Miele NJ, et al. Coronary anatomy in patients who present with non-Q wave myocardial infarction differs from unstable angina pecctoris: A Report from TIMI 3B. *Circulation* 1994;90: I–438. Abstract.
42. Davies SW, Marchant B, Lyons JP, et al. Coronary lesion morphology in acute myocardial infarction: Demonstration of early remodelling after streptokinase treatment. *J Am Coll Cardiol* 1990;16:1079–1086.
43. Veen G, Meijer A, Werter CJPJ, et al. Dynamic changes of culprit lesion morphology and severity after successful thrombolysis for acute myocardial infarction: An angiographic follow up study. *J Am Coll Cardiol* 1994;23:147A.
44. Haft JI, al-Zarka AM. The origin and fate of complex coronary lesions. *Am Heart J* 1991;121:1050–1061.
45. Nakagawa S, Hanada Y, Koiwaya Y, et al. Angiographic features in the infarct-related artery after intracoronary urokinase followed by prolonged anticoagulation. Role of ruptured atheromatous plaque and adherent thrombus in acute myocardial infarction, in vivo. *Circulation* 1988;78:1335–1344.
46. Chen L, Chester MR, Huang J, et al. Progression of ischaemia-related stenoses in unstable angina. *Circulation* 1994;90:I–438. Abstract.
47. Van Axen PJ, Emeis JJ. Organization of experimentally induced arte-

rial thrombosis in rats from two weeks until ten months. The development of an arterioscleroc lesion and the occurence of rethrombosis. *Artery* 1983;11:384–399.

48. Freeman MR, Williams AE, Chisholm RJ, et al. Intracoronary thrombus & complex morphology in unstable angina. Relation to timing of angiography and in hospital cardiac events. *Circulation* 1989;80:17–23.

49. Sherman CT, Litvack F, Grundfest W, et al. Coronary angioscopy in patients with unstable angina pectoris. *N Engl J Med* 1986;5:913–919.

50. White CJ, Ramee SR, Mesa J, et al. Percutaneous coronary angioscopy in patients with restenosis after coronary angioplasty. *J Am Coll Cardiol* 1991;17:46B–49B.

51. Ambrose JA. Coronary arteriographic analysis and angiographic morphology. *J Am Coll Cardiol* 1989;13:1492–1494. Editorial.

52. Vetrovec GW, Cowley MJ, Overton H, et al. Intracoronary thrombus in syndromes of unstable myocardial ischemia. *Am Heart J* 1981;102: 1202–1208.

53. Mandlekorn JB, Wolf NM, Singh S, et al. Intracoronary thrombus in nontransmural myocardial infarction in unstable angina pectoris. *Am J Cardiol* 1983;52:1–6.

54. Cowley MJ, DiSciascio G, Rehr RB, et al. Angiographic observations and clinical relevance of coronary thrombus in unstable angina pectoris. *Am J Cardiol* 1989;63:108E–113E.

55. Ambrose JA, Winters SL, Arora RR, et al. Angiographic evolution of coronary morphology in unstable angina. *J Am Coll Cardiol* 1986;7: 472–478.

56. Ambrose JA, Tannenbaum MA, Alexopoulos D, et al. Angiographic progression of coronary artery disease and the development of myocardial infarction. *J Am Coll Cardiol* 1988;12:56–62.

57. Little WC, Constantinescu M, Applegate RJ, et al. Can coronary angiography predict the site of a subsequent myocardial infarction in patients with mild to moderate coronary artery disease? *Circulation* 1988;78:1157–1166.

58. Giroud D, Jian ML, Urban P,et al. Relation of the site of acute myocardial infarction to the most severe coronary arterial stenosis at prior angiography. *Am J Cardiol* 1992;69:729–732.

59. Nobuyoshi M, Tanaka M, Mosaka H, et al. Progression of coronary atherosclerosis: Is coronary spasm related to progression? *J Am Coll Cardiol* 1991;18:904–910.

60. Brown BG, Zhao XQ, Sacco DE, et al. Lipid lowering and plaque regression;New insights into prevention of plaque disruption and clinical events in coronary disease. *Circulation* 1993;87:1781–1791.

61. Webster MWI, Chesebro JH, Smith HC, et al. Myocardial infarction and coronary artery occlusion: A prospective 5-year angiographic study. *J Am Coll Cardiol* 1990;15:218A.

62. Brown BG, Gallery CA, Badger RS, et al. Incomplete lysis of thrombus in the moderate underlying atherosclerotic lesion during intracoronary infusion of streptokinase for acute myocardial infarction: Quantitave angiographic observations. *Circulation* 1986;73:653–661.

63. Hackett D, Davies G, Maseri A. Pre-existing coronary stenoses in patients with first myocardial infarction are not necessarily severe. *Br Heart J* 1988;9:1317–1323.

64. Serruys PW, Arnold AER, Brower RW, et al. Effect of continued rt-PA adminstration on the residual stenosis after initially successfull recanal-

ization in acute myocardial infarction: A quantitative coronary angiography study of a randomized trial. *Eur Heart J* 1987;8:1172–1181.

65. Porter TR, D'Sa A, Turner C, et al. Myocardial contrast echocardiography for the assessment of coronary blood flow reserve: Validation in humans. *J Am Coll Cardiol* 1993;21:349–355.

66. Stiel GM, Stiel LSG, Schofer J, et al. Impact of compensatory enlargement of atherosclerotic coronary arteries on angiographic assessment of coronary artery disease. *Circulation* 1989;80:1603–1609.

67. Moise A, Lesperance J, Theroux P, et al. Clinical and angiographic predictors of a new total coronary occlusion in coronary artery disease: Analysis of 313 non-operated patients. *Am J Cardiol* 1984;54:1176–1181.

68. Neil WA, Wharton TP, Fluri-Lundeen J, et al. Acute coronary insufficiency: Coronary occlusion after intermittent ischemic attacks. *N Engl J Med* 1980;2:1157–1162.

Chapter 8

Coronary Angiography in the Acute Coronary Syndromes

Mervyn S. Gotsman, MD, Chaim Lotan, MD,
Morris Mosseri, MD, Yonathan Hasin, MD,
Shimon Rosenheck, MD, A. Teddy Weiss, MD,
and Yoseph Rozenman, MD

Introduction

The acute coronary syndromes are ischemic states that develop over a short period of time. They include the sudden natural progression of native coronary atheroma with the development of unstable angina or acute myocardial infarction, or iatrogenic disease that is induced by acute percutaneous revascularization or after coronary artery bypass surgery.

Unstable Angina

Primary unstable angina has been defined as the new onset of angina pectoris, exacerbation of existing stable angina pectoris, or angina pectoris at rest or after acute myocardial infarction.[1] Pathologically there is rupture or a fissure of an atheromatous plaque with or without superadded thrombus formation.[2,3] Angioscopy shows this ulcerated plaque with a small layer of overlying thrombus.[4] Two angiographic patterns have been described.[5,6] The first is a plaque with irregular or ulcerated surfaces, as evidence of underlying rupture (Figure 1). Pedunculated fresh thrombus is uncom-

This research was supported by a grant from the National Council for Research and Development, Israel and GSF Munchen, Germany.

From: Fuster V, (ed.) *Syndromes of Atherosclerosis: Correlations of Clinical Imaging and Pathology.* Armonk, NY: Futura Publishing Company, Inc.: © 1996.

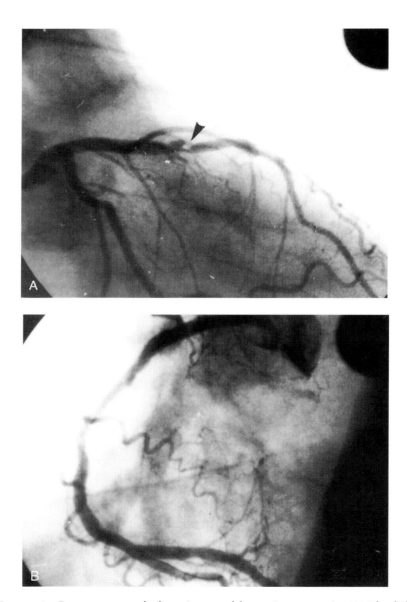

FIGURE 1. *Coronary morphology in unstable angina pectoris. (**A**) The left anterior descending coronary (LAD) artery in the cranial right anterior oblique view demonstrating typical angiographic appearance of an ulcerated plaque (arrow). (**B**) There is only mild atheroma in the right coronary artery (RCA) seen in the left anterior oblique view. The patient elected to be treated medically and was free of symptoms for 1 year. A thallium exercise test was negative. One year later the patient was admitted again with unstable angina.*

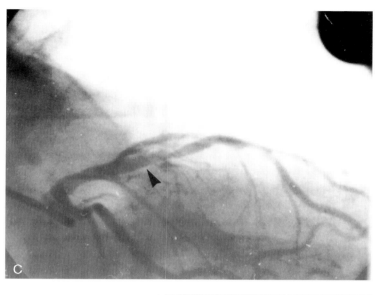

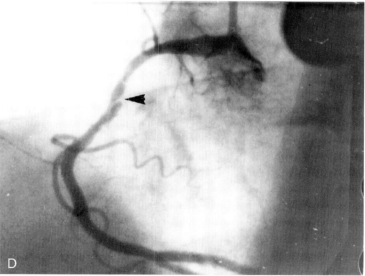

FIGURE 1 *continued* (*C*) Coronary angiography in the same views as in the previous year show healing of the ulcerated plaque in the LAD (arrow), and (*D*) a new ulcerated plaque in the RCA (arrow).

mon at angiography. The second is indistinguishable from the plaque seen in stable angina and the distinction can only be made on the basis of clinical history or sequential angiography. The classical angiographic pattern of a patient with unstable angina consists of one or two lesions in an otherwise almost normal arterial tree and sequential studies have shown that these occur in sites of the arterial wall that were almost normal previously (Figure 1).[7] The lesions respond readily to angioplasty, but there is an increased incidence of complications and restenosis is more common than in longstanding chronic disease.[8,9] Presumably, thrombotic activity in the region of the plaque, or the presence of soft thrombogenic lipid, collagen, and von Willebrand factor act as dynamic progenitors of thrombus generation, which induces excessive cellular proliferation in the healing process. A minority of patients have hard lesions that are difficult to dilate and in them, the longstanding noncompliant underlying plaque, presumably with superficial endothelial dysfunction and decrease flow at a high shear rate leads to superadded thrombus formation causing increased stenosis.[10] First principles suggest that thrombolytic therapy, by lysing superadded thrombus should improve prognosis. The TIMI III Trial, however, which examined lytic therapy in unstable angina pectoris, showed no additional therapeutic value of intravenous thrombolytic therapy.[11] A smaller subset of patients have extensive triple vessel disease. Natural progression of atheroma simply increases the severity of the angina pectoris.

Acute Myocardial Infarction

Acute myocardial infarction is frequently associated with total obstruction of the infarct related coronary artery (80%).[12] Pathological studies show an underlying plaque, usually ruptured, with superadded and propagated thrombus and occasional distal emboli.[13,14] Coronary angiography in the acute stage shows complete obstruction of the artery (Figure 2), often progressing backwards to a bifurcation where there is a clear, abrupt interruption of the coronary artery lumen. Angiographic studies made 60–90 minutes after intravenous or intracoronary lytic therapy then show a thin, new channel that has formed in the obstructing thrombus and blood flow trickles into the distal artery.[15,16] With time, the lumen widens as the clot is lysed further and flow through the lesion gradually increases (from TIMI grade 0 [no flow] to TIMI grade 3 [normal flow]) as lysis of the thrombus continues.[17,18] Angiography done during lysis demonstrates this gradual erosion of the clot leaving an

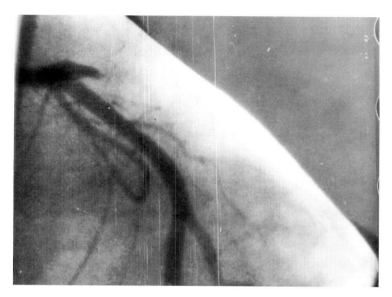

FIGURE 2. *Total proximal occlusion of the left anterior descending coronary artery in a patient with acute myocardial infarction. Complete cutoff of the artery without distal opacification of this artery.*

irregular crater (Figure 3). After successful lysis, a partially occluding lesion remains in the coronary artery. This is frequently eccentric, but may also be concentric. In a few patients the underlying plaque rupture, crater or dissection is obvious, but in the majority of patients, residual thrombus covers the ruptured plaque so that the arterial wall has a smooth inner contour. Studies made 1 week after the acute episode in a group of 308 patients with acute transmural myocardial ischemia and impending myocardial infarction treated with high-dose intravenous thrombolytic therapy showed that the patients had an average of 2.4 lesions each.[19,20] Four-fifths of the arteries were patent, 104 (34%) had a ruptured plaque, 22 (7%) had an ulcerated plaque and in 189 (62%) the lesions were eccentric (Figure 4). The lesions were proximal and related to bifurcations. This study gave insight into the possible pathogenetic mechanisms of formation of the initial atheromatous plaque. The lesions were at branch points and bends, at flow dividers where alteration in laminar flow increased eddies and the formation of backwashes with stagnation of blood flow (Figure 5). Low endothelial shear stress altered endothelial cellular function with decreased secretion of nitric oxide and anticoagulant function. Macrophage adhesion and accretion in the low flow backwashes

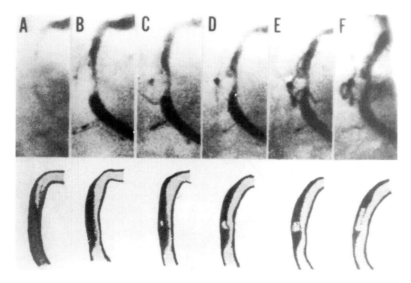

FIGURE 3. *Sequential angiograms of the right coronary artery in a patient with acute myocardial infarction during the course of thrombolytic therapy. The clot in the artery is lysed and the lumen of the artery widens. Reprinted with permission from Reference 18.*

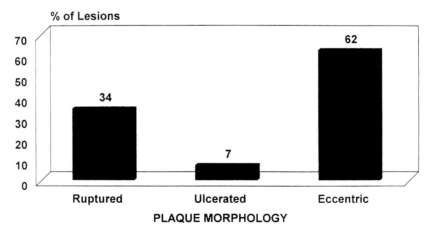

FIGURE 4. *Plaque morphology of the culprit lesion in a group of patients who underwent coronary angiography 1 week after streptokinase administration for acute myocardial infarction.*

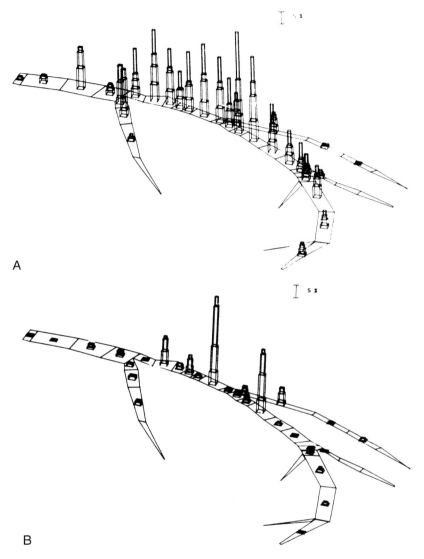

FIGURE 5. *(A) Distribution of coronary lesions in the left anterior descending coronary artery in patients with stable angina, and (B) in patients after thrombolysis for acute myocardial infarction. In the post lysis group lesions are proximal and closely related to bifurcations (2.4 lesions per patient). In the stable angina group, proximal location close to bifurcations is more common but lesions are more widely distributed in the artery (5.7 per patient). Reprinted with permission from Reference 20.*

with a prolonged transit time permitted attachment to vascular cell adhesion molecules. If and when the small plaque ruptures, reduced flow permits the formation of a stable thrombus. This study contrasts with our previous study[19] of 302 consecutive patients with stable angina pectoris who underwent coronary angiography. They had a similar distribution of lesions, but they were more disseminated with a mean of 5.7 lesions per patient (Figure 5).

Reocclusion of the culprit lesion in patients with successful thrombolysis occurs in 8% of patients in the subsequent week and in another 12% in the subsequent 2 years.[21] Clinically this is often silent. In our own series of patients, severe residual stenosis was associated with silent reocclusion of the artery within 3 months.[22] Repeat angiographic studies again show a complete cut-off of the artery. In lesions between 40% to 60% residual stenosis, the lesion often improved suggesting further clot resorption.

If the patient is studied routinely 2–3 months after the infarct, and the artery is completely occluded, the distal end of the lesion appears as an irregular "rats tail" with slow flow of blood through the newly formed recanalized arterial passages (Figure 6), often with well-developed antegrade bridge collaterals. In some, the distal vessel fills via newly formed collaterals from the nonoccluded vessel.

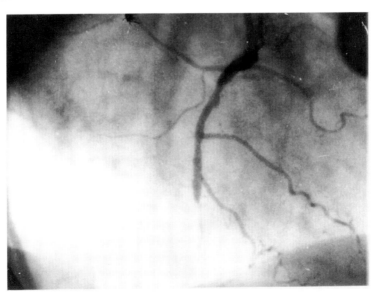

FIGURE 6. *Total occlusion of the right coronary artery 3 months after acute myocardial infarction. The distal end of the artery is irregular.*

Balloon Angioplasty

Percutaneous transluminal coronary angioplasty (PTCA) uses a balloon to dilate a coronary artery, stretching a normal artery and damaging endothelial cells. The artery usually recoils and returns to its previous luminal size after a few days. Extensive damage of the endothelium in animals causes marked intimal proliferation. If the atheromatous plaque is eccentric, then the result of balloon dilatation depends on the relative compliance or elasticity of the plaque segment and the normal arterial wall.[23] If the plaque is noncompliant, it is displaced laterally by the increased intraluminal pressure and the normal part of the coronary artery is dilated. If the normal artery is very elastic, it does not retain its new form, long-term remodeling does not occur, the wall recoils, and the artery returns to its previous shape and diameter. In these patients, symptoms return within a month and the angiographic picture is unchanged at second angiography. If the atheromatous plaque is circumferential, then the entire noncompliant circumference may be dilated. Recoil may occur immediately, but if reconstriction does not occur, then long-term remodeling maintains a larger arterial lumen.[24]

Cracking of the arterial intima at a vulnerable site is the classic mechanism of dilatation.[23–25] The atheromatous lesion indents the inflated dilating balloon and imparts to it an hourglass appearance. The indentation snaps suddenly when the endothelium ruptures and then, the atheromatous material is either squeezed and compressed, and the entire media dilated. A fissure appears at the interface of differential compliance of the arterial wall and this creates a plane of cleavage similar to the formation of a geological rift valley. The crack leaves a free arterial intima that is then squeezed and sealed against the dilated media. The entire artery is dilated. The exposed subintima is potentially thrombogenic. If the intimal flap is sessile or mobile, or blood flow is compromised, or if the lesion is very thrombogenic, thrombus forms. These conditions mimic those found in the spontaneously ruptured coronary arterial plaque, the basis of coronary artery obstruction in acute myocardial infarction. Why then, does acute obstruction not occur after most balloon angioplasties? Three factors prevent arterial occlusion: rapid coronary blood flow once the narrowing is relieved; therapeutic anticoagulation[8,26,27] (heparin, aspirin, the new antithrombin hirudin and antagonists of the IIB IIIA receptors); and squeezing and sealing of the flap against the native arterial wall to create a smooth contour so that eddies and backwashes are prevented. We believe that balloons that are slightly smaller in diameter than the natural size of the normal coronary artery slow initial inflation and prolonged inflation periods; long balloons reduce the incidence of significant dissection. Once a dissection occurs, it can be short, long and filiform, or spiral. Contrast media penetrates the subintima and fills the dissected plane of cleavage: single plane angiograms may be misleading. If the dissection is seen en face, it is invisible, and the coronary artery appears to be adequately dilated. In profile, the contrast medium extravasates into the media and shows a clear linear extra luminal shadow (Figure 7). Intracoronary ultrasound is a sensitive technique of demonstrating minute dissections.

If the flap is thrombogenic, thrombus accumulates, coronary blood flow decreases and the artery gradually obstructs and closes within minutes to hours. This may occur with the guidewire in situ, but frequently appears after the wire has been removed. The patient experiences chest pain, ST segment elevation and re-injection of contrast medium shows total occlusion of the coronary artery. In severe cases, left ventricular function is compromised, stroke volume falls, and hemodynamic compromise occurs. A small group of patients who were studied the day after successful angioplasty showed that in some patients, the previous narrowing returned,

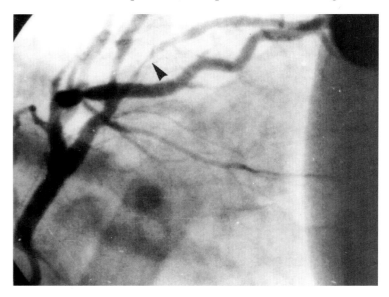

FIGURE 7. (A) Left anterior descending artery in the cranial right anterior oblique view in a patient with unstable angina. A long irregular narrowing in the middle segment of the artery is demonstrated (arrow). The patient was treated by inflation of a long balloon to relieve the obstruction.

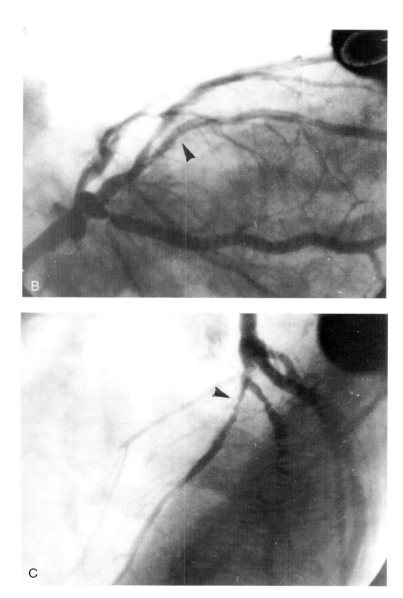

FIGURE 7 *continued.* *(B) Coronary dissection was seen vaguely in the same view (arrow). (C) An orthogonal view demonstrates severe narrowing of the arterial lumen (arrow).*

probably a consequence of acute elastic recoil after dilatation or ocassionally due to clot accretion.

Bifurcation Lesions

Many atheromatous lesions are located at bifurcations of the major coronary arteries. The classic sites are the junction of the left anterior descending artery and its first diagonal branch, the main circumflex artery and one of its major marginal branches, or in the right coronary artery where the major branches occur (infundibular artery, right ventricular, acute marginal, first interventricular branches).

If a single balloon is used to dilate the parent artery, the cholesterol plaque can be squeezed into the origin of the contiguous branch and susequently cause lateral obstruction. A double balloon technique is the method of choice for good dilatation (Figure 8), but it complicates angioplasty. The double balloon technique needs two guidewires, extra manipulation of the guidewire through the atheromatous plaque into the branch and then the simultaneous use of two balloons. Simultaneous inflation of the two balloons of-

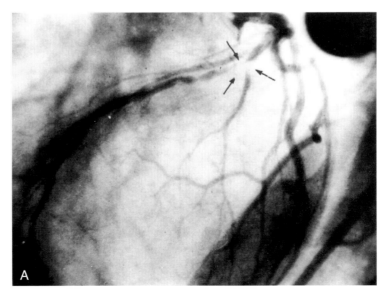

FIGURE 8. (A) Coronary lesion at the bifurcation of the left anterior descending coronary artery and the first diagonal branch in the cranial left anterior oblique view (arrows).

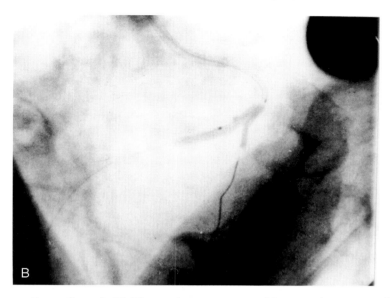

FIGURE 8 *continued*. (B) *The patient was treated by simultaneous infla-tion of two balloons (kissing balloon technique). Successful dilatation of both branches was achieved.*

ten causes overdilatation of the parent artery proximally with dis-section of the bifurcation.

The predilection for atheroma at branch points is related to the flow characteristics of the branching coronary artery—high flow at the bifurcation creates a vortex with low shear stresses in the branch dividers. LDL molecules attach themselves more readily to the endothelial adhesion molecules in the low flow regions and are not washed away. Similarly if the plaque ruptures, platelet adhe-sion is enhanced in these areas of reduced flow.

Rotational Ablation

Rotational ablation uses a diamond-coated drill, 1.25–2.5 mm in diameter that rotates on a wire in the coronary artery at 200,000 revolutions per minute. It is ideal for patients with calcification of the inner portion of the atheromatous plaque because it differen-tially abrades noncompliant calcified tissue.[28,29] It reams out calci-fied coronary atheroma, does not cut normal arterial wall, but may damage normal intima. Small microemboli are created and may block the distal vascular bed. Intimal abrasion often induces coro-

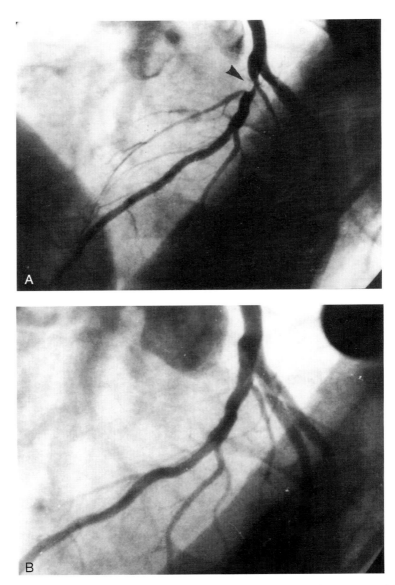

FIGURE 9. (**A**) Eccentric narrowing (arrow) in the proximal segment of the left anterior descending coronary artery (cranial left anterior oblique view) in a patient with unstable angina. (**B**) The patient was successfully treated with directional coronary atherectomy.

nary artery spasm. Rotational ablation creates a smooth-walled arterial lumen. A burr is selected that is smaller in size than the normal coronary arterial diameter; larger diameter burrs may
perforate the artery. Therefore, patients often require subsequent
low-pressure balloon inflation. Intense arterial spasm, intimal
damage, and clot formation may cause subsequent occlusion of the
artery, but the results are excellent in patients with rigid calcified
atheromatous plaques.

Directional Coronary Atherectomy

A cylindrical cutting knife is housed within a guarded cone
that has a lateral aperture. It is advanced to the site of the
atheroma, and by dilatation of a small balloon, the atheroma is
pressed into the conal aperture and can be cut by the rotating cylindrical knife (Figure 9).[30,31] This leaves a clear sharp surface that re-
endothelializes. Intracoronay ultrasound has shown that the
coronary arteriographic results are often fallacious and may overestimate the final arterial lumen. Atherectomy rarely creates frac-
tured sessile intimal flaps and leaves a smooth surface. Restenosis
is not uncommon,[32,33] although in our own series recurrent lesions
were unusual. The device has a large outer diameter (5–7F) and the
nose cone is relatively stiff. It requires a 9–10F guiding catheter. Its
use is restricted to proximal, large, nontortuous, and noncalcified
coronary arteries.

Restenosis

Restenosis is another acute lesion that occurs within 1–6
months of coronary artery intervention.[34,35] Two mechanisms account for restenosis. The first (two thirds of patients) consists of
simple recoil with retraction and contraction of the arterial lumen
due to asymmetric initial dilatation of the artery.[24] The normal segment simply recoils and returns to its former state. The second
mechanism is a consequence of intimal proliferation.[36] Thrombus
forms on the intimal surface and is rich in platelets that secrete
platelet-derived and other growth factors, which induce medial
muscle myocyte migration into the intima, proliferation and
change of the phenotypic profile of the myocyte to a fibroblastic
form. Interstitial matrix forms, usually under the stimulation and
control of tissue growth factor-β. The patients angina returns after
2–3 months, the effort test that had normalized, again becomes is-

chemic, and a thallium cardiac scan confirms the presence of an ischemic area. Angiographically, the pattern of the arterial lumen resembles the previous obstruction in extent, severity, and shape so
that it is often identical to the original atheromatous plaque. Presumably flow determines mechanisms of remodeling and the shape
of the restenotic plaque.

Atheromatous lesions normally progress very slowly in normal
arteries. We found that in arteries intubated for PTCA, new lesions
may appear suddenly. Old lesions tend to progress less rapidly and
regress more frequently in the PTCA artery compared with the non-
PTCA artery. For lesions located in the angioplasty artery, progression
is more common, regression less common, and the appearance of
new lesions more common in arteries with restenosis compared
with the nonangioplasty artery or to arteries without restenosis.
Mechanical trauma to the artery during angioplasty is probably responsible for the appearance of more new lesions. We believe that
a change in flow rate and pattern, especially in arteries without
restenosis, explains the tendency for less progression and more regression in these arteries.[37]

Stent Implantation

Expandable metal stents act as an inert scaffolding of the coronary artery and are useful in many situations. In the past, they were
used primarily to treat acute dissection with imminent occlusion
(Figure 10).[38] The indications for use have been expanded, and currently, these stents are inserted as primary treatment in a large
artery, usually more than 3 mm in diameter, where the artery is
likely to recoil or where restenosis has occurred.[39,40] The angiographic lumen is usually smooth after stent implantation, but intracoronary ultrasound has shown that in many instances the stent
is poorly applied to the underlying intima, leaving a potentially
thrombogenic space between the stent and arterial wall.[41] The dilatation may also be eccentric and non-cylindrical because of differential compliance of the artery. This is an index of inadequate
intra-arterial dilatation. Incomplete apposition, or expansion, or an
irregularity of the inner surface of the stent leads to thrombosis
and subacute occlusion of the artery 6–10 days after implantation.
Intensive anticoagulation was used to prevent subacute occlusion,
but this prolongs hospital stay and may cause bleeding in the groin
or the site of catheterization.[42,43] Intracoronary ultrasound guided
delivery or high-pressure delivery of stents with good apposition
and the use of the newer platelet inhibitors prevents subacute

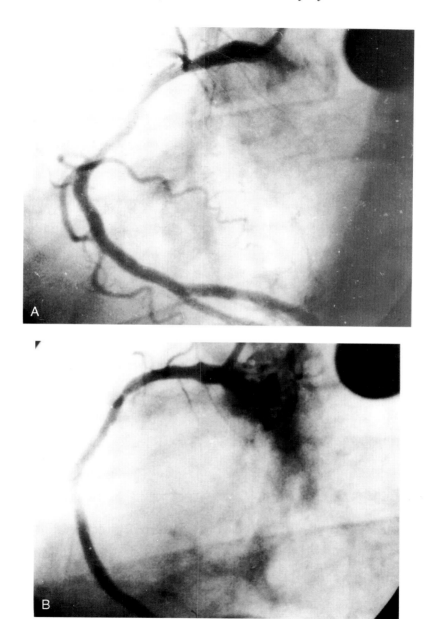

FIGURE 10. *(A) Proximal dissection of the right coronary artery after bal-loon dilatation of an ulcerated lesion in the middle segment of the artery (patient shown in Figure 1). (B) The original lesion and the dissection site were covered by two Palmaz-Shatz coronary stents.*

thrombosis so that intensive anticoagulation might not be necessary.[44,45] The angiographic luminogram is unreliable; an apparently perfect lumen may be irregular, often with eccentric deployment and expansion of the stent. Subacute occlusion presents with acute prolonged anginal pain, change in the ST segment, and total occlusion at angiography. Treatment is by repeat balloon dilatation. Late restenosis also occurs with slight loss of luminal diameter, usually due to ingrowth of new intimal tissue rather than arterial recoil. Treatment is by subsequent dilatation.

Long lesions or long dissections in a large coronary artery can be treated by two or more serial stents, often with overlapping of the ends, so that the entire arterial lumen is supported on a metal lattice. New stents with heparin impregnation may release heparin slowly for 1–2 weeks and reduce the need for anticoagulation without incurring the risk of subsequent subacute closure. Biodegradable stents have been shown to be fibrogenic.

Coronary Artery Bypass Grafts

Venous bypass conduits have an interesting natural history. A small percentage fail immediately after implantation due to a technically poor anastomosis or arterial outflow or vein handling, so that flow decreases and the vein closes.[46] Others have an abnormal pathological endothelium; the vein is potentially thrombogenic and clot forms in the new high-pressure environment. Angiographically the conduit shows a symmetrical narrowing of the graft lumen (Figure 11) and the venous conduit closes. By the end of the first year after implantation 20% have occluded. Pathological studies show progressive fibrous hyperplasia, whereas angiographic studies have shown that the vein gradually narrows and then occludes.[47] These patients present with angina pectoris shortly after bypass surgery, having had a short symptom-free period. Therapeutic balloon dilatation dilates the fibrous vein with long-term remodeling; good long-term results are obtained. Another delayed process appears clinically 7–10 years after vein implantation, usually in patients in whom risk factor modification was not achieved.[48,49] Atheroma forms in the artery, but pathologically it is different from conventional arterial disease. It consists of soft friable cauliflower-like atheromatous masses. The angiographic picture is characteristic (Figure 12). The atheroma gradually occludes the graft, usually with superadded thrombosis, with or without underlying rupture or destabilization of the atheromatous material. Angina returns, the exercise stress test and thallium scan become

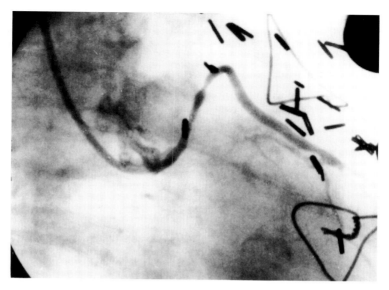

FIGURE 11. *Typical appearance of early saphenous vein graft lesion in a patient with angina 4 months after coronary artery bypass surgery. Two localized narrowings are demonstrated in the proximal segment of the vein graft to the first diagonal branch of the left anterior descending coronary artery (right anterior oblique view).*

positive and angiography shows these bulky, irregular lesions within the vein graft. A common site of predilection is immediately beyond the ostium of the aortic anastomosis, in relation to a side branch where a clip is visible, or near a natural valve. Others occur at sharp angulations or between arteries in sequential grafts. Ultimately thrombus forms, probably on an ulcerated exposed surface, and when flow decreases to a critical level, the vein is obstructed. Several angiographic patterns are diagnostic: atheroma narrows the lumen and presents as an irregular filling defect, initially localized, but more widespread as the disease progresses. The vein develops into a long, thin irregular tube with poor flow of contrast medium. Complete obstruction of a mid-portion of the graft occurs. Later it leaves a blind stump with a cul de sac without flow in the obstructed graft. If the graft is freshly occluded, high-dose intravenous or direct intragraft thrombolysis gradually restores blood flow and exposes the underlying atheromatous lesion. Twenty-four to 48 hours later, after most of the clot has been lysed, it is possible to dilate the vein with a balloon or extract the atheroma using a transluminal extraction coronary device.[50] Restenosis rates are

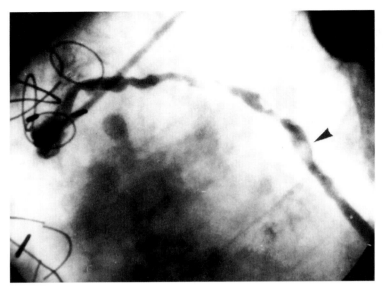

FIGURE 12. *Typical appearance of late disease in a saphenous vein graft. The patient was admitted with unstable angina pectoris 9 years after coronary artery bypass surgery. The vein graft to the obtuse marginal is severely degenerated with filling defects suggestive of overlying thrombus (arrow).*

high; occasionally the vein recoils, or atheroma reforms in the affected segment. The pattern of restenosis resembles the initial predilatation lesion. Recent observations have shown that implantation of a stent can restore a good lumen with the development of a smooth neo-intima. Many believe that chronically narrow grafts require replacement, the large atheromatous mass is friable and emboli liberated during angioplasty can obstruct the distal arterial bed.

The internal mammary and other arterial grafts are used extensively because of their improved patency rates. The internal mammary artery is an excellent conduit, providing all its side branches have been ligated and that the parent trunk supplies the target artery. The artery is narrow so that the distal anastomotic site is small and constriction may occur at this point. Stenosis at this site can be dilated with a balloon.

Coronary artery atheroma progresses after bypass surgery[51,52] and the most common event is proximal closure of the native grafted artery, which is usually silent. It seems that an alternative preferential flow through the graft reduces flow through the native coronary artery and narrowing of the atheromatous segment predisposes either to more atheroma formation or silent generation of a clot with obstruction of the artery. Many patients, 10–12 years after successful coronary artery bypass grafting, have occluded native proximal coronary arteries and are totally dependent on venous or arterial grafts. Progression of the disease in the native arteries or grafts may also cause unstable angina or acute myocardial infarction. Return of angina 7–10 years after coronary artery obstruction is a medical emergency. A graft has been obstructed and requires immediate opening by thrombolysis or balloon angioplasty.

Coronary Angiography and Other Diagnostic Modalities

Coronary angiography has become the mainstay of the diagnosis of coronary artery lesions. The history, while specific for ischemia, does not indicate the number of lesions, their site, or extent of disease. Stress testing is not possible in the acute situation, but dipyridamole thallium SPECT indicates the site of ischemia and also fibrosis. Coronary angiography is therefore the gold standard for anatomic diagnosis. Coronary angiography, however, is only a luminogram. Multiple projections show profiles of the coronary arteries from different angles, but the picture is often incomplete and an eccentric 80% lesion in one view may reveal a normal coronary artery in another. A very short stenosis in a site that is not perpendicular to the beam of the x-ray may not be diagnosed because of overlapping shadows. Coronary artery ultrasound has emerged as a much more accurate diagnostic procedure that shows the true thickness of the arterial wall and often indicates the pathological basis of the lesion. Soft plaques give clear shadows, fibrous plaques merge with the media, but calcification shows echo dense areas with penumbric shadows and are diagnostic. Intracoronary ultrasound is also invaluable after stent implantation.

Coronary ultrasound is being used to complement coronary angioplasty, but the latter requires invasive intubation of the coronary arteries. We hope that noninvasive techniques (fast computed tomography or nuclear magnetic resonance or gated echocardiography), may replace coronary angiography and intracoronary ultrasound as a simpler, precise method of diagnosing the acute coronary syndromes.

Conclusions

Acute coronary syndromes are common and diagnosis by coronary angiography, while limited to an anatomic luminogram, is the simplest currently available diagnostic modality. A good coronary angiogram shows the anatomic abnormality and serves as a pathological basis for subsequent diagnosis and treatment.

References

1. Braunwald E. Unstable angina. A classification. *Circulation* 1989;80(2): 410–414.
2. Fuster V, Badimon L, Badimon JJ, et al. The pathogenesis of coronary artery disease and the acute coronary syndromes (first of two parts). *N Engl J Med* 1991;326:242–250.
3. Fuster V, Badimon L, Badimon JJ, et al. The pathogenesis of coronary artery disease and the acute coronary syndromes (second of two parts). *N Engl J Med* 1991;326:310–318.
4. Mizuno K, Satomura K, Miyamoto A, et al. Angioscopic evaluation of coronary artery thrombi in acute coronary syndromes. *N Engl J Med* 1992;326:287–291.
5. Freeman MR, Williams AE, Armstrong PW. Intracoronary thrombus and complex morphology in unstable angina. *Circulation* 1989;80: 17–23.
6. Ambrose JA, Winters SL, Stern A, et al. Angiographic morphology and the pathogenesis of unstable angina pectoris. *J Am Coll Cardiol* 1985;5:609–616.
7. Ambrose JA, Tannenbaum MA, Alexopoulos D, et al. Angiographic progression of coronary artery disease and the development of myocardial infarction. *J Am Coll Cardiol* 1988;12:56–62.
8. Tenaglia AN, Stack RS: Angioplasty for acute coronary syndromes. *Ann Rev Med* 1993;44:465–479.
9. Myler RK, Shaw RE, Stertzer SH, et al. Unstable angina and coronary angioplasty. *Circulation* 1990;82;II-88–II-95.
10. Badimon L, Badimon JJ. Mechanism of arterial thrombosis in non-parallel streamlines: Platelet thrombi grow on the apex of stenotic severely injured vessel wall. Experimental study in the pig model. *J Clin Invest* 1989;84:1134–1144.
11. The TIMI IIIB Investigators. Effects of tissue plasminogen activator and a comparison of early invasive and conservative strategies in unstable angina and non-Q wave myocardial infarction: Results of the TIMI IIIB Trial. *Circulation* 1994;89:1545–1556.
12. DeWood MA, Spores J, Notske R, et al. Prevalence of total coronary occlusion during the early hours of transmural myocardial infarction. *N Engl J Med* 1980;303:897–902.
13. Davies MJ, Thomas AC. Plaque fissuring—the cause of acute myocardial infarction, sudden ischaemic death, and crescendo angina. *Br Heart J* 1985;53:363–373.
14. Gertz SD, Kragel AH, Kalan JM, Braunwald E, Roberts WC, and the TIMI Investigators: Comparison of coronary and myocardial morphologic findings in patients with and without thrombolytic therapy during fatal first acute myocardial infarction. *Am J Cardiol* 1990;66:907–909.
15. Terrosu P, Vibba GV, Contini GM, et al. Angiographic features of the coronary arteries during intracoronary thrombolysis. *Br Heart J* 1984;52:154–163.

16. Wu D, Matsuda M, Takemura G, et al. Cineangiographic and pathological features of the infarct related vessel in successful and unsuccessful thrombolysis. *Br Heart J* 1989;61:385–389.
17. Serruys PW, Arnold AER, Brower RW, et al. Effects of continued rt-PA administration on the residual stenosis after successful recanalization in acute myocardial infarction—A quantitative coronary angiography study of a randomized trial. *Eur Heart J* 1987;8:1172–1181.
18. Nakagawa S, Hanada Y, Koiwaya Y, et al. Angiographic features in the infarct-related artery after intracoronary urokinase followed by prolonged anticoagulation. *Circulation* 1988;78:1335–1344.
19. Halon DA, Lewis BS, Gotsman MS. Localization of lesions in the coronary circulation. *Am J Cardiol* 1983;52:921–926.
20. Gotsman MS, Rosenheck S, Nassar H, et al. Angiographic findings in the coronary arteries after thrombolysis in acute myocardial infarction. *Am J Cardiol* 1992;70:715–723.
21. Vogt A, von Essen R, Tebbe U, et al. Frequency of achieving optimal reperfusion with thrombolysis in acute myocardial infarction (analysis of four German trials). *Am J Cardiol* 1994;74:1–4.
22. Koren G, Luria MH, Gotsman MS, et al. Early treatment of acute myocardial infarction with intravenous streptokinase: A high risk syndrome. *Arch Intern Med* 1987;147:237–240.
23. Waller BF, Pinkerton CA, Orr CM, et al. Restenosis 1 to 24 months after clinically successful coronary balloon angioplasty: A necropsy study of 20 patients. *J Am Coll Cardiol* 1991;17:58B–70B.
24. Mintz GS, Pichard AD, Kent KM, et al. Intravascular ultrasound comparison of restenotic and de novo coronary artery narrowings. *Am J Cardiol* 1994;74:1278–1280.
25. Rozenman Y, Gilon D, Nassar H, et al. Creation and healing of severe coronary dissection by the use of oversized balloon for the treatment of restenosis after an initially successful angioplasty. *Cathet Cardiovasc Diagn* 1994;31:34–36.
26. Topol EJ, Califf RM, Weisman HF, et al. Randomised trial of coronary intervention with antibody against platelet IIb/IIIa integrin for reduction of clinical restenosis: Results at six month. *Lancet* 1994;343:881–886.
27. van den Bos AA, Deckers JW, Heyndrickx GR, et al. Safety and efficacy of recombinant hirudin (CGP 39 393) versus heparin in patients with stable angina undergoing coronary angioplasty. *Circulation* 1993;88: 2058–2066.
28. Warth DC, Leon MB, O'Neil W, et al. Rotational atherectomy multicenter registry: Acute results and 6-month angiographic follow-up in 709 patients. *J Am Coll Cardiol* 1994;24:641–648.
29. Stertzer S, Rosenblum J, Shaw RE, et al. Coronary rotational ablation: Initial experience in 302 procedures. *J Am Coll Cardiol* 1993;21:287–295.
30. Hinohara T, Selmon MR, Robertson GC, et al. Directional atherectomy: New approaches for treatment of obstructive coronary and peripheral vascular disease. *Circulation* 1990;81(Suppl IV):IV-79–91.
31. Fishman RF, Kuntz RE, Carrozza JP Jr, et al. Long-term results of directional coronary atherectomy: Predictors of restenosis. *J Am Coll Cardiol* 1992;20:1101–1110.
32. Topol EJ, Leya F, Pinkerton CA, et al. A comparison of directional atherectomy with coronary angioplasty in patients with coronary artery disease. *N Engl J Med* 1993;329:221–227.
33. Adelman AG, Cohen EA, Kimball BP, et al. A comparison of directional

atherectomy with balloon angioplasty for lesions of the left anterior descending coronary artery. *N Engl J Med* 1993;329:228–233.

34. Califf RM, Fortin DF, Frid DJ, et al. Restenosis after coronary angioplasty: An overview. *J Am Coll Cardiol* 1991;17:2B–13B.

35. Holmes DR, Schwartz RS, Webster MWI: Coronary restenosis: What have we learned from angiography? *J Am Coll Cardiol* 1991;17:14B–22B.

36. Liu MW, Roubin GS, King SB: Restenosis after coronary angioplasty. Potential biologic determinants and role of intimal hyperplasia. *Circulation* 1989;79:1374–1387.

37. Rozenman Y, Gilon D, Lotan C, Gotsman MS: Progression of coronary artery disease after successful balloon angioplasty: Relation to the angioplasty artery and to restenosis. Annual meeting of the Israeli Cardiac Society, Tel-Aviv, Israel, 1994.

38. George BS, Voorhess WD, Roubin GS, et al. Multicenter investigation of coronary stenting to treat acute or threatened closure after percutaneous transluminal coronary angioplasty: Clinical and angiographic outcomes. *J Am Coll Cardiol* 1993;22:135–143.

39. Schatz RA, Baim DS, Leon MB, et al. Clinical experience with Palmaz-Schatz coronary stent: Initial results of a multicenter study. *Circulation* 1991;83:148–161.

40. Savage MP, Fischman DL, Schatz RA, et al. Long term angiographic and clinical outcome after implantation of a balloon expandable stent in the native coronary circulation. *J Am Coll Cardiol* 1994;24:1207–1212.

41. Goldberg SL, Colombo A, Nakamura S, et al. Benefit of intracoronary ultrasound in the deployment of Palmaz-Shatz stents. *J Am Coll Cardiol* 1994;24:996–1003.

42. Nath FC, Muller DWM, Ellis SG, et al. Thrombosis of flexible coil coronary stent: Frequency, predictors and clinical outcome. *J Am Coll Cardiol* 1993;21:622–627.

43. Rozenman Y, Lotan C, Mosseri M, et al. Relation of thrombotic occlusion of coronary stents to the indication for stenting, stent size, and anticoagulation. *Am J Cardiol* 1995;75:84–85.

44. Colombo A, Hall P, Almagor Y, et al. Results of intravascular ultrasound guided coronary stenting without subsequent anticoagulation. *J Am Coll Cardiol* 1994;23:335A.

45. Morice MC, Bourdonnec C, Biron Y, et al. Coronary stenting without coumadin. Phase II. *J Am Coll Cardiol* 1994;23:335A.

46. Grondin CM, Lesperance J, Bourassa MG, et al. Serial angiographic evaluation in 60 consecutive patients with aorto-coronary artery vein grafts 2 weeks, 1 year and 3 years after operation. *J Thorac Cardiovasc Surg* 1974;67:1–6.

47. Kalan JM, Roberts WC. Morphological findings in saphenous veins used as coronary arterial bypass conduits for longer than one year: Necropsy analysis of 53 patients, 123 saphenous veins. *Am Heart J* 1990;119:1164–1184.

48. Campeau L, Enjalbert M, Lesperance J, et al. Atherosclerosis and late closure of aortocoronary saphenous vein grafts: Sequential angiographic studies 2 weeks, 1 year, 5 to 7 years, and 10 to 12 years after surgery. *Circulation* 1983;68(II):1–9.

49. Campeau L, Enjalbert M, Lesperance J, et al. The relationship of risk factors to the development of atherosclerosis in saphenous vein bypass grafts and the progression of disease in the native circulation. A study 10 years after surgery. *N Engl J Med* 1984;311:1329–1332.

50. Lotan C, Mosseri M, Rozenman Y, et al. Combined mechanical and thrombolytic therapy for totally occluded bypass grafts: Short and long term results. *Br Heart J* 1995;74:455–459.
51. Pasternak R, Cohn K, Selzer A, et al. Enhanced rate of progression of coronary artery disease following aorto-coronary saphenous vein bypass surgery. *Am J Med* 1975;58:166–170.
52. Chasin WL, Sanmarco ME, Nessim SA, et al. Accelerated progression of atherosclerosis in coronary vessels with minimal lesions that are bypassed. *N Engl J Med* 1984;311:824–828.

Panel Discussion I

Overview of Pathology: Clinical Considerations of Atherosclerosis with Emphasis on Coronary Artery Disease

Dr. Valentin Fuster: In coronary disease, plaques that tend to rupture are small but very soft due to a high lipid content; this is, in part, why they rupture. In carotid disease, the plaques that rupture are severely stenotic and often calcified. What's the mechanism? Is it the same? Dr. Glagov, maybe you can start.

Dr. Seymour Glagov: Well, I intend to show in my talk this afternoon what's going on in carotid plaques and I will show you quite graphically that one of the problems is the proximity to the lumen or to the fibrous cap of either calcification or the lipid core. These are two very, very important findings in our plaques. These are the plaques that disrupt, and it depends, really, on plaque complexity and plaque size, but the proximity of these processes to the lumen is extremely important. The processes that are going on in the plaque to generate either calcification or accumulation of a lipid pool, and the rate at which these things are happening determines the proximity to the lumen. These are very important factors and, of course, the triggering mechanisms have to do with factors that we don't fully understand because the hemodynamics change with plaque size. As soon as you have a very narrow lumen, you have a bruit, and as soon as you have a bruit you're talking about vibrations, and these triggering mechanisms need very detailed investigation in terms of the distribution of these stresses and eventually the strains within the plaque. Carotid pathology has to do with plaque disruption; stenosis has to do with plaque size; and plaque size has to do with plaque complexity; those are the key features.

Dr. Fuster: The carotid arteries carry high flow under a very high kinetic energy. One wonders if the carotid flow in itself is an important trigger in the rupture of a plaque that is severely stenotic, in contrast with the coronary flow, mostly diastolic, which has low kinetic energy. Maybe Dr. Sherman or Dr. Fallon may comment on this.

Dr. David G. Sherman: Well, I have no idea what the answer is. The things that come to my mind are, certainly, from the clinical standpoint. If the patient has the same degree of stenosis and they have symptoms, that puts them into a much different category in terms of their subsequent risk. So, one of the questions is whether or not the fact that a person has had a transient ischemic attack (TIA) or a minor stroke is, in fact, a marker that they have a larger core or a thinner fibrous cap and the lesion is more likely to rupture.

Dr. John T. Fallon: I think the thing that's interesting is that in the carotid [artery], at least, the symptomatology is very closely related to the degree of stenosis and not to the degree of ulceration. Although if you compare symptomatic versus asymptomatic plaques, you will find that the degree of complexity again is related to the degree of stenosis. And people, for many years, have tried to relate asymptomatic ulceration to risk of stroke, and haven't been able to do it. It's the degree of stenosis that is the predictor. And if you look at the aorta you will see very large ulcerated lesions routinely at autopsy, in patients who have always been entirely asymptomatic. So it's very interesting to think about the question of how plaques erode and ulcerate and remain entirely asymptomatic and where does all that atheromatous material that then embolizes or washes out go? Now the spectrum for symptomatology is much less in the carotid because you'd recognize a TIA or a small embolus much faster than let's say an embolus to the lower extremities. But, it's really remarkable how much you can ulcerate and presumably embolize and remain asymptomatic and nonthrombotic.

Dr. Fuster: Dr. Falk, a few years ago you wrote a paper saying that the coronary plaques that tend to rupture are severely stenotic. Today, you were saying that the plaques that tend to rupture are small. I wonder if you are thinking as an angiographer now, despite being a pathologist, while in the past you thought as a pathologist. Pathologists all say that the plaques that lead to infarcts are severely stenotic, while the angiographers, say that such plaques are rather small.

Dr. Erling Falk: I don't think that this is what I wrote some years ago. I examined coronary thrombi or I examined the entire coronary tree in 49 patients who died of ischemic heart disease. In these 49 patients, I found 103 ruptured plaques, and only 40 of these ruptured plaques were associated with an occlusive luminal thrombus. So, in 63, there was no occluding thrombus. Ruptures occur constantly and probably are responsible for rapid growth, but which are asymptomatic because they cause no significant flow reduction. So I asked the question, why do some plaques rupture and give rise to occlusive thrombosis, while others do not give rise to occlusive thrombosis but only to rapid plaque progression without occlusion? Then, I measured the degree of stenosis at the site of plaque disruption, and I found that the degree of stenosis was a major determinant for the outcome of plaque disruption. The more severe the stenosis, the higher was the risk that a plaque rupture would give rise to occlusive thrombosis. If there was no stenosis of the rupture site, the rupture site would just heal with a mural thrombus and organization. And so, the outcome of plaque disruption depends on flow abnormality and on the degree of stenosis; the more severe the stenosis, the higher is the risk that this plaque disruption will give rise to vessel occlusion. And I think it also fit many other observations. We know that rapid flow and high shear forces activate platelets and promote thrombosis, opposite to what's going on in the venous system. In the arterial system, the more severe the stenosis, the higher the shear forces and the higher the risk that plaque disruption will go on to thrombosis. However, as you have published, we know that it is the mild or moderately stenotic lesions which most frequently give rise to acute myocardial infarction and to clinical symptoms. We also know by sequential angiography that it is the most severe stenoses that more frequently progress to total occlusion.

Dr. Fuster: And no symptoms.

Dr. Falk: Exactly, they do it without symptoms. Probably because the most severe stenoses are protected by collateral vessels, while the less severe stenoses, although they rupture much less frequently and are less predisposed to occlusive thrombosis, on the few instances that this happens, there are no collateral vessels to protect and it is then when myocardial infarction occurs. So I don't see any disagreement because I studied coronary occlusion.

Dr. Fuster: Dr. Chandler, you are a pioneer of the concept that the progression of coronary atherosclerotic disease depends very much on thrombus formation and organization of the thrombus, as we heard this morning. My question is, do you think this is the main mechanism by which a stenotic lesion of 40% or 50% goes to 90%? Or, you think it's still maybe a slow process of growing. I would like to get a sense from you about the two possibilities of how the atherosclerotic plaque grows.

Dr. A. Bleakley Chandler: The contribution of thrombus to the growth of a plaque—and by that I mean the incorporation of thrombus into a plaque and its conversion to connective tissue so that it is no longer recognizable as thrombus—creates the first problem of saying how big a contribution is this because the thrombi, after a while, are no longer recognizable as thrombi. But even so, many studies over several years have shown that one can identify thrombi in anywhere from 40% to 45% of atherosclerotic plaques. At the same time, one only has to ask how many of these plaques have thrombi that have been completely organized so that the remnants are no longer there. So I think thrombosis is a major contributor. The rate at which this happens is very difficult to estimate in human lesions. I think we're not yet at that stage where we can say from invasive and noninvasive studies how rapidly thrombi organize. I do think we can say, from experimental studies, that it is extremely rapid; but for example, we have studied in the rabbit and the dog the evolution of occlusive coronary and pulmonary thrombi, and found that thrombi can become completely organized and converted to plaques in as short a period as three weeks. This brings to mind one other aspect that is now becoming well recognized but was questioned for many years. And that is, what happens to an occlusive thrombus in relation to its natural history. Quite often the thrombus undergoes partial lysis and retraction and becomes eccentric, creating a single lumen. We think of a re-canalized thrombus as having multiple lumens. But, in fact, what often happens is that an occlusive thrombus can be rearranged so that a single lumen is reformed.

Dr. Fuster: Dr. Wissler and Dr. Stary, very briefly, do you believe that thrombosis is a major contributor to plaque growth?

Dr. Robert W. Wissler: Very briefly, after the age of 35, probably. But, at least in the first 35 years, we have yet to see a really sizable thrombus in relation to many of these advanced plaques. And since our trichrome very sensitively identifies remnants of old thrombi, I think there isn't much evidence in these young people, even though some of them have rather advanced disease. I would say, though, that we mustn't forget that fibrin and fibrinogen are found in very early stages of plaque formation. I think we need to explore much more thoroughly what the contribution of that substance is within the plaque, and not in a thrombotic form.

Dr. Herbert. C. Stary: I do have fairly good data on thrombosis in aortic lesions. In the age group rangin from 20 to 29 years, 24% of the grossly raised lesions that we find in the aorta contain thrombus or thrombotic remnants. In the age group ranging from 30 to 39 years, the frequency is already twice as high. However, the thrombotic deposits are mostly very small in these relatively young people. They accelerate lesion growth but they do not obstruct the lumen, or not much.

Dr. Fuster: I'm asking these questions because one of the challenges in the future may be to develop more targeted antithrombotic drugs that can be safe and much more powerful in preventing mural thrombosis. In fact, there's a lot going on in this area with the use of new oral antithrombotic agents. That, is a new approach to prevent the progression of the atherosclerotic plaque.

Dr. Colin J. Schwartz: Just one small comment. I, of course, agree wholeheartedly with Bleakley Chandler, that mural thrombosis contributes very substantially to the growth of plaques in the later stages of plaque development. I have little doubt about that. Our own experience shows that. But, I would just like to make a point. If one accepts this, it is not surprising then that the coronary disease risk factor profile has changed in the last few years. I think it's just worth drawing everybody's attention to the fact that we now have risk factors that relate to disturbances in hemostasis and thrombosis emerging as independent predictive factors. I refer to Tom Meade's excellent studies from Northwick Park in terms of hyperfibrinogenemia, the many studies that have indicated that plasminogen activator inhibitor-1 is a predictive risk factor and, of course, factor VII. So I think that this whole field is moving in the direction of abnormal hemostasis risk profile as a part of the complex clinical picture.

Dr. Fuster: I would like to ask a question related to the issue of extracellular lipid accumulation. Dr. McGill, you have some experience with this. I always thought that the early stages of lipid accumulation were cellular dependent. In other words, the accumulated extracellular lipid, in a way, was derived from foam cells that had initially taken up lipoprotein and stored it. In the later stages of the disease, let's say in type IV or type Va lesions with a lot of extracellular lipid in a core, that lipid material could actually be a transudate from the plasma into the vessel wall rather than having been derived from cells. I would just like to ask this because in the future treatment, it's going to be essential. If we talk about antioxidants, for example, it's quite different because we are really talking about a cellular component being involved. If we are talking about lowering lipid levels, then it's a transudation aspect. I would like to hear what your views are.

Dr. Henry C. McGill, Jr: I think Dr. Stary presented very convincing evidence that the first lesion you see, in children, is intracellular lipid in macrophages. And then he showed very convincingly how these increase in number and then appear to spill their lipid as extracellular lipid, and that accumulates in the the advanced lesions. Then you wonder how you are ever going to mobilize this. That's something we need more information about. One of the interesting, very new findings I think, is a discovery that 27-hydroxylase can convert cholesterol into very polar and mobile 27-hydroxyl cholesterol. The enzyme is in macrophages too; in fact, it's a mitochondrial enzyme present in many cells other than the liver. This just might be one of a number of ways in which the macrophages around this core of lipid could mobilize the otherwise relatively immobile crystallized cholesterol. We need to look for other possible ways. Maybe we can find a way to stimulate 27-hydroxylase, activate it and accelerate the mobilization. There are just lots of exciting new openings here that we might try to explore.

Dr. Fuster: This is why I am asking the question because pharmacologically, in terms of mobilizing the lipid, it's going to be quite different depending on how we understand where this extracellular lipid comes from.

Dr. McGill: So far it certainly appears that lowering LDL is a major contributor to lipid mobilization. Now the question is, can we find other ways to accelerate the mobilization.

Discussant A from the Audience: Mr. Chairman, I think it's a numbers game. The world is filled with millions of people who have 30% and 40% lesions and only tens of thousands of people who have 90% lesions. And so, it's a numbers game. If the incidence of myocardial infarction is 1% among a population of people with 40% lesions, but there are millions of them, we will see a lot more infarcts in that group than if the incidence of stroke and myocardial infarction is 20% among people with 90% lesions. Does that make sense?

Dr. Fuster: I think your concept is correct. There are many studies indicative that the more severely stenotic lesions are in the coronary arteriogram, the more likely that numerous smaller lesions are present that may lead to an infarct. So, if you have a normal coronary arteriogram, the chances of having an infarct I think is very, very small. But if you have three-vessel coronary disease the chances are much higher. That is, the severity of the disease is a marker, that there are many small lesions that are dangerous, although perhaps only one will lead to myocardial infarction.

Dr. Falk: If you look at the totality of atherosclerotic lesions that exist, a very small percentage of them are actually symptomatic. All you have to do is look at the autopsy data or look at any patient who's 100 years old in the autopsy suite. They all have atherosclerotic lesions that have never had symptoms. You can find very complex lesions, ulcerated lesions, and so on. So if you look at the totality of lesions that exist in the world, a very small percentage of them actually produce symptoms. And, of course, the more severe the stenosis, the greater the risk of angina but not necessarily of infarction.

Dr. Fuster: Dr. Ambrose, as an angiographer, what is your view about this discussion of small, dangerous lesions versus severely stenotic, less dangerous lesions.

Dr. John A. Ambrose: The problem is not knowing the denominator of the equation and how many of these small or moderate lesions are available that can undergo this process of disruption with clinical events. The answer is probably millions of lesions. But, the fact of the matter is that large infarcts we now think, at least in the majority of cases, seem to be related to a process occurring in a mild to moderate lesion as Drs. Fuster and Falk have mentioned. At that stage there are no collaterals to limit or prevent infarction. However, we know that when a lesion, perhaps small, ruptures and complicates with thrombus, it can become very severely stenotic and symptomatic, for example, with unstable angina. These acute stenotic lesions are active, they are thrombogenic, they may go on to occlusion. If we don't treat those patients, very often a substantial percentage will develop myocardial infarction.

Discussant B from the Audience: A comment brought up by many speakers has been that we need a way to identify the culprit lesion or the vulnerable lesion. Dr. Falk mentioned in his talk that early in development of lesions, platelet deposition plays a role, and that platelets that are loosely attached wash off downstream. If they get to the venous system certainly we can sample and identify those platelets. There are markers that will tell whether they are activated or not. P-selectin and flow cytometry have been used as markers to identify circulating activated platelets. If that's true and they do exist, then I think we have a very simple way to determine that a culprit lesion is present in the patient. Then we can use imaging techniques to show where the culprit lesion is and decide what to do about it.

Dr. Fuster: Severely stenotic lesions are de-endothelialized and platelets are activated but, as we mentioned today, they are not "dangerous" plaques. What I'm saying is that these markers are absolutely nonspecific. You are really dealing with a field in which whatever you measure is very difficult to accurately predict.

Discussant B from the Audience: I agree that old platelet tests just don't work this way, but flow cytometry may provide a different picture. But there is a second question I want to raise. How long before the occurrence of the acute myocardial infarction is the platelet having this recurrent thrombosis, lysis, in terms of platelets, not in terms of fibrinogen or thrombin? Is that a process that goes on for weeks before patients have their event? Or is it a process that goes on for hours before the event? This, I think, is the critical question. We are not talking about sensitivity of platelets; we're talking about platelets that are activated by circulating agonists in the patient.

Discussant C from the Audience: I remember Dr. Fuster telling me about 10 or 12 years ago, when he had been so interested looking at different platelet testing, how difficult it was to assess platelet activation. And that advice always kind of reverberates in the back of my mind. In addition, I don't think that cytometry is the most sensitive or the best technique because I think, depending on how you gate the machine and so forth, you can get variable results. Concerning your question, I don't think anyone has an answer on how long thrombosis has been going on before myocardial infarction occurs. If you believe that myocardial infarction occurs very commonly after awakening or assuming the upright position, you might assume that if a plaque disrupts and there is the millieu in the blood for the event to occur, that it may occur acutely but I don't think there's a lot of data on this.

Dr. Mervyn S. Gotsman: I would like to just give you some tangential information. It has nothing to do with the P-selecting. If we look epidemiologically at time intervals between possible triggers and acute myocardial infarction, then often there are acute emotional episodes or acute physical episodes, sometimes after a 24- to 36-hour delay, in which the patient has chest pain, the pain disappears, the pain returns, and we have this waxing and waning onset of the myocardial infarction. In fact, so few patients are thrombolized because they start with pain early—about 30% of patients have warning signs within 24–36 hours before the infarct.

Dr. Falk: I don't think it's reasonable to believe that in the future we will be able to find systemic markers for this disease because it's a universal disease. It's going on in many vascular beds, and if the disease is progressing we know it is related to endothelial dysfunction, to endothelial activation. In endothelial activation you will have expression of adhesion molecules. We know some of these adhesion molecules are shed into the circulation. Progressive disease is also associated with platelet activation, activation of the coagulation system, and we now have very fine markers of very low, ongoing activation of coagulation. So I think maybe in the future we will be able to monitor disease activity by using these kinds of systemic markers. They are not specific, I know that. But, for example, C reactive protein is nonspecific and still a very sensitive marker of inflammation. And if you rule out that there's inflammation in other parts of the body, maybe you can use this marker to say something is going on in the vasculature.

Discussant D from the Audience: I'm surprised at how little has been said about the role of intramural hemorrhage in the plaques playing a role in acute vascular events. My question is justified by Dr. Falk's interpretation of the slide he showed of coagulated blood at three different stages. It's been known for over a hundred years that clot which forms in a flowing column of blood occurs by the deposition of platelets, formation of fibrin, and trapping of a few blood cells, the so-called salmon-colored clot. This is quite different from the clot which forms in a test tube, where blood stops flowing and where all of the blood elements are homogeneously distributed. In the plaque he showed, there were two sites where there were lines of Zahn and there was laminated thrombus. But in the wall of the plaque, there was blood with its elements homogeneously distributed. This is characteristic of a hematoma that forms within tissue. And in the carotid bifurcation it has been possible to demonstrate, from specimens that have been photographed in situ at the operating table before any dissection of the plaque has been done, that massive, grossly visible hematomas will occur in carotid plaques, entirely within a fibrous core with no sign of a lipid pool or any plaque degeneration. I therefore wonder how much of what is called thrombus in the pathologic specimens is indeed hematoma that is occurring within the plaque? And therefore I would welcome some comments.

Dr. Falk: If you have a ruptured plaque surface, then you will also have some degree of hemorrhage into the soft lipid and then you will always have some degree of thrombosis where thrombogenic material has been exposed. In fact, I call this a hemorrhage into the plaque through the ruptured surface. Others, such as Michael Davies in London, call this an intraplaque thrombus. Within the plaque there are a lot of erythrocytes and some fibrin, while in the lumen where you have flow, there is platelet-rich thrombus. I would prefer to call what you have in the vessel wall a hemorrhage and what you have in the lumen a thrombus.

Dr. Chandler: I think also one might point out that there are two types of hematomas within the wall as far as the origin. One, as Dr. Falk has described, is a dissection into the wall. The other is a hemorrhage from the vascularization of a plaque. Indeed, Winternitz, Thomas and LeCompte published a book in 1938 in which they wrote about the importance of intramural hemorrhage in plaque growth. Whether or not what we say is thrombus contributing to the growth of a plaque really is thrombus and not a simple hemorrhage is indeed a difficult question to answer. And I can only say that one approach has been to define these thrombic remnants, not only by their nature, that is fibrin, fibrinogen, and platelet content, but by their lamination occurring in strata within the plaque suggesting layers of thrombus.

Discussant E from the Audience: We have several investigators on the panel who have done animal experiments. My question is, do we have an animal model in which atherosclerotic lesions progress to rupture and thrombosis? And if not, why not?

Dr. Fuster: In the pig model on a high-cholesterol diet, lesions develop in the trifurcation of the aorta that eventually go through ulceration but you do not see thrombus. And the reason is the high flow; it really washes out the thrombus.

Dr. Schwartz: One of the real problems is that nearly all of the experimental models of atherosclerosis are not thrombotic models as well. And my experience is that it's very hard to get a good thrombosis model spontaneously. But, I would like to just comment that many years ago McLetchie did some very interesting work and we followed this up at Oxford in MacFarlane's laboratory. The use of Russell viper venom injected subcutaneously in animals produces the most significant thrombi in all sorts of parts of their vascular tree and lesions are produced that can be followed sequentially as they undergo organization and atheromatous and fibrouslike lesions. So, that's about the only model I know that, in fact, consistently will produce thrombosis without an invasive approach. However, this is not a model of plaque rupture.

Dr. Fuster: Dr. Fallon, do you know of any model of ulceration and thrombosis?

Dr. Fallon: I know about one. For the last half year I have looked at a pig model and the people who have developed the pig model are here today—Dr. Jan Rapacz and Judith Hasler-Rapacz from Madison, Wisconsin. In their pig model, the pigs have genetically very high cholesterol levels and in the course of 2 or 3 years they have advanced lesions in the coronary artery. They have lipid with core formation, with fibrous cap rupture, thrombosis and hemorrhage into the lesion. However, it takes several years before the advanced lesions develop and the pigs weigh 300 kg.

Dr. Wissler: The Rapacz's have, along with Margaret Prescott, published convincing evidence that that particular genetically induced swine model does develop thrombosis and plaques with all the characteristics of human plaque. The rhesus monkey also will do that as we have reported but they are almost prohibitive now as a species for investigation.

Dr. Jan Rapacz: I would like to make a comment regarding the size of the swine model with familial hypercholesterolemia (FHC), the first animal model which develops thrombosis and plaques with all the characteristics of human plaques without the intervention of vascular injury or diet-induction. In addition to the original large pigs, we have now half size or smaller animals which weigh about 140 kg at 3 years of age and have plasma cholesterol reaching 400 mg/dL. We hope that in two or more generations the downsized FHC swine will be 60–70 kg at 18 months of age with well expressed lesions.

Dr. Fuster: The minipig?

Dr. Rapacz: It's not yet minipig. It takes generations, I don't have any funding to accelerate the achievement of the essential characteristics in the new model.

Discussant F from the Audience: We have heard so far that the plaques causing unstable angina are predominantly lipid-rich plaques that disrupt and thrombose. However, we have found in some preliminary work with angioscopy that there is a fair number of patients with unstable angina who have actually nondisruptive plaques which are white and smooth. In fact, the TIMI 3 data show that angiographic complexity of the culprit lesions is present only in about <50% of these patients. I guess my question is, do you think that we're being too simplistic about lumping all the patients with unstable angina together and the possibility that there is the subset of patients with unstable angina in which the culprit lesions are more vasoreactive than thrombogenic.

Dr. Fuster: As a member of the recent panel on unstable angina guidelines, I can state that the group agreed with Braunwald's classification suggesting that, in perhaps more than 25% of patients with unstable angina, the problem is an increase in oxygen demand, which is transient in a patient who has stable disease. The fact that the patient has angina does not necessarily mean that it's a catastrophe in the coronary artery. The artery can be stable but the patient may be going through an emotional state that may increase oxygen demand, or have other noncoronary conditions such as anemia, hyper- or hypothyroidism, or that may contribute to the angina without implying plaque rupture.

Chapter 9

Cerebrovascular Disease:
A Pathologist's View

Seymour Glagov, MD, Hisham S. Bassiouny, MD,
Nobuhide Masawa, MD,
Yasuhiro Sakaguchi, MD, Don P. Giddens, PhD,
and Christopher K. Zarins, MD

Introduction

The syndromes associated with cerebrovascular arterial disease may be grouped in several characteristic clinical entities. These include 1) stroke, which is the partial or total loss of motor and/or sensory function due to infarction and/or hemorrhage that destroys a region of the brain. Although the resulting necrosis is irreversible, the degree of restoration of function is determined by the extent of the injury, the state of intracranial and extracranial circulation, and the potential for recovery or for transfer of function to preserved regions; 2) transient ischemic attack, which is the temporary and reversible sudden loss and spontaneous recovery of motor and/or sensory function of short duration due to focal arrest of intracranial circulation usually by embolization; and 3) mental deterioration, which is the loss of cognitive function, usually gradual and attributable to extensive and diffuse compromise of intracranial circulation, with or without evidence of associated loss of localized motor and/or sensory function.

Underlying anatomically demonstrable vascular abnormalities that may result in one or another of these ischemic syndromes (Table 1) include atherosclerosis, either intracranial or extracranial, leading to gradual stenosis or to intermittent or sudden occlusions associated with plaque disruption and local thrombosis

From: Fuster V, (ed.) *Syndromes of Atherosclerosis: Correlations of Clinical Imaging and Pathology.* Armonk, NY: Futura Publishing Company, Inc.: © 1996.

TABLE 1

Arterial Abnormalities in Cerebrovascular Disease

Atherosclerosis: extracranial, intracranial.
Abnormal Configurations and Positions: extrinsic compression, kinking.
Abnormal Structure or Composition: fibromuscular dysplasia, dissection, aneurysm, arteriovenous malformations.
Physical Injury, Inflammations, Interventions: local, proximal or distal repercussions.
Cardiac or Aortic Disease: embolization due to endocarditis, mural thrombi, or aortic arch disease.

and/or to distal embolization. Stenosis and plaque disruptions caused by atherosclerosis are the most common underlying causes of the syndromes noted above. Other less common causes include abnormal vascular configurations caused by abnormalities of location, origin, or trajectory, leading to extended or intermittent reductions or arrests of flow, often related to changes in position or associated with extrinsic compression by neoplasms, adjacent bones, or muscles. Abnormalities of wall structure or tensile strength including fibromuscular dysplasia, aneurysm formation, arteriovenous malformations, or archetectural disruptions such as those associated with medial dissection are possible causes. Other abnormalities may be due to physical trauma, inflammatory reactions, or complications of vascular interventions that result in configurational distortions, disruptions, ulcerations or thromboses that cause sudden or gradual vessel obstructions locally or proximal or distal to the region of abnormality. Cardiac or aortic sources of obstructive embolization include dislodged infected thrombi as in endocarditis, or bland thrombi in the event of atrial fibrillation or ventricular aneurysm, or of debris from severe thoracic aortic disease as in Takayasu's arteritis.

Prominence of Atherosclerotic Disease at the Carotid Bifurcation

Atherosclerotic plaques around the carotid bifurcation account for more than 40% of the significant stenoses that come to the attention of the clinician in relation to potential or manifest cerebrovascular symptoms. Vertebral artery plaques account for about 20%, while intracranial atherosclerosis, including involvement of the carotid siphon, the basilar artery, and the middle cerebral artery together account for fewer than 20% of cerebrovascular stenoses.[1] The ready accessibility of the carotid bifurcation for angiographic as well as noninvasive ultrasonic and magnetic resonance imaging and for characterization of blood flow by color Doppler ultrasonic techniques allows clinical evaluations of the degree of stenosis, plaque configuration and composition, and of corresponding effects on flow and on artery wall mechanical properties. Such information, together with the clinical evaluation of symptoms may permit estimates with respect to prognosis and to likely outcomes of interventions.

Most significant is the growing evidence for the efficacy of carotid endarterectomy as therapy for transient ischemic attacks and mild strokes, and for the prevention of both transient ischemic attacks and stroke in asymptomatic individuals with tightly stenotic ($\geq70\%$) atherosclerotic lesions.[2] Imaging and flow measurements at the carotid bifurcation are in current widespread use for early detection of lesions, for assessment of progression and regression in relation to risk factors, and for the identification of features that connote plaque stability or instability. In view of the overwhelming prominence of symptomatic and potentially symptomatic atherosclerotic cerebrovascular disease due to plaques at the carotid bifurcation; the accessibility of the region for clinical monitoring of early and advanced atherosclerotic disease; for therapeutic intervention; and for access to endarterectomy specimens suitable for correlation with clinical symptoms as well as with diagnostic imaging and hemodynamic findings, we will confine our discussion to the natural history of atherosclerotic lesions at this site.

Detection of Minimal Asymptomatic Lesions at the Carotid Bifurcation

Detection of early plaque formation at the carotid bifurcation usually depends on ultrasonic measurements of artery wall thickness, ie, intima plus media,[3] and of possible corresponding changes in mural mechanical properties. Because of the usual focal and eccentric location of sites of plaque initiation at the carotid bifurcation in relation to geometric transitions,[4,5] the selection of precise regions to be interrogated is critical. The transition from common carotid to internal carotid artery, the proximal internal carotid, and the sinus are regions where conditions of flow separation and reduced and oscillating wall shear stress favor the formation of detectable early intimal thickenings. In keeping with the axial distribution of the predisposing flow field features, the distribution of early plaques in this location tends to be helical (Figure 1).[6] Intimal deposits tend to occur at the flow divider side of the bifurcation in the distal common carotid artery proximal to the bifurcation division, veering laterally and posteriorly just proximal to the division, in the region opposite the flow divider in the proximal internal carotid and sinus. These then tend to develop medially in the distal internal carotid. The flow divider aspects at the bifurcation division, immediately proximal internal carotid, and at the sinus level are relatively spared.[4-6] Modifications of this pattern are, however, likely to correspond to differences in the flow field in relation to individual geometric variations. Thus, any single axial location and direction of examination by ultrasound may not identify the site of maximal intimal thickening. To detect the maximum wall thickness due to early plaque formation, interrogation of the carotid bifurcation is therefore best performed over a range of incident angles and axial locations whenever possible.

Although dystrophic calcium deposits may occur in moderately advanced plaques that have not yet resulted in stenosis, the extent to which minimal asymptomatic atherosclerosis can be detected or quantified on the basis of calcification remains to be defined.[7,8] The extent to which early atherosclerosis at the carotid bifurcation may serve as a surrogate for plaque formation at sites such as the coronary arteries also awaits further investigation.[9] Growing evidence suggests, however, that abdominal aortic and coronary atherosclerosis tend to precede the formation of carotid bifurcation disease. As a rule, therefore, manifest plaques at the carotid bifurcation indicate that disease is also likely to be present in the coronary or peripheral circulation, but the relative severity of atherosclerosis in these locations may be quite variable.

A possible confounding problem in relating absolute values of wall thickness to atherogenesis derives from the usual relationship between wall thickness and artery diameter. Media thickness and composition are determined by wall tension for normal homologous vessels in mammals, but also for specific vessel segments and branches.[10] Evidence has been forthcoming that nonatherosclerotic intimal thickening, as well as early atherosclerotic plaques may contribute to tensile support as wall tension increases with increased diameter.[11] Calculations of tensile stress based on measurement of media thickness alone may yield elevated values compared with regions without intimal thickening. If intimal thickness is included in estimates of total wall thickness, tensile stress tends to normalize to levels that prevail where no intimal thicken-

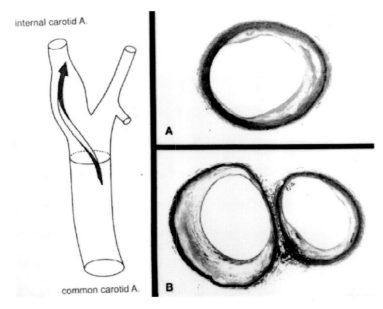

FIGURE 1. *Axial and circumferential distribution of early intimal lesions at the carotid bifurcation. In the left panel, the helical arrow indicates that, on the average, maximum intimal thickening tends to be on the flow divider side in the subadjacent common carotid artery, toward the opposite wall just proximal to the division and in the proximal internal branch and sinus, and then veers toward the posterior wall in the distal internal carotid artery segment. In the right upper panel (**A**), a section from the common carotid artery at some distance proximal to the flow divider shows the lesion to be at the flow divider side. In the right lower panel (**B**) a section from the same specimen was taken at the level of the bifurcation, reveals that both internal (larger cross section) and external (smaller cross section) carotid arteries are involved. The lesion in the internal carotid artery is opposite the flow divider. Adapted with permission from Reference 6.*

ing is evident. Thus, it may be appropriate to normalize intima-media thickness in relation to diameter for any given individual and location, particularly if such data are used for epidemiologic comparisons of absolute thickness in relation to risk factors. Such considerations may also be appropriate for sequential studies, because early plaque formation at the carotid bifurcation results in artery enlargement and alterations in tensile stress distribution even in the absence of reduction in lumen diameter.

Evaluation of Progression and Regression: Associated Changes in Plaque Configuration and Lumen Diameter

Studies of human atherosclerotic plaques have furnished a reasonably consistent morphological classification of the characteristic transitions in lesion morphogenesis. The microanatomic features have been documented in several recent reviews furnished by the Committee on Vascular Lesions of the American Heart Association.[12,13] Many of the features of plaque evolution suggest underlying adaptive modeling mechanisms that tend to preserve functional integrity in the face of progressive lesion development.[14] Lipid accumulates initially within a focal eccentric thickening of the wall, usually but not always, in relation to an intimal fibrocellular proliferative response containing smooth muscle cells. Erosion of the subjacent media may be noted, but the intimal reaction adjacent to the media is often characterized by fibrosis as well, including both collagen and elastin fibers. As the plaque progresses, a fibrocellular reaction becomes increasingly evident at the luminal subendothelial aspect of the enlarged intima. Thus, the lipid and the associated products of tissue degeneration and necrosis, the lipid necrotic core, tends to be segregated to a mid-intimal zone by deep and superficial fibrocellular reactions (Figure 2). The superficial fibrous zone often procedes to differentiate into a compact fibrocellular structure, the fibrous cap, which is often similar in both thickness and architecture to the underlying media or to the media of the uninvolved region of the vessel opposite the lesion. These modifications result in stratification of the lesion components. In association with the erosive changes in the media, plaques bulge outward into the adventitial aspect.[15] The plaque is thereby effectively sequestered from the lumen at this stage (Figure 2). In the absence of deforming complications by plaque disruptions, fissuring, hematoma formation, or thrombus deposition, the lumen surface remains regular and the cross-sectional lumen contour remains circular or oval.[16] The smooth muscle cells in the subendothelial fibrous cap region may be presumed to differentiate and synthesize connective tissue fibers in keeping with the imposed pulsatile stresses that tend to be concentrated near the lumen surface.[17,18] The fibrous cap may, however, become less sharply defined and replaced by fibrous tissue containing both collagen and elastin fibers (Figure 3A), often in layers suggesting episodic deposition. Lipid cores tend to resolve, becoming myxomatous at first (Figure 3C), with the subsequent appearance of focal calcium deposits and vas-

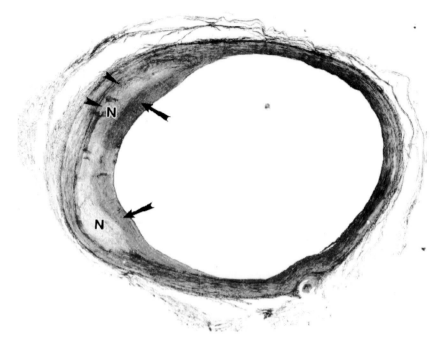

FIGURE 2. *An early plaque in the internal carotid artery near the level of the sinus shows the usual modeling features. The lipid necrotic core (N) is contained between the media and the fibrous cap (arrows). The lumen contour is round or slightly oval, but the outer contour is oval in relation to the outward bulge beneath the lesion. There is evidence of focal erosion of the media (arrowheads), but there is also evidence of nearby reactive fibrosis on the lumen side of the media. Adapted with permission from Reference 21.*

cular channels. Fibrosis and calcification in these regions progress and become increasingly prominent as the lesion increases in size. Lipid necrotic cores may, however, be evident immediately beneath the fibrous subluminal region, often in relation to focal or extended thinning or complete erosion of the subluminal fibrous tissue (Figure 3B). Associated foam cells, lymphocytes, and less frequently plasma cells and giant cells may be evident in relation to these features (Figure 4). Thus, large lesions tend to be complex, ie, comprised of juxtaposed regions of differing and contrasting composition. Large lesions that are highly stenotic also tend to be complicated, with regions of disruption, thrombosis, or hematoma in evidence.[19] Nevertheless, neither lesion size nor lesion composition necessarily correspond to degree of stenosis because erosion of

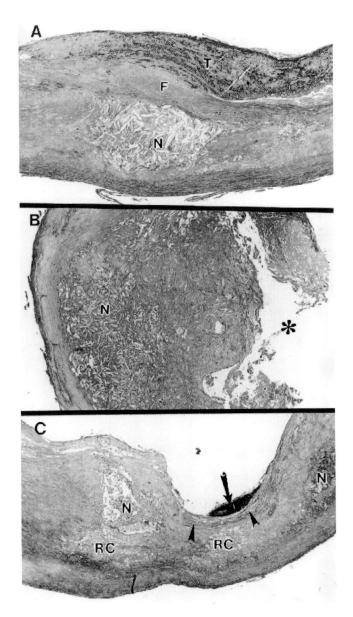

FIGURE 3. *Multiple level sections of a carotid bifurcation endarterectomy specimen of a symptomatic patient with marked stenosis. A variety of morphological features are noted.* **A:** *Just proximal to the bifurcation an organizing thrombus (T) is noted on a zone of fibrosis (F) that may have replaced a fibrous cap. An underlying lipid necrotic region (N) is evident.*

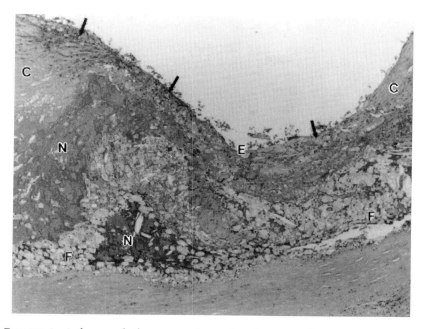

FIGURE 4. *A focus of plaque neoformation in an endarterectomy specimen from a symptomatic patient. The fibrous cap (C) is eroded (E) and mainly absent in relation to the lumen surface (arrows). Foam cells (F) and lipid necrotic core material (N) are prominent. Adapted with permission from Reference 19.*

the media and/or plaque disruption or reorganization may result in marked changes in vessel diameter.

A particularly significant process that may limit evaluation of plaque size by angiography is the finding that arteries enlarge as plaques form, tending to preserve a lumen of adequate cross section even in the presence of relatively large intimal plaques.[16,20]

FIGURE 3 *Continued. B:* *More distally, an extensive erupting lipid necrotic core (N) containing some admixed blood is evident. No fibrous cap is evident. The lumen side of the ulceration is marked by an asterisk. **C:** A surface depression at a more distal level of the internal carotid branch shows a fresh thrombus (arrow) deposited on a zone in which subluminal matrix fibers have been organized (arrowheads) presumably representing the healing of a previous ulceration. Lipid necrotic zones (N) are evident within the plaque as well as myxomatous regions that correspond to resolving lipid cores (RC). Adapted with permission from Reference 21.*

That artery enlargement is a consequence of plaque formation and is not merely a consequence of initial differences in artery size, is indicated by the fact that in any given artery segment, lumen cross-sectional area and other dimensions are usually similar for involved and uninvolved or reference segments. Although initially demonstrated in human coronary arteries, studies of interval axial sections at the carotid bifurcation indicate that artery enlargement and protracted preservation of lumen diameter is evident in relation to both early and moderately advanced lesions, ie, artery size increases with plaque area (Figure 5).[11] Since plaque enlargement

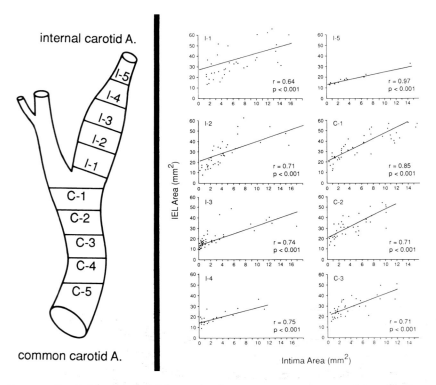

FIGURE 5. *Evidence for plaque enlargement as plaques form at the carotid bifurcation. In the left panel, a carotid bifurcation is represented diagrammatically with the levels of sampling at 0.5-cm intervals indicated. A series of graphs, each corresponding to a level of sampling, indicates a close correspondence between the area encompassed by the internal elastic lamina (IEL area), an index of artery size, and intimal area. Adapted with permission from Reference 11.*

is associated mainly with the outward bulging of the artery wall beneath an eccentric lesion (Figures 1 and 2),[15] lumen contour tends to remain circular whereas the outer contour of the vessel becomes oval. Although there is evidence that plaque morphogenesis may become fixed at any stage of evolution or even revert to a previous or simpler stage, new lesions may develop on an apparently previously stabilized plaque.[13] The sequence of changes in secondary or even tertiary superimposed plaques may be incomplete as compared with the primary lesion or may recapitulate the entire process. With advance of the disease, circumferential extension and extention into the lumen may proceed, but the lesion tends to remain predominantly eccentric with a concave lumen surface (Figures 1 and 2).

Thus, modeling of arteries with plaques can be defined as the manifestation of the adaptive-reactive tissue responses that determine size, configuration, composition, and patency in relation to the interaction between atherogenic and mechanical factors. The features of the modeling reactions, which occur during plaque development and influence interpretations of plaque progression and regression, are summarized in Table 2. In any patient over a given time interval, individual plaques within a given cerebrovascular bed or at the carotid bifurcation may be unchanged, appear to progress to greater stenosis or to show evidence of reduced stenosis, or become complicated by lumen irregularities that connote ulceration and/or thrombosis. In general, plaques at the carotid bifurcation, examined in postmortem material or in sequential clinical studies, appear to manifest the usual range of morphological variation and modeling. The likely determinants of the modeling reactions are listed in Table 3.

TABLE 2

Processes Underlying Changes in Wall Thickness, Intima Thickness, Lumen Dimensions and Lumen Configuration

Modeling and Remodeling Responses to Wall Shear and Tensile Stresses
Atherosclerotic Plaque Progression, Regression and Neoformation
Artery Enlargement During Atherogenesis
Wall Erosion by Atherosclerosis
Ulceration of Plaques
Resolution of Necrotic Core and Calcification
Organization of Plaque Thrombus Formation and Hematoma

TABLE 3

Likely Determinants of Plaque Modeling

Atherogenic (Metabolic)
Episodic progression, regression, disruption; healing
and compensatory reactions.
Age of onset; individual susceptibility.
Changes in life style: diet, smoking, exercise.
Superimposition of hypertension, diabetes.
Hemodynamic (Mechanical)
Local differences in hemodynamic risk.
Individual differences in hemodynamic risk.
Individual differences in tissue response to physical stresses.
Changing mechanical properties of plaque.
Changing hemodynamics as plaques enlarge.

Features Indicative of Manifest
or Imminent Plaque Disruption

Much of our information about the composition and complication of advanced plaques is derived from the examination of
highly stenotic endarterectomy specimens. Although tight stenoses
correspond to large complex plaques, it should be emphasized that
images of lumen diameter on angiograms provide information regarding comparative degrees of lumen narrowing, but do not provide an accurate appraisal of lesion cross-sectional area, or
composition volume.[11,16,20] This limitation is due to the compensatory enlargement of arteries where plaques form as noted above,
to changes in lumen size caused by modifications of plaque modeling and composition, to the occurrence of plaque disruptions and
ulcerations, to erosions of the underlying media, and to the formation and organization of thrombi. Focal irregularities and depres-
sions at the lumen surface do not necessarily portend the presence
of current ulcerations, because examination of many human endarterectomy specimens and corresponding angiograms indicate
that these may be regions of healing where previous thrombi or ulcerations may have occurred (Figures 3A and 3C). Neither the degree of calcification, nor the outer vessel contour are reliable
indices of plaque progression, degree of stenosis, or complication.

Although severe atherosclerotic disease at the carotid bifurcation frequently presents clinically as transient ischemic attacks or

stroke, marked degrees of stenosis can be detected in the absence of such symptoms. Vibrations created by turbulent flow distal to tight stenoses create vibrations detectable as bruits on physical examination and draw attention to marked stenoses. Flow instabilities and increases in velocity characteristic of stenoses can be confirmed using ultrasonic methods. Angiography and magnetic resonance imaging provide information on lumen configuration. As noted above, tight stenoses are associated with the presence of large plaques and large plaques are complex and tend to be complicated by ulceration, calcification, hematoma, and thrombus formation even when manifest symptoms are not present clinically.[7,19] Preemptive excision of such lesions and comparison with those removed because of symptoms have permitted studies that provide insights into the nature of the changes associated with the onset of symptoms, ie, impressions based on clinical observations may be critically evaluated from actual specimens. These include comparative estimates of lesion and lumen configuration, lesion composition, and lumen surface continuity and integrity. Determination of the chemical composition of highly stenotic lesions have failed to reveal any significant differences between symptomatic and asymptomatic plaques (Table 4). Specimens with little or only moderate stenosis and not associated with evidence of clinical symptomatology may be obtained at autopsy and compared with findings in stenotic endarterectomy specimens. In view of the axial variation in lesion composition and complication, such correlations require detailed sequential sampling. Our own studies are based on sections of the entire bifurcation taken at 0.5-cm intervals, ie, on 6–10 sections of each specimen.[6,11,19,21] We have compared the morphological evidences of plaque complication in endarterectomy specimens of highly stenotic plaques ($\geq$80%) with those identified in postmortem material in which stenoses was mild or moderate (<50%). For the highly stenotic endarterectomy plaques, those associated with clinical symptoms were compared with those without clinical symptoms and with the moderately stenotic plaques (Table 5). One or more of the complicating features was noted in most of the specimens. Evidence of a necrotic core was present in 58% of the highly stenotic specimens and in only 12% of those with little or moderate narrowing. Ulceration was evident in 53% of the highly stenotic specimens, but in only 6% of the moderately stenotic samples. Hematoma, usually within an associated necrotic core or evidence of previous hemorrhage or hematoma in the form of collections of siderophages was noted in 73% of the highly stenotic, but in only 41% of the moderately narrowed asympto-

TABLE 4

Chemical Composition of Carotid Bifurcation Plaques[*]

Composition	High-Grade Carotid Stenosis	
	Asymptomatic (n=14)	Symptomatic (n=31)
DNA (ng)	206±50	182±28
Phospholipid (μg)	15.5±2.8	15.2±1.7
Total cholesterol (μg)	77.2±13.5	92.7±18.4
Free cholesterol (μg)	36±7.0	45±9
Cholesterol ester (μg)	41.4±6.9	47.4±10.1
Triglycerides (μg)	2.4±0.5	2.6±0.3
Free fatty acids (μg)	1.5±0.3	1.5±0.3
Collagen (μg HP)	11.3±1.1	10±0.9
Apoprotein A (ng)	0.29±0.05	0.21±0.04
Immunoglobulin G (ng)	1.05±0.3	0.75±0.16
Complement factor C_3 (ng)	0.76±0.3	0.43±0.06
Fibrinogen (μg)	0.23±0.06	0.14±0.02
Acid lipase activity (μm α-naphthol/min)	73.7±28	56±14.01
Cholesterol esterase activity (CPM/min)	1,974±802	1,092±237
ACAT activity (CPM/min)	6,494±2262	5,317±982
Collagenase activity (CPM/min)	285±84	190±37
Elastase activity (CPM/min)	579±88	346±51

[*]All values expressed per mg wet weight; None of the differences between asymptomatic and symptomatic plaques are significant

TABLE 5

Morphology of Stenotic Carotid Bifurcation Plaques
(percent of plaques with each feature)

	Highly Stenotic (>80%)		Moderate Stenosis (<50%)
	Symptomatic	Asymptomatic	Asymptomatic
Necrotic Core	61%	50%	12%[+]
Ulceration	58%	43%	6%[*+]
Hematoma	68%	86%	41%[*]
Calcification	90%	71%	53%[§]

[*]$P<0.05$ compared with asymptomatic and symptomatic highly stenotic plaques;

[+]$P<0.01$ compared with highly stenotic plaques;

[§]$P<0.05$ compared with highly stenotic plaques.

matic plaques. Calcification was a common finding, noted in 84% of the tight stenoses and 53% of the moderately narrowed arteries. These differences were significant at the $P<0.05$ to $P<0.01$ level for each finding. Thus, plaques associated with tight stenoses were more complicated than those with moderate stenoses. When only the asymptomatic highly stenotic plaque were compared with the asymptomatic moderately stenotic post-mortem specimens, the comparisons gave similar results. Necrotic core was evident in 50% of those with tight stenosis and in 12% of those with little or moderate stenosis. Ulceration was present in 43% of the highly stenotic and only 6% of the moderately stenotic plaques. Hematoma was evident in 86% of the tightly stenotic and 41% of the moderately stenotic. Calcification was present in 71% of the tightly stenotic and in 53% of the moderately stenotic. There were no significant differences between highly stenotic symptomatic and highly stenotic asymptomatic plaques with respect to the incidence of these complications.

Lumen and plaque features in advanced stenotic plaques that correlate best with specific cerebrovascular symptomatic manifestations include recent or remote evidences of plaque disruption, fissuring, hematoma or thrombus deposition (Figure 3). Problems of clinical interpretation from images arise from difficulties in relation to the modeling changes in plaque size, configuration, and composition during progression or regression of advanced lesions as noted above, and in relation to the healing and remodeling processes following previous plaque disruptions, hematoma formation, or thrombosis (Figures 3A and 3C) and in relation to the neoformation of plaques on apparently stable or resolving lesions (Figure 4). At the histologic level, the specific features in endarterectomy specimens that connote underlying plaque instability and correlate well with symptom production include: 1) erosion, focal narrowing, or absence of the fibrous cap with or without an immediately subjacent lipid necrotic core, foam cells, or an associated inflammatory cellular infiltrate, with or without demonstrable thrombus deposition; 2) the presence of manifest fissuring or ulceration with or without evident thrombus deposition; 3) the presence of hematoma within the plaque, usually in the form of blood within a necrotic core often in direct relationship to a focal surface disruption and/or the presence of clusters of siderophages, suggesting previous resolved hemorrhage or hematoma; 4) secondary lesion formation (neoformation) on an older plaque as indicated by juxtalumenal foam cell and lipid core accumulations and/or focal inflammatory cell infiltration within or on an underlying apparently stable plaque; and 5) the juxtaposition of regions of presumably different composition and elastic modulus associated with the above mentioned features. Putative features connoting resistance to disruption or indicative of recent or imminent disruption are summarized in Table 6. Foci of symptom-producing plaque disruption, immediate or remote, may however be quite small, appearing at one or more places in a given endarterectomy plaque and limiting detection by most current imaging methods. A diagrammatic representation of an extensive advanced plaque with marked stenosis at the carotid bifurcation is shown in Figure 6. The histologic sections shown in Figure 3 were all taken at different levels of the same type of highly stenotic specimen with a large complex plaque and each could have been the basis of the transient ischemic attacks suffered by the patient. Intervening sections failed to show complications which could be associated with symptoms. A high degree of echolucency, corresponding to an extensive lipid necrotic core with or without hematoma as shown in Figure 3B and detectable by ultrasonic imaging, has been offered as a criterion of plaque susceptibility to disruption.[22] In our own studies, recent findings suggest that the proximity of the echolucent region to the fibrous cap or lumen may be a better positive correlate of symptom production than either the extent of echolucency or calcification. Recent studies also suggest that plaque cross-sectional composition, including irregularities of fibrous cap thickness as well as the distribution of lipid core and calcification in relation to the fibrous cap, determine the precise location of the region of peak tensile

---

TABLE 6

Morphological Correlates of Plaque Integrity

Features Implying Resistance to Disruption
Uniform plaque fibrosis on cross section
circular, regular lumen contour
Demarcated fibrous cap of uniform thickness: absence
of focal erosions or inflammation

Features Associated with Disruption
Large plaque with marked stenosis
Juxtaposed regions
of contrasting composition: calcification, necrotic core,
fibrosis, hematomas
Lumen irregularities and asymmetries: thromboses, cavitations
Focal fibrous cap thinning or defects: Erosions
and inflammation; neoformation of atherosclerosis within,
upon or beneath fibrous caps or at lumen surface
Close proximity to fibrous cap or lumen surface
of necrotic core or calcification

internal carotid A.

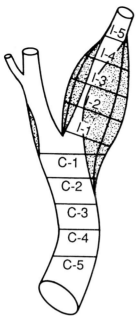

common carotid A.

FIGURE 6. *A diagrammatic representation of a carotid bifurcation with a large plaque in the usual distribution and a tight stenosis. The specimens from which our knowledge of pathological changes underlying symptoms are derived are mainly of this type. The sections in Figure 3 have been taken from one such specimen. Sections with moderate stenosis are usually available only from postmortem material, usually from patients without previously known symptoms. Adapted with permission from Reference 21.*

stress. Thus, the occurrence of plaque complications is probably directly related to individual metabolic and tissue reactive factors that determine plaque neoformation architecture, composition, and consistency (Table 3), and therefore, determine plaque fragility, and to mechanical and geometric factors that determine the distribution, magnitude, and variation in shear and tensile stresses that may induce disruption in susceptible lesions.

Therefore, predictions of imminent plaque instability from images depends on accurate detection, identification, and quantitative appraisal of plaque features, and particularly on their distribution within the plaque. Problems arising in establishing reliable morphological criteria are listed in Table 7. Consistent criteria are likely to emerge as resolution, sensitivity, and specificity of clinical imaging modalities improve.[21] Improvements in resolution of clinical imaging modalities, including capabilities for three-dimensional reconstruction of both diagnostic images and plaques may be expected to provide increasingly detailed evaluation of the atherosclerotic process and the factors governing its instability.[7,23]

TABLE 7

Clinical Evaluation of Carotid Plaques: Problems Arising in
Establishing Reliable Morphological Criteria

Geometric Factors
Circumferential asymetry of plaque localization
Axial and circumferential variation in plaque size and
  composition
Plaque Evolution
Uncertain predicability of plaque evolution
Disruptions may occur in apparently stable plaques
Sites of actual or potential disruption often very small
Uncertain nature of lumen irregularities
Technological
Current limits (specificity, sensitivity) of imaging modalities

Conclusion

The major cerebrovascular syndromes, stroke and transient ischemic attack, are associated with advanced atherosclerosis at the
carotid bifurcation. Therapeutic decisions, as well as the interpretations of data obtained in clinical trials depend largely on an accurate appreciation of atherosclerotic plaque morphogenesis at
this location as observed by diagnostic imaging and flow measurement techniques. Lesions can be evaluated by noninvasive ultrasonic methods and are amenable to therapeutic endarterectomy.
Examinations of this region are therefore used for early detection
of plaque formation, for evaluation of lesion progression and regression and for detection of features that suggest plaque instability. Excised plaques furnish material for verification of clinical
findings and may be studied to provide insights into the natural history of complex and complicated lesions. Clinical detection of minimal, asymptomatic carotid intima-media thickening requires
interrogation at regions at high risk for plaque induction in relation
to geometry and associated flow field properties. Although lesions
tend to form opposite the flow divider where wall shear stress is
low and oscillates in direction, maximum thickness corresponding
to early lesions tends to follow a helical distribution from the common carotid to the distal internal carotid in keeping with the axial
flow field pattern. Sequential changes in lumen contour and in
plaque size and composition often reflect complicating and modeling processes as well as plaque progression and regression. Clinical
detection of imminent, recent, or remote plaque disruption and fis-

suring depend on the identification of corresponding microanatomic features. These include lumen irregularities, cross-sectional distribution of plaque components and evidences of fibrous cap thinning or absence associated with adjacent necrotic core or plaque neoformation. Sites of symptom-producing fissures and disruptions may be extremely small and are noted to occur in large, highly stenotic plaques in both symptomatic and asymptomatic individuals subjected to carotid endarterectomy. Improvements in both sensitivity and specificity of the available imaging modalities are likely to permit more precise identification and evaluation of significant prognostic indicators.

References

1. Fields WS. Symptomatic extracranial vascular disease: Natural history and medical management. In: Veith FJ, Hobson RW, Williams RA, et al. eds. *Vascular Surgery: Principles and Practice*. New York: McGraw-Hill, Inc; 1994:611–622.
2. Moore WS, Barnett HJM, Beebe HG, et al. Guidelines for carotid endarterectomy. A multidisciplinary consensus statement from the Ad Hoc Committee, American Heart Association. *Circulation* 1995;91:566–579.
3. Tang R, Mercuri M, Bond MG. B-mode ultrasound imaging for detecting and monitoring peripheral atherosclerosis. *Am J Cardiac Imaging* 1992;6:333–338.
4. Zarins CK, Giddens DP, Bharadavaj AK, et al. Carotid bifurcation atherosclerosis: Quantitative correlation of plaque localization with flow velocity profiles and wall shear stress. *Circ Res* 1983;53:502–514.
5. Ku DN, Zarins CK, Giddens DP, et al. Pulsatile flow and atherosclerosis in the human carotid bifurcation: Positive correlation between plaque localization and low and oscillating shear stress. *Arteriosclerosis* 1985;5:292–302.
6. Masawa N, Glagov S, Zarins CK. Quantitative morphologic study of intimal thickening at the human carotid bifurcation. I. Axial and circumferential distribution of maximum intimal thickening in asymptomatic uncomplicated plaques. *Atherosclerosis* 1994;107:137–146.
7. Hatsukami TS, Thackray BD, Primozich JF, et al. Echolucent regions in carotid plaque: Preliminary analysis comparing three-dimensional his-tologic reconstructions to sonographic findings. *Ultrasound Med Biol* 1994;20:743–749.
8. Giachelli CM, Bae N, Almeida M, et al. Osteopontin is elevated during neointima formation in rat arteries and is a novel component of human atherosclerotic plaques. *J Clin Invest* 1993;92:1686–1696.
9. Megnien JL, Sene V, Jeannin S, et al. Coronary calcification and its relation to extracoronary atherosclerosis in asymptomatic hypercholesterolemic men. The PCV METRA Group. *Circulation* 1992;85:1799–1807.
10. Clark JM, Glagov S. Transmural organization of the arterial wall: The lamellar unit revisited. *Arteriosclerosis* 1985;5:19–34.
11. Masawa N, Glagov S, Zarins CK. Quantitative morphologic study of in-

timal thickening at the human carotid bifurcation: II. The compensatory enlargement response and the role of the intima in tensile support. *Atherosclerosis* 1994;107:147–155.

12. Stary HC, Chandler AB Glagov S, et al. A definition of initial, fatty streak and intermediate lesions of arteriosclerosis. *Circulation* 1994;89:2462–2478.

13. Stary HC, Chandler AB, Dinsmore RE, et al. Difinition of advanced types of atherosclerotic lesions and a histological classification of atherosclerosis. *Arterioscler Throm Vasc Biol* 1995;15:1512–1531.

14. Glagov S, Bassiouny HS, Giddens DP, et al. Intimal thickening: Morphogenesis, functional significance and detection. *J Vasc Invest* 1995;1:2–14.

15. Ko C, Glagov S, Zarins CK. Structural basis for the compensatory enlargement of arteries during early atherogenesis. Proceedings of the 3rd International Workshop on Vascular Hemodynamic (Bolgna 1991). Borgatti E, ed. Centro Scientifico Editore; 1992:157–161.

16. Glagov S, Weisenberg E, Kolettis G, et al. Compensatory enlargement of human atherosclerotic coronary arteries. *N Engl J Med* 1987;316: 1371–1375.

17. Cheng GC, Loree HM, Kamm RD. Distribution of circumferential stress in ruptured and stable atherosclerotic lesions. A structural analysis with high pathologic correlation. *Circulation* 1993;87:1179–1187.

18. Lee RT, Grodzinsky AJ, Frank EH. Structure-dependent dynamic mechanical behavior of fibrous caps from human atherosclerotic plaques. *Circulation* 1991;83:1764–1170.

19. Bassiouny HS, Davis H, Masawa N, et al. Critical carotid stenosis: Morphological and chemical similarity between symptomatic and asymptomatic plaques. *J Vasc Surg* 1989;9:202–212.

20. Zarins CK, Weisenberg E, Kolettis G, et al. Differential enlargement of artery segments in response to enlarging atherosclerosis plaques. *J Vasc Surg* 1988;7:386–394.

21. Glagov S, Masawa N, Bassiouny H, et al. Morphologic bases for establishing end-points for early plaque detection and plaque stability. *Int J Cardiac Imaging* 1995;4:1–7.

22. Geroulakos G, Ramaswami G, Nicolaides A, et al. Characterization of symptomatic and asymptomatic carotid plaques using high-resolution real-time ultrasonography. *Br J Surg* 1993;80:1274–1277.

23. Masawa N, Yoshida Y, Yamada T, et al. Three-dimensional analysis of human carotid atherosclerotic ulcer associated with recent thrombotic occlusion. *Pathol Int* 1994;44:745–752.

Chapter 10

Morphology of Atherosclerotic Plaque at the Carotid Artery Bifurcation:
Mechanism of Thromboembolic Cerebrovascular Disease

Jesse Weinberger, MD

Introduction

Atherosclerotic disease at the carotid artery bifurcation has long been recognized as a source of ischemic cerebrovascular disease.[1] A controversy exists as to whether cerebral ischemia is caused by hemodynamic reduction in brain perfusion or occlusion of intracranial vessels by distal embolization of atherosclerotic debris from the cervical carotid artery. The brain has extensive collateral circulation from the circle of Willis and from branches of the external carotid artery that anastomose to intracranial vessels such as the ophthalmic artery. Therefore, most individuals can tolerate complete occlusion of one carotid artery or even both carotid arteries without sustaining cerebral infarction.[2] The finding of cholesterol emboli in the ipsilateral retina of patients with carotid artery bifurcation atheroma suggests an embolic mechanism of cerebral ischemia.[3] Further evidence for an embolic mechanism was demonstrated by Moore,[4] who described patients with cerebral infarction ipsilateral to nonobstructive ulcerated plaques at the extracranial carotid artery bifurcation.

The results of recent trials of the efficacy of carotid endarterectomy in preventing stroke have renewed interest in the importance of the degree of stenosis as the critical factor in precipi-

From: Fuster V, (ed.) *Syndromes of Atherosclerosis: Correlations of Clinical Imaging and Pathology.* Armonk, NY: Futura Publishing Company, Inc.: © 1996.

tating cerebral ischemia.[5,6] The North American Symptomatic Carotid Endarterectomy Trial (NASCET) has documented beneficial effect of carotid endarterectomy compared with medical therapy with aspirin in preventing stroke in patients with >70% stenosis of the internal carotid artery who are symptomatic for transient cerebral ischemic attacks or transient monocular blindness (amaurosis fugax).[5] The Asymptomatic Carotid Artery Stenosis Study (ACAS) has a documented beneficial effect of carotid endarterectomy compared with medical therapy with aspirin in preventing stroke in patients with >60% diameter stenosis of the internal carotid artery who are asymptomatic.[6] These studies suggest that hemodyamic factors play a significant role in producing carotid stroke. Earlier studies by Busuttil et al[7] also support the importance of hemodynamic obstruction in the etiology of carotid stroke. These investigators found that patients with carotid stenosis >70% who had reduction in distal perfusion pressure measured at the ophthalmic artery (the first intracranial branch of the carotid artery) had a 20% risk of stroke whereas patients with an equivalent carotid stenosis and normal ophthalmic artery pressure had only a 2% risk of stroke.[6]

Previous studies have used intra-arterial contrast angiography to measure the degree of internal carotid artery stenosis and evaluate the shape and position of atherosclerotic plaque in the extracranial carotid artery bifurcation. More recent studies have used real-time B-mode ultrasonography with duplex Doppler ultrasound to image plaque in the carotid artery bifurcation and assess hemodynamics simultaneously by measurement of Doppler frequency shifts, which are proportional to the velocity of blood flow. Angiography produces a silhouette of the atheroma in the bifurcation, outlined by the contrast medium. B-mode sonography provides an image of the actual plaque in relation to the wall of the artery from which the morphological configuration and consistency can be directly observed. Information from B-mode sonography can thus be used to elucidate the mechanisms of thromboembolic stroke caused by atheroma at the carotid artery bifurcation.

Imaging of Carotid Plaque Histology

Imparato et al[8] were the first to correlate symptoms of cerebral ischemia with the histologic constituents of atheroma at the carotid artery bifurcation. These investigators examined 376 specimens of carotid bifurcation plaques obtained during endarterectomy. They noted a correlation between the presence of intramural hemorrhage and ipsilateral ischemic symptoms. Hemorrhage was present in 34.2% of 275 symptomatic plaques and in only 20.8% of 101 asymptomatic plaques, a significant difference ($P<0.02$). Ulceration was present in 48% of symptomatic plaques and 40.6% of asymptomatic plaques, indicating no significant correlation between plaque ulceration and thromboembolism.[9]

Lusby et al[10] also noted an association between intraplaque hemorrhage at the carotid artery bifurcation and ipsilateral symptoms of cerebral ischemia. They found intraplaque hemorrhage in 92.5% of 57 symptomatic lesions and only 27% of 26 asymptomatic lesions. They found that the recesses seen on angiographic outline of plaques did not correlate with intimal disruption, but mounds of plaque extending into the lumen were associated with intimal disruption and hemorrhage into plaque.[8]

Reilly[11] and Lusby et al[10] were able to categorize carotid plaque morphology using real-time B-mode ultrasonography. Using sonography, they analyzed 50 carotid artery bifurcations prior to carotid endarterectomy and characterized 14 plaques as homogeneous and 36 plaques as heterogeneous. The homogeneous plaques were uniformly found to contain collagenous fibrous material, although 3 had a small hemorrhagic component of <2 mm. There were no ulcerations in the homogeneous lesions. Major intraplaque hemorrhage was found in 30 of the 36 heterogeneous lesions, with very low echodensity areas corresponding to blood. In the remaining 6 heterogeneous lesions, the plaque was composed predominantly of lipid, cholesterol, loose stroma, and proteinaceous deposits. The lipid component probably accounted for the low echogenicity, but was not as lucent as blood.[11]

There was also an association between the ultrasound appearance of plaques and ipsilateral symptomatology. All 7 lesions from stroke patients and 22 of 30 lesions from patients with transient cerebral ischemic attacks were heterogeneous and contained intraplaque hemorrhage.[11] Only 4 of 13 asymptomatic patients had evidence of recent hemorrhage into plaque, 6 had fibrous plaque and 3 had evidence of prior resolving hemorrhage.[11] There was no correlation with symptomatology and ulceration or percentage of luminal stenosis.[11]

Steffen et al[12] categorized carotid bifurcation plaques as to the degree of heterogeneous changes, as well as the degree of stenosis. The categories of plaque were: type 1—predominantly echolucent raised lesion with thin "eggshell" cap of echogenicity; type 2—echogenic lesions with substantial areas of echolucency; type 3—predominantly echogenic with small areas of echolucency deeply localized and occupying less than aone fourth of the plaque; type 4—uniformly dense echogenic lesions; and type 5—no plaque seen, increased wall density or normal (Figures 1A through 1D).[12,13] There was a preponderance of echolucent type 1 and 2 lesions in the symptomatic arteries (67%) and a preponderance of echodense type 3 and 4 lesions in asymptomatic arteries (86%).[12]

Langsfeld et al[13] performed a prospective sonographic study imaging carotid plaques in the asymptomatic carotid artery of 289 patients who had contralateral carotid endarterectomy and an additional 260 carotid arteries in 130 asymptomatic patients who did not have carotid endarterectomy. The mean period between initial and follow-up scans was 15 months with a range of 0 to 48 months. The carotid lesions were categorized as type 1 to type 4 by the method outlined by Steffen et al.[12] Most plaques remained the same or became more echodense on follow-up study, with 25% becoming more echolucent or heterogeneous. Symptoms occurred ipsilateral to 10.7% of the asymptomatic arteries, but there was no definite correlation between change in plaque morphology or increasing degree of stenosis and the occurrence of symptoms.[12] There was a significant association between development of symptoms and the presence of heterogeneous plaque on the initial B-mode scan ($P<0.02$),[13] suggesting that heterogeneous plaques are more prone to subsequent thromboembolic events.

Johnson et al[14] analyzed 297 carotid artery bifurcations prospectively with B-mode sonography over a 3-year period. Plaques were classified as calcified (highest density), dense, or soft (lowest density). Lesions were also characterized as to whether they were hemodynamic (>75% stenosis) or not hemodynamic. Only 4 of 37 hemodynamic calcified plaques became symptomatic, whereas none of the 53 nonstenotic calcified plaques became symptomatic. There were 42 hemodynamic dense plaques, 26 of which became symptomatic, whereas only 5 of 76 nonstenotic dense plaques became symptomatic for transient ischemic attack. There were 42 hemodynamic soft plaques, 39 of which became symptomatic, 8 with strokes. Even among nonstenotic soft plaques, the risk of events was high with 10 of 47 becoming symptomatic. The presence of soft plaque was the greatest predictor of future thromboembolic events irrespective of the degree of stenosis.[14]

The presence of soft or echolucent heterogeneous plaque at the carotid artery bifurcation is associated with a 47% increased risk of symptoms compared to echodense or homogeneous plaque.[13] Echolucency or heterogeneity is associated with both intraplaque hemorrhage and intraplaque lipids.[11] Mercuri and Bond[15] have

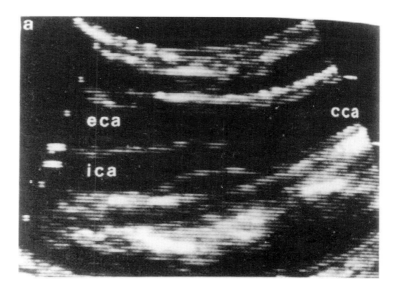

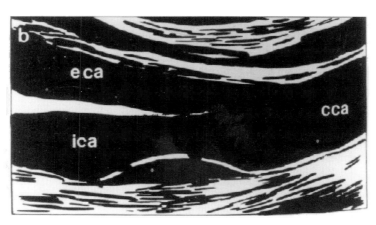

FIGURE 1. CATEGORIZATION OF PLAQUE MORPHOLOGY BY ULTRASONOGRA-PHY. **A:** *Type I. Echolucent raised lesion with thin cap, correlating with recent intraplaque hemorrhage. eca indicates external carotid artery; ica, internal carotid artery; cca, common carotid artery. Reprinted with permission from Reference 12.*

been able to differentiate lipid deposition from hemorrhage in vitro with B-mode ultrasound by examining strips of human aorta in a water bath and performing quantitative video-densitometry. However, B-mode ultrasound has not been able to definitively differentiate lipid material from hemorrhage in vivo.

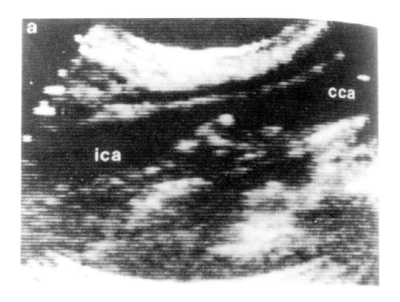

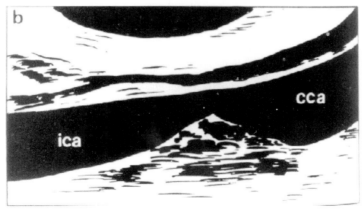

FIGURE 1 *continued.* **B:** *Type II. Echogenic lesion with substantial areas of echolucency (thrombus) near luminal surface. eca indicates external carotid artery; ica, internal carotid artery; cca, common carotid artery. Reprinted with permission from Reference 12.*

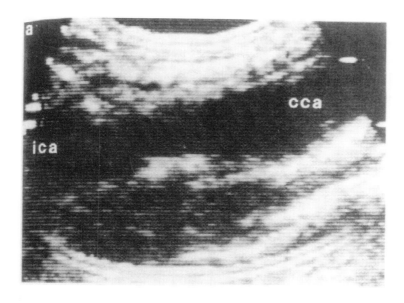

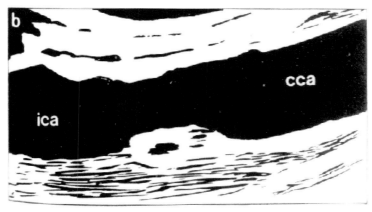

FIGURE 1 *continued. C:* Type III. Echogenic lesion with small areas of lucency localized deep in the plaque. eca indicates external carotid artery; ica, internal carotid artery; cca, common carotid artery. Reprinted with permission from Reference 12.

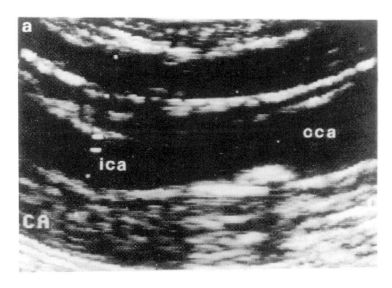

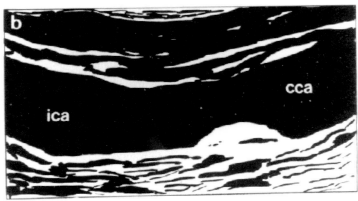

FIGURE 1 *continued. D:* Type IV. Uniformly dense echogenic lucency, consistent with simple fibrous or calcified plaque. eca indicates external carotid artery; ica, internal carotid artery, cca, common carotid artery. Reprinted with permission from Reference 12.

Imaging of Carotid Plaque Configuration

In addition to the echogenicity of carotid plaque material, the configuration of plaque in relation to the arterial wall can identify lesions that are more prone to proliferation and thromboembolism. Weinberger and Robbins[16] noted two types of plaque configuration: nodular plaques (Figure 2) that formed a spherical shape, and mural plaques (Figure 3) that grew along the curvature of the carotid sinus or internal carotid artery in a crescentic shape. Correlation of the results of B-mode sonography in 742 carotid arteries with presenting symptoms at the time of the study revealed that mural plaques were associated with a higher incidence of ipsilateral symptoms than nodular plaques. Lesions were characterized as to whether or not they were hemodynamically obstructive using Doppler sonography.[17] Hemodynamic lesions were associated with a 43.9% incidence of ipsilateral symptoms. Nonobstructive nodular plaques were associated with a 23.4% incidence of ipsilateral symptoms and mural plaques were associated with a 32.1% incidence of ipsilateral symptoms. Taking into account that normal bifurcations

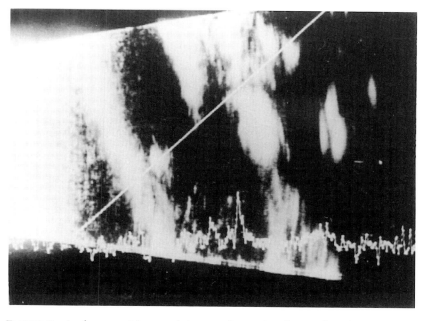

FIGURE 2. *A plaque with a nodular configuration located in the curvature of the carotid sinus below the origin of the internal carotid artery. The plaque is homogeneous and is composed of simple fibrous plaque. Reprinted with permission from Reference 16.*

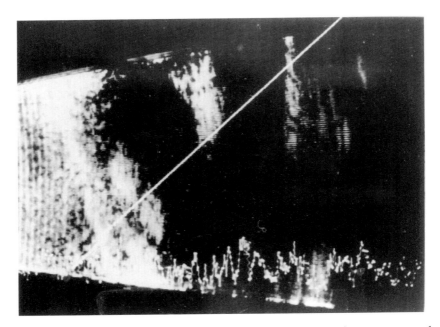

FIGURE 3. *A mural plaque forming a crescent pattern in the curvature of the carotid sinus below the origin of the internal carotid artery. Echolucencies are seen within the plaque and scalloped borders appear on the surface of the plaque. The morphology is consistent with recent plaque hemorrhage. Reprinted with permission from Reference 16.*

were associated with a 14.5% incidence of ipsilateral symptoms, statistical analysis demonstrated that nonobstructive nodular plaques had an equivalent incidence of symptoms as a normal bifurcation while mural plaques had an equivalent incidence of ipsilateral symptoms as hemodynamic lesions.[16] The angiographic appearance of mural plaques was similar to the clinically relevant nonobstructive ulcerated plaques described by Moore[4] and were analogous in configuration to the clinically relevant crescentic plaques described by Ambrose et al[18] in coronary angiography of symptomatic lesions.

Histologic examination of 54 carotid plaques removed at endarterectomy showed that mural plaques had a 72% incidence of recent organizing hemorrhage (Figure 4),whereas nodular plaques had only a 23% incidence of organizing hemorrhage.[19] Intraluminal thrombus was seen only in mural plaques with recent hemorrhage (Figure 5). The mural plaques without recent organizing hemorrhage had evidence of degenerative changes suggestive of old hemorrhage or thrombosis. Thus, recent organizing hemorrhage

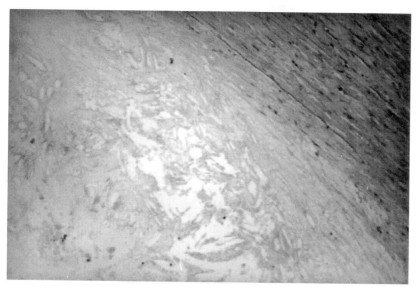

FIGURE 4. *Section from a proliferative mural plaque (H & E × 100) show-ing recent plaque hemorrhage with red blood cells in the plaque and cholesterol clefts. Reprinted with permission from Reference 19.*

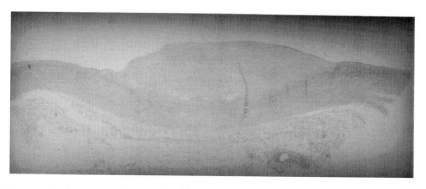

FIGURE 5. *Section of a simple fibrous plaque (H & E × 100) seen on ul-trasonography as a nodular plaque. Reprinted with permission from Ref-erence 19.*

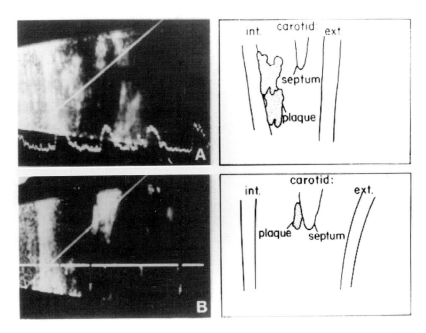

FIGURE 6. *Ultrasonographic image of a proliferative mural plaque of the type seen in Figure 4, with low echodensity areas, clefts, and soft echodensities suggesting intraluminal thrombus overlying the plaque as described in Reference 19.*

was again responsible for the difference in symptomatology of mural and nodular plaques. Recent hemorrhage accounted for the sonographic configuration of the mural plaque, and the appearance of carotid bifurcation plaque could be a marker to identify lesions with recent hemorrhage (Figure 6).

Sequential sonographic imaging of 246 carotid bifurcation plaques in 123 patients, comparing initial and follow-up studies showed a significantly higher incidence of symptoms ipsilateral to plaques that enlarged (25%) than plaques that remained unchanged or diminished in size (8%) (Figure 7).[20] While plaques that became hemodynamically obstructive had a higher incidence of ipsilateral symptoms (40%) than nonobstructive plaques (13%), plaques that grew in a mural configuration (Figure 8) had a higher incidence of symptoms (40%) than plaques that grew and maintained a nodular configuration (12%), independent of hemodynamic factors.[20] The study indicated that acute hemorrhage into plaque that produced growth in a mural configuration resulted in thromboembolic phenomena that caused symptoms of cerebral ischemia.[20]

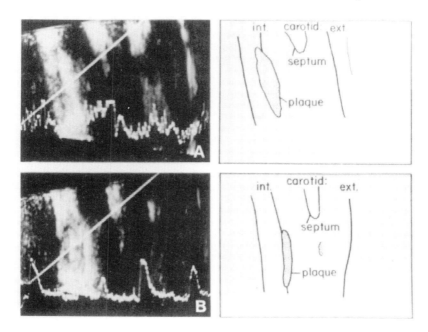

FIGURE 7. *A mural plaque visualized in a patient with an asymptomatic bruit that diminished in width and degree of stenosis over a 6 month follow-up period. The raised portion of the plaque has flattened and lucent areas have filled in. Morphological examination of plaques such as this have shown evidence of prior hemorrhage with retraction of intraplaque thrombus and deposition of hemosiderin.[19] Reprinted with permission from Reference 20.*

Plaque Ulceration and Crevices

Crevices and indentations in plaques can be visualized with real-time B-mode ultrasonography (Figure 9), but these plaque irregularities do not coincide with pathological evidence of intimal disruption and ulceration.[21,22] Bluth et al[21] found no features in heterogeneous plaques that could predict pathological correlation with intimal ulceration. O'Leary et al[22] found a 60% accuracy of B-mode in predicting pathological evidence of intimal ulceration, with a sensitivity of 39% and a specificity of 72%. One difficulty in establishing plaque ulceration on B-mode sonography is that there may be a thin layer of intimal or fibrous cap over what appears to be an ulcer that is difficult to visualize. Color flow Doppler sonography has been proposed as a way of delineating whether there is an echolucent cap over a potential ulcer by defining whether the

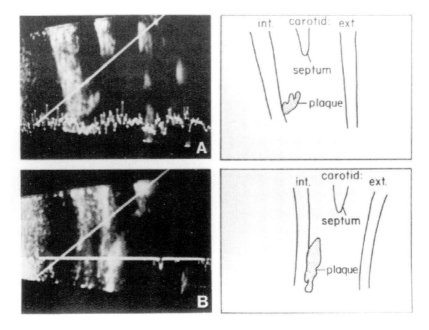

FIGURE 8. *An asymptomatic nodular plaque seen in a patient with a transient ischemic attack (TIA) from a contralateral carotid stenosis. The patient had a TIA ipsilateral to this lesion 3 months later, and follow-up sonography at that time showed that the plaque had lengthened and assumed a mural configuration. The nodular plaque seen originally is atypical because it showed evidence of crevices in the plaque. This may have led to plaque fissuring and intraplaque thrombus. Reprinted with permission from Reference 20.*

color map of Doppler flow penetrates into the irregular surface or not. However, Mohr et al[23] were not able to differentiate histologic plaque ulceration by this color flow method.

In many instances, crevices in the plaque may not penetrate all the way to the intimal surface. This can occur particularly when a piece of plaque material has been evulsed from the plaque without disrupting the junction between the intimal wall and the plaque. In Figure 10, a portion of the plaque has been expressed by manual compression of the artery, resulting in an ipsilateral transient ischemic attack. The resulting crevice does not penetrate to the intimal surface. Most of the plaque has been removed by the manual compression, and the patient remained asymptomatic after this event. In this instance, the B-mode image can be used to predict that because most of the plaque material has been ex-

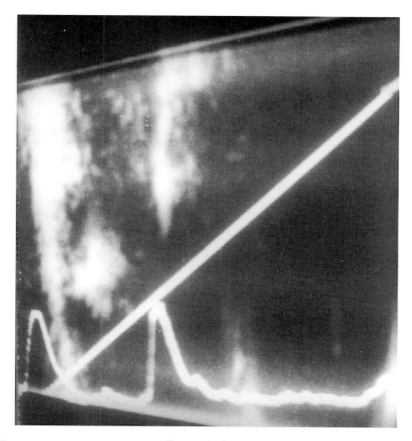

FIGURE 9. *A crevice in a small mural plaque seen with ultrasonography. Crevices do not necessarily correspond to ulceration, but may serve as a nidus for thrombus because they expose blood to tissue factor from the endothelial wall.*

truded, the patient is at relatively low risk of subsequent thromboembolic events.

The presence of irregularities or craters in heterogeneous plaques may still represent a potential risk for future thromboembolic events, particularly if the crater extends all the way to the intimal surface. These crevices expose the intimal surface containing tissue factor to blood, which can form a nidus for induction of thrombus formation and platelet aggregation.[24–26] This can lead to subintimal dissection with hemorrhage and evulsion of plaque material and thrombus, producing thromboembolism.[24–27] The small plaque shown in Figure 8, which had subsequent en-

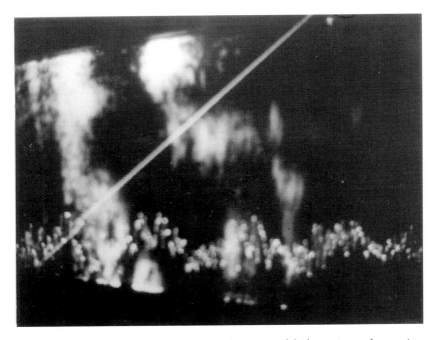

FIGURE 10. *A mural plaque seen in the carotid bifurcation of a patient who had a focal seizure of the opposite arm during compression of the carotid artery. A crater is seen in the plaque, suggesting that plaque material has been evulsed by the carotid compression. Extrusion of plaque may be the mechanism for some thromboembolic events. There is only moderate plaque remaining, indicating that no surgical treatment is necessary.*

largement into a mural configuration and became symptomatic, had evidence of crevice formation. This may be predictive of plaques that are prone to further growth and thrombus formation, but prospective studies to confirm this have not as yet been performed.

The inability of B-mode ultrasonography to identify intimal ulceration does not detract from the prognostic value of plaque morphology studies. It appears to be sufficient to be able to differentiate heterogeneities in plaques in order to discriminate lesions that are prone to future clinically relevant thromboembolism.[12–14] Furthermore, intimal ulceration has not been found to be as important a factor as intraplaque hemorrhage in the initiation of thromboembolic cerebrovascular disease,[8,9] and hemorrhagic plaques can readily be identified by real-time B-mode ultrasonography.[11–14,16–18]

Intimal Wall Thickness

The categorization of carotid bifurcation atheroma into heterogeneous plaques or mural plaque configuration is subjective. Attempts have been made to quantify carotid bifurcation atherosclerosis on a reproducible basis by measurement of intimal wall thickness at standardized points along the common and internal carotid arteries.[28] This method was first designed to identify the earliest atherosclerotic lesion of intimal wall thickening from lipid accumulation in population studies of atherosclerotic vascular disease.[29] The method has been extended to include measurement of thickness of atherosclerotic plaques protruding into the lumen of the artery (Figure 11).[30] Surface heterogeneities have been quantified by the variability of the wall thickness measurements along the plaque.[30] Correlation has been established between the degree of carotid artery wall thickness and the occurrence of clinical thromboembolic cerebrovascular events.[31]

There are several limitations to the wall thickness method. Measurements are made at finite standardized locations along the carotid artery, and significant accumulations of plaque may not be included in the analysis. The method can only reproducibly measure plaques in the internal carotid artery with an accuracy of 50%,[31] which weighs the measurement of wall thickness towards the common carotid artery, where atherosclerosis is less likely to form. The configuration of plaque in relation to the vessel wall is not taken into account. Most importantly, while irregularities in the surface of the plaque can be measured, heterogeneities and lucencies below the surface cannot be identified. It is these intraplaque lucencies that have had the greatest correlation with clinically significant thromboembolic events.[11-14] Therefore, morphological studies of plaque constitution and configuration are still necessary, in addition to studies of wall thickness, to define the role of extracranial carotid atherosclerosis in the etiology of cerebrovascular disease.

The Correlation of Hemodynamics with Plaque Morphology

Intraplaque hemorrhage and plaque heterogeneity that can be visualized by real-time B-mode ultrasonography at the bifurcation of the extracranial carotid artery have been established as independent risk factors for thromboembolic cerebrovascular disease.[8-14,16,17]

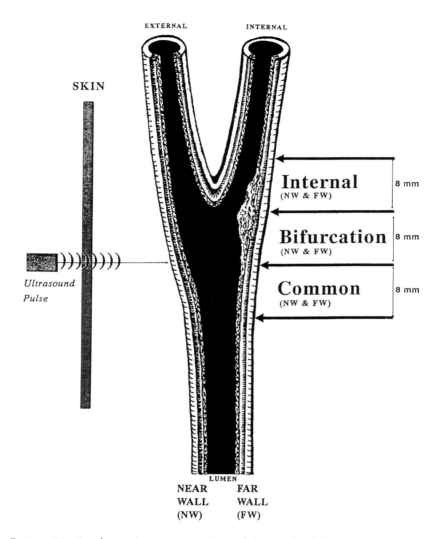

FIGURE 11. *A schematic representation of the methodology of measuring intimal-medial wall thickness. Exophytic plaque is included in the measurement. Reprinted with permission from Reference 30.*

Yet, in all of these studies, hemodynamically critical lesions with >75% stenosis have been associated with a higher incidence of ipsilateral symptoms than nonobstructive lesions. Intraplaque hemorrhage into nonobstructive plaques may result in thromboembolic events that present more often as transient ischemic attacks, while hemodynamic lesions are more likely to result in cerebral infarction,[16] particularly if distal perfusion pressure is reduced.[7]

Hemodynamic lesions may be more prone to intraplaque hemorrhage. Imparato et al[9] detected intraplaque hemorrhage only in hemodynamic lesions with >75% stenosis. The shear stresses created by stenotic lesions of the internal carotid artery may lead to plaque rupture and hemorrhage,[32,33] analogous to the findings in stenotic coronary arteries of patients with crescendo angina and acute myocardial infarction.[34,35] Eddy currents and retrograde flow in the bifurcation proximal to the stenosis (Figure 12) may be responsible for dissection of blood into the junction of the plaque and the intimal wall, resulting in intraplaque hemorrhage. In one case, a patient with crescendo episodes of amaurosis fugax (transient monocular blindness) was observed to have a complete heterogeneous plaque dissecting off the wall of the carotid bifurcation just below the origin of the internal carotid, which was highly stenotic (Figure 13). The patient immediately underwent carotid endarterectomy, where the surgeon observed a degenerative plaque with thrombus dissecting off of the wall of the artery and squeezing out of the origin of the internal carotid artery. This is probably the mechanism for major thromboembolism of plaque and thrombus from the extracranial carotid artery to cause hemispheric cerebral infarction from occlusion of large distal intracranial arteries, which in this case was aborted by endarterectomy prior to extrusion of the plaque.

The recent multicenter trials of carotid endarterectomy have documented a beneficial effect of surgery in both symptomatic[5] and asymptomatic[6] patients with significant internal carotid artery stenosis. In the case of patients who are symptomatic, the carotid plaques are clearly in an active phase because they have expressed themselves clinically by generating symptoms of transient cerebral ischemia or cerebral infarction. Carotid endarterectomy virtually eliminates further clinical events in these patients once the perioperative period is over.[5] Patients treated with aspirin 650 mg twice daily continue to have a significantly higher incidence of recurrent cerebrovascular events for about 18 months after endarterectomy, at which time few further events occur and the incidence of new events parallels the surgical group.[5] This suggests that after a certain time, the plaques heal or regress and become inactive. This would correspond to the lesions seen on B-mode ultrasonography that show regression (Figure 7),[20] and contain degenerative changes and hemosiderin consistent with previous resorbing thrombus.[19] Plaque morphology studies may be helpful in determining which patients with asymptomatic carotid stenosis have

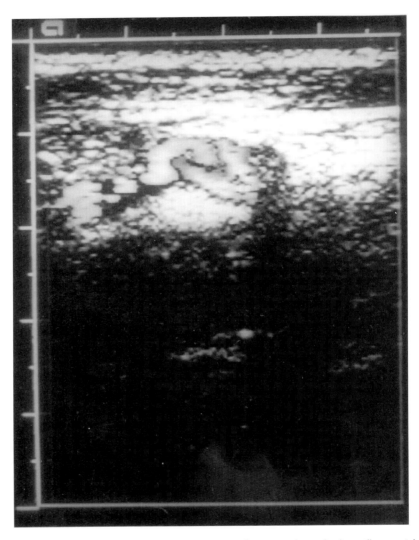

FIGURE 12. *Color flow Doppler sonography reveals turbulent flow with reversal in the carotid bifurcation below the origin of internal carotid artery proximal to a high-grade stenosis of the internal carotid artery. The shear forces created by this swirl of antegrade and retrograde flow can set up shear forces that can dissect beneath the proximal edge of plaque and cause plaque rupture with embolization.*

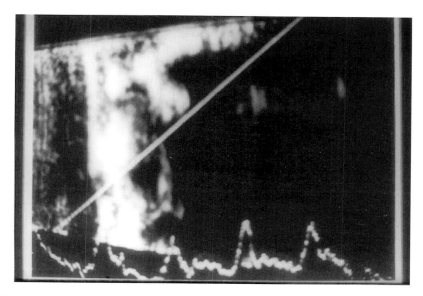

FIGURE 13. *A large plaque extending along the length of the carotid sinus with a high-grade stenosis of the origin of the internal carotid artery is seen shearing off the wall of the carotid bifurcation in a patient with repetitive episodes of amaurosis fugax. Carotid endarterectomy was performed 30 minutes after sonography. Degenerative plaque was seen squeezing out of the origin of the internal carotid artery. This is probably the mechanism of major thromboembolism to the intracranial carotid arteries that results in massive hemispheric stroke.*

potentially active plaques that are more prone to future thromboembolism[13,14] and which are chronic and have already passed through the active phase.[19,20] Identification of heterogeneities and crevices in plaques confined mainly to the carotid sinus that are not causing hemodynamic stenosis of the internal carotid artery may also have clinical relevance in determining which patients might benefit from carotid endarterectomy.[4]

Conclusion

The morphology of atherosclerotic plaque at the carotid artery bifurcation can be imaged with real-time B-mode ultrasonography. The constitution and configuration of plaque correlates with recent intraplaque hemorrhage and clinical symptomatology. The sonographic appearance of the plaque can be used to judge whether a plaque is in an active or chronic phase and whether it is prone to produce significant thromboembolism. This can be helpful in clinical decision making as to the best method of treatment, either medical or surgical, in a patient with carotid artery stenosis. Plaque morphology and measurements of carotid artery wall thickness can be used to assess the effects of medical therapies of atherosclerosis such as lipid-lowering agents to determine if they can produce regression of plaque.[36] The study of carotid plaque morphology is a valuable tool for evaluation of the mechanisms of atherosclerotic vascular disease.

References

1. Fisher CM, Gore I, Okabe N, et al. Atherosclerosis of the carotid and vertebral arteries—Extracranial and intracranial. *J Neuropathol Exp Neurol* 1965;6:245–252.
2. Doniger DE. Bilateral complete carotid and basilar artery occlusion in a patient with minimal deficit: Case report and discussion of diagnostic and therapeutic implications. *Neurology* 1963;13:673–677.
3. Fisher CM. Transient monocular blindness associated with hemiplegia. *Arch Ophthalmol* 1952;47:167–203.
4. Moore WS, Hall AD. Importance of emboli from carotid bifurcation in pathogenesis of cerebral ischemic attacks. *Arch Surg* 1970;101: 708–711.
5. North American Symptomatic Carotid Endarterectomy Trial Collaborators. Beneficial effect of carotid endarterectomy in symptomatic patients with high-grade carotid stenosis. *N Engl J Med* 1991;325: 445– 453.
6. Ececuive Committee for the Asympomatic Carotid Atherosclerosis Study. Endarterectomy for asymptomatic carotid artery stenosis. *JAMA* 1995;273:1421–1428.
7. Busuttil RW, Baker JD, Davidson RK, et al. Carotid artery stenosis: Hemodynamic significance and clinical course. *JAMA* 1981;245: 1438–1441.
8. Imparato AM, Riles TS, Gorstein F. The carotid bifurcation plaque: Pathologic findings associated with cerebral ischemia. *Stroke* 1977;10: 238–245.
9. Imparato AM, Riles TS, Mintzer K, et al. The importance of hemorrhage in the relationship between gross morphologic characteristics and cerebral symptoms in 376 carotid artery plaques. *Ann Surg* 1983;197: 195–203.
10. Lusby RJ, Ferrell LD, Ehrenfeld WK, et al. Carotid plaque hemorrhage: Its role in production of cerebral ischemia. *Arch Surg* 1982;117:1479–1488.
11. Reilly LM, Lusby RJ, Hughes I, et al. Carotid plaque histology using real-time ultrasonography: Clinical and therapeutic implications. *Am J Surg* 1983;146:188–193.
12. Steffen CM, Gray-Weale AC, Byrne KE, et al. Carotid artery atheroma: Ultrasound appearance in symptomatic and asymptomatic vessels. *Aust N Z J Surg* 1989;59:529–534.

13. Langsfeld M, Gray-Weale AC, Lusby RJ. The role of plaque morphology and diameter reduction in the development of new symptoms in asymptomatic carotid arteries. *J Vasc Surg* 1989;9:548–557.

14. Johnson JM, Kennelly MM, Decesare D, et al. Natural history of asymptomatic carotid plaque. *Arch Surg* 1985;120:1010–1012.

15. Mercuri M, Bond MG. B-mode ultasound characterization of atherosclerosis. *J Cardiovasc Technol* 1992;10:277–291.

16. Weinberger J, Robbins A. Neurologic symptoms associated with nonobstructive plaque at carotid bifurcation: Analysis by real-time B-mode ultrasonography. *Arch Neurol* 1983;40:489–492.

17. Weinberger J, Biscarra V, Weitzner I, et al. Noninvasive carotid artery testing: Role in management of patients with transient ischemic attacks. *NY State J Med* 1981;81:1463–1468.

18. Ambrose JA, Winters SL, Arora RR, et al. Angiographic evolution of coronary artery morphology in unstable angina. *J Am Coll Cardiol* 1986;7:472–478.

19. Weinberger J, Marks SJ, Gaul JJ, et al. Atherosclerotic plaque at the carotid artery bifurcation: Correlation of ultrasonographic imaging with morphology. *J Ultrasound Med* 1987;6:363–366.

20. Weinberger J, Ramos L, Ambrose JA, et al. Morphologic and dynamic changes of atherosclerotic plaque at the carotid artery bifurcation: Sequential imaging by real time B-mode ultrasonography. *J Am Coll Cardiol* 1988;12:1515–1521.

21. Bluth EI, McVay LV III, Merritt CRB, et al. The identification of ulcerative plaque with high resolution duplex carotid scanning. *J Ultrasound Med* 1988;7:73–76.

22. O'Leary DH, Holen J, Ricotta JJ, et al. Carotid bifurcation disease: Prediction of ulceration with B-mode US. *Radiology* 1987;162:523–525.

23. Steinke W, Hennerici M, Rautenberg W, et al. Symptomatic and asymptomatic high-grade carotid stenoses in Doppler color-flow imaging. *Neurology* 1992;42:131–138.

24. Lassila R. Inflammation in atheroma: Implications for plaque rupture and platelet-collagen interaction. *Eur Heart J* 1993;14(Suppl K):94–97.

25. Sakariassen KS, Barstad RM. Mechanisms of thromboembolism at arterial plaques. *Blood Coagul Fibrinolysis* 1993;4:615–625.

26. Pawashe AB, Golino P, Ambrosio G, et al. A monoclonal antibody against rabbit tissue factor inhibits thrombus formation in stenotic injured rabbit carotid arteries. *Circ Res* 1994;74:56–63.

27. Badimon L, Badimon JJ, Cohen M, et al. Vessel wall-related risk factors in acute vascular events. *Drugs* 1991;42(suppl 5):1–9.

28. Bond MG, Barnes RW, Riley WA, et al. High-resolution B-mode ultrasound scanning methods in the Atherosclerosis Risk in Communities (ARIC) cohort. *J Neuroimaging* 1991;1:68–73.

29. Riley WA, Barnes RW, Bond MG, et al. High-resolution B-mode ultrasound reading methods in the Atherosclerosis Risk in Communities (ARIC) cohort. *J Neuroimaging* 1991;1:168–172.

30. Espeland MA, Hoen H, Byington R, et al. Spatial distribution of carotid intimal-medial thickness as measured by B-mode ultrasonography. *Stroke* 1994;25:1812–1819.

31. Davis VG, Bond MG, Furberg CD. Reproducibility of noninvasive ultrasonic measurement of carotid atherosclerosis: The Asymptomatic Carotid Artery Plaque Study. *Stroke* 1992;23:1062–1068.

32. Zarins CK, Giddens DP, Bharadvaj BK, et al. Carotid bifurcation atherosclerosis: Quantitative correlation of plaque localization with flow velocity profiles and wall shear stress. *Circ Res* 1983;53:502–514.

33. Ku DN, Zarins CK, Giddens DP, et al. Pulsatile flow and atherosclerosis in the human carotid bifurcation: Positive correlation between plaque localization and low and oscillating shear stress. *Arteriosclerosis* 1985;5:292–302.

34. Falk E. Unstable angina with fatal outcome: Dynamic coronary thrombosis leading to infarction and/or sudden death. Autopsy evidence of recurrent mural thrombosis with peripheral embolization culminating in total vascular occlusion. *Circulation* 1985;71:600–708.

35. Davies MJ, Thomas AC. Plaque fissuring—The cause of acute myocardial infarction, sudden ischemic death and crescendo angina. *Br Heart J* 1985;53:363–373.

36. Blankenhorn DH, Selzer RH, Mack WJ, et al. Evaluation of colestipol/niacin therapy with computer derived coronary endpoint measures. *Circulation* 1992;86:1701–1709.

Chapter 11

Imaging of Carotid Artery Lesions: A Surgeon's View

Ted R. Kohler, MD

Introduction

Stroke is the third leading cause of death in the United States, accounting for 150,000 deaths annually.[1] An additional 450,000 to 600,000 persons suffer from nonfatal, often debilitating strokes. The most common cause of stroke is embolization from atherosclerotic carotid arteries.[2,3] Recent large clinical trials have determined that carotid endarterectomy significantly reduces the risk of stroke in symptomatic and asymptomatic patients with high-grade stenosis of the internal carotid artery. However, 74% of symptomatic patients with high-grade stenoses in the control (unoperated) groups who do not undergo surgery remain stroke-free during 2-year follow-up. These patients presumably had stable plaques and would not have benefitted from endarterectomy. Surgery could be withheld in this group if noninvasive studies were able to differentiate between stable and potentially unstable plaques. Instability involves disruption of the fibrous plaque, local hemodynamic factors, and certain plaque characteristics such as the thickness of the fibrous cap, presence of intraplaque hemorrhage, the extent of central necrosis, and the composition of the matrix. Some of these features can be detected on ultrasound imaging. Duplex ultrasound scanning of the carotid bifurcation is widely used as a relatively inexpensive noninvasive screening examination for carotid disease. Based on velocity information, it can identify a > 70% carotid artery stenosis with an overall accuracy of 90%. Attempts to predict plaque behavior based on features seen on B-mode imaging have not been as successful. This chapter reviews the pathophysiology of

From: Fuster V, (ed.) *Syndromes of Atherosclerosis: Correlations of Clinical Imaging and Pathology.* Armonk, NY: Futura Publishing Company, Inc.: © 1996.

cerebrovascular disease, the role of carotid endarterectomy, and the usefulness of noninvasive evaluation. The potential role of noninvasive testing of plaque morphology is discussed.

The Embolic Theory

Knowledge of the pathogenesis of embolic stroke provides the basis for evaluation of noninvasive diagnostic testing. Although the degree of carotid artery diameter reduction is used as the criterion for selecting patients for carotid endarterectomy, the primary cause of stroke is embolism rather than flow reduction. Noninvasive tests that can accurately assess plaque morphology may improve our ability to predict which lesions are likely to cause neurological events.

The embolic theory of cerebrovascular ischemia emerged in the mid-1900s when it was noted that patients with cerebral symptoms had a much higher incidence of high-grade lesions and occlusions than did asymptomatic patients. Fisher[4] was among the first to realize the importance of carotid bifurcation atherosclerosis. He described ulceration of the plaque, hemorrhage within the plaque, mural thrombus, and thrombus formation distal to extremely tight carotid lesions. Fisher noted that total occlusion of the internal carotid artery may be silent, but found that hemiplegia was the most common clinical picture encountered and usually progressed slowly in a stuttering fashion over days or was preceded by prodromal warnings consisting of fleeting attacks of paralysis, paresthesia, dysphasia, or monocular blindness. Fisher postulated that " . . . it is even conceivable that some day vascular surgery will find a way to by-pass the occluded portion of the artery during the period of ominous fleeting symptoms."

Compelling evidence for embolization in the territory of the carotid artery came from Hollenhorst's observation of atherosclerotic debris in the fundus of patients with cerebrovascular symptoms.[5] Hollenhorst found that 63% of patients with retinal emboli had symptoms or signs of cerebral ischemia, and in 79% of patients with both cerebral symptoms and retinal findings, crystals were lodged in the ipsilateral eye. Zukowski and colleagues[6] reported that 88% of patients presenting with transient ishemic attacks (TIA) had evidence of ipsilateral cerebral infarction on computerized tomography. At this time it was noted that infarcts were particularly common in patients whose carotid lesions were ulcerated.

The prevalence of ulceration in carotid artery plaques was observed by Julian and co-workers in 1963, who also noted that the presence of ulceration is often difficult to detect on angiography.[7] Drake and Drake[8] noted that 90% of patients with cerebrovascular insufficiency had stenotic lesions that presumably caused their symptoms. In a study of carotid endarterectomy specimens, Sterpetti and colleagues[9] found that ulceration and mural thrombus were the only morphological findings statistically correlated with the presence of hemispheric symptoms. However, during the early development of carotid endarterectomy, it was thought that the major benefit of the operation was improvement in blood flow rather than removal of a source of embolism. The hypotensive crisis theory proposed that brief episodes of hypotension together with cerebrovascular occlusive disease cause vascular insufficiency and cerebral symptoms. This theory was gradually debunked when investigators found that hypotension caused symptoms of generalized ischemia rather than focal neurological deficits and that cerebral symptoms usually cease after carotid artery occlusion.

Moore[10,11] emphasized the importance of emboli rather than flow reduction as a cause of cerebral events. The results of carotid endarterectomy in 49 symptomatic patients with irregular or ulcerated carotid plaques, but no significant luminal narrowing were reported. The fact that most of the patients had no further neurological symptoms following the surgery was taken as evidence supporting the embolic theory of cerebrovascular disease. Further evidence that symptoms of carotid disease are not caused by reduced flow comes from the observation that clamping of the carotid artery is well tolerated. Less than 10% of conscious patients undergoing endarterectomy under local anesthesia develop neurological symptoms when the carotid artery is clamped.[12,13]

The Importance of Plaque Morphology

Advanced lesions of carotid atherosclerosis are typically eccentric with a central core that accumulates free lipid, cholesterol crystals, and areas of calcification (Figure 1). Focal calcification is commonly seen in the necrotic cores, but also frequently involves acellular fibrous regions of the plaque. Cholesterol in advanced plaques is derived from dying foam cells or from conversion of low-density lipoproteins (LDL) within the matrix. Although the media is typically uninvolved, it may become thin in regions of prominent intimal thickening. Capillaries grow into these lesions, but they may not provide adequate nutrient supply to the central core, which leads to necrosis. Most intraplaque hemorrhage is due to dis-

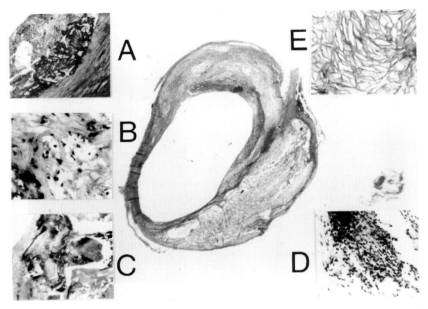

FIGURE 1. *Photomicrograph of a segment of diseased internal carotid artery. The inserts are magnified views of (counterclockwise): (A) a small area of intraplaque hemorrhage nestled between loose necrosis and fibrous plaque; (B) a small group of lipid-laden foam cells; (C) nodules of calcified plaque surrounded by loose necrosis; (D) a cluster of inflammatory cells; (E) cholesterol clefts imbedded in a matrix of prior hemorrhage. (Courtesy of the University of Washington Department of Pathology.)*

ruption of the fibrous cap. Typically the lesions are rich in platelets and fibrin and therefore are really areas of thrombosis rather than hemorrhage (Figure 2). The plaque cap consists mainly of connective tissue matrix, smooth muscle cells, and lipid-laden macrophages. Factors contributing to cap disruption include hypertension, stenosis, decreased collagen in the cap, decreased width of the cap, and the presence of a large soft lipid core. Macrophage infiltration near the shoulder region, where disruption most commonly occurs, may contribute to weakening of the cap by releasing proteases (elastase and collagenase) that break down the extracellular matrix. The concentration of macrophages appears to be higher in caps of plaques that ulcerate and in regions where fissures occur.[14–16] Analysis of plaques that have undergone disruption and thrombosis have revealed the presence of both macrophages and T lymphocytes.[17] Macrophages can contribute to thrombosis by releasing tissue fac-

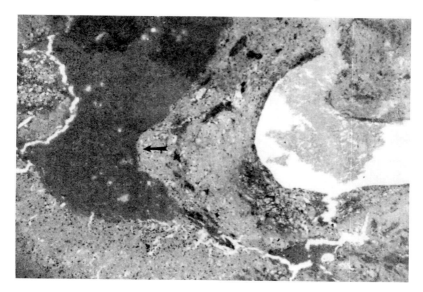

FIGURE 2. *Histologic section of carotid plaque containing intramural hemorrhage (arrow). This region has fibrin and platelet deposits with evidence of surrounding tissue reaction. Reprinted with permission from Reference 59.*

tor and possibly plasminogen activator inhibitor-1.[17] Large amounts of messenger ribonucleic acid (mRNA) for tissue factor is located in the plaque core around cholesterol crystals.[18] Surface thrombosis also occurs as the blood is exposed to the necrotic core and its highly thrombogenic interstitial collagen and tissue factor. Plaque fissuring is common, and healing of these lesions may contribute to plaque enlargement.[17]

Hemorrhage into the substance of the plaque is often a prominent feature in unstable plaques. Bleeding may result either from rupture of the overlying fibrous cap or from rupture of one of the thin-walled, capillary-like vessels that are prevalent in these plaques. This is the likely explanation for hemorrhage that is seen beneath an intact fibrous cap. These penetrating vessels appear to be derived from the vasa vasorum in the adventitia, however, some may arise directly from the arterial lumen. They may play an important role in supporting growth of the developing plaque. Thrombus or hemosiderin are often found in the vicinity of these vessels, suggesting that they often disrupt, causing hemorrhage. However, it may be that organizing blood products stimulate the ingrowth of these vessels into the plaque. Angiogenic activity has been found in atherosclerotic plaques.

While carotid atherosclerosis is a common cause of cerebral ischemia, the majority of patients with atherosclerosis are asymptomatic. In 1960, Martin[19] reported that 40% of patients over 50 years
of age had at least a 50% stenosis of one or more extracranial cerebral vessels at autopsy, and the majority had been asymptomatic.
Lesions usually produce symptoms when they become unstable
due to fissuring or cracking of the fibrous cap of the plaque. This
causes release of necrotic debris from the lipid core and exposes
blood to lipid, tissue factor, and collagen resulting in further
thrombosis. This phenomenon has been particularly well studied in
coronary artery disease where it is assumed to initiate unstable
angina and acute myocardial infarction. Fuster and colleagues[20]
have reviewed the role of plaque rupture in coronary artery disease.
Plaques with large lipid collections are particularly prone to rupture. Rupture of plaques is a principle component of ischemic coronary syndromes. Thrombus that forms after plaque disruption may
lead to decreased perfusion and an unstable coronary syndrome or
may organize and cause accelerated luminal narrowing. The extent
of myocardial damage depends on the size of the vessel affected,
the duration of occlusion, the extent of collateral flow, and the ability of the fibrinolytic system to dissolve the thrombus. Plaque disruption is particularly prevalent in coronary arteries of patients
who have died of myocardial infarction.

Breakdown of the fibrous cap of carotid lesions undoubtedly is
an important element in producing cerebral symptoms. Plaque hemorrhage and disruption are more frequent in carotid endarterectomy specimens from patients who have had symptoms than from
those who were asymptomatic.[21,22] Eccentric plaques with soft lipid
cores are more prone to rupture. Finite element analysis of stress
forces on plaques reveal increased force in the shoulder region of
the plaque.[16] The high velocity of blood flow at the site of severe vessel narrowing causes a reduction in intraluminal blood pressure by
the Bernoulli effect. Reduction of intraluminal pressure on the
plaque may contribute to bleeding from vessels within it.[23]

The Role of Endarterectomy

In the mid-1980s, carotid endarterectomy became the most increasingly used surgical procedure in the United States. In 1987, an
estimated 150,000 procedures were performed at an average cost of
$13,000 per operation.[24] The rapid increase in the number of pro-
cedures combined with reports of unusually high complication
rates led many physicians to question the role of carotid en-

darterectomy in the prevention of stroke.[25,26] As a result, several randomized clinical trials investigated the role of carotid endarterectomy in stroke prevention. The findings of the North American Symptomatic Carotid Endarterectomy Trial (NASCET) and the European Carotid Surgery Trial (ECST) were released simultaneously in 1991. These results demonstrated the efficacy of carotid endarterectomy for stroke prevention in patients with TIA or stroke with recovery and a >70% diameter-reducing stenosis by conventional angiography.[27–29] Because most symptomatic plaques are high-grade lesions, the NASCET trial had too few patients to analyze the results in the 30% to 69% carotid-narrowing category. The ECST group found that patients with <30% narrowing did not benefit from surgery.

Many retrospective studies have suggested a role for carotid endarterectomy in preventing neurological events in asymptomatic patients with high-grade lesions.[30–32] Results are now available from two major prospective trials involving asymptomatic patients. The Veterans Affairs Cooperative Study Group randomly assigned 444 asymptomatic male patients with a >50% diameter reducing lesion to receive either aspirin or aspirin plus carotid endarterectomy.[33] The incidence of all ipsilateral neurological events (TIA, amaurosis fugax, or stroke) was significantly reduced in the surgical group (8.0% vs. 20.6%, $P<0.001$). Although the reduction in ipsilateral stroke alone was not significant (4.7% vs. 9.4%), 3 of the 10 strokes in the surgical group were a result of angiography and could have been prevented by a diagnostic routine that eliminated this test. The larger Asymptomatic Carotid Atherosclerosis Study found a significant benefit of endarterectomy in asymptomatic patients. This study group randomly assigned 1662 asymptomatic patients with >60% carotid stenosis to either surgery or medical management. The surgical group had a significantly lower 5-year incidence of ipsilateral stroke or stroke death than the medically-treated group (4.8% vs. 10.8%, $P<0.01$).

The Role of Ultrasound

Diagnostic Accuracy for Classification of Degree of Stenosis

Duplex scanning has become a reliable method for determining the degree of carotid stenosis, and many clinicians have suggested that the use of this test, either alone or in conjunction with computerized tomography scan or magnetic resonance imaging

(MRI), may be sufficient prior to carotid endarterectomy.[34–41] The NASCET Trial raised some question about the accuracy of duplex scanning. This method requires experienced and dedicated vascular technologists for accuracy, and unfortunately, the participating centers in the NASCET group did not use standardized equipment or methods for the ultrasound studies. Experienced laboratories have reported excellent results with duplex scanning. For the use of velocity data alone the sensitivity of duplex scanning has always been >95%. Its specificity is 94%. We have reported our results with this technique extensively, including four separate validation studies.[42–48]

Several authors have suggested that conventional angiography is not necessary when a high-quality duplex scan demonstrates an appropriate lesion in a symptomatic patient.[34,36–41,49,50] We have reported both a retrospective and a prospective study of the need for arteriography in patients who were considered candidates for carotid endarterectomy on the basis of a duplex scan.[35,51] Prospectively, we studied 111 consecutive patients. In 95 of these cases the members of the vascular section recorded their management plan after reviewing the results of the duplex scan. In these 95 patients, the duplex scan was diagnostic in 88 (95%). Diagnostic errors with duplex scanning occurred as follows: 1) disease was not limited to the carotid bifurcation; 2) the examination was technically difficult and satisfactory Doppler waveforms could not be obtained; 3) in some cases it is difficult to distinguish carotid occlusion from a high-grade stenosis. Each of these conditions is evident when the duplex scan is performed, therefore, the need for further testing is apparent as soon as this study is completed. Conventional angiography supplies the necessary anatomic information in these cases, but it may be supplanted by other noninvasive methods such as magnetic resonance angiography.

Potential Role of Ultrasound in Evaluating Plaque Morphology

Ultrasound images display regions of differing acoustic impedance with an axial resolution of approximately 0.5 mm. The ability to define the composition of plaques precisely based on echogenicity is limited. Calcification can be identified by its bright reflections and acoustic shadowing, but other important plaque components such as lipid pools, necrotic regions, and hemorrhage have similar acoustic properties. Over the last decade several investigators have tried to correlate aspects of the B-mode image of carotid plaques with histologic features. Based on our current understanding of the factors that cause plaque rupture, the features that are most likely to predict instability include surface ulceration, thickness of the fibrous cap, and the presence of hemorrhage and lipid in the plaque. One of the ultrasound features that is easiest to determine is whether or not the echo reflections from the plaque appear homogeneous or heterogeneous (Figure 3). It has been assumed that heterogeneous regions with mixed echoes and anechoic regions correspond to complex plaques, which have combined features of lipid pools, necrosis, and cholesterol clefts. Homogeneous regions, which have a uniform appearance on ultrasound, are thought to correspond to fibrous regions containing smooth muscle cells and matrix. In one prospective study of patients with $> 60\%$ diameter reducing carotid lesions, patients with heterogenous lesions had significantly more cerebral vascular events and deaths than those whose plaques were homogeneous.[52] Plaques that are large enough to obstruct the lumen generally have advanced complex morphology. This is consistent with our own experience that most plaques that are surgically removed are heterogeneous, even when obtained from asymptomatic patients. Therefore, it is unlikely that distinguishing homogenous from heterogeneous morphology will be clinically useful.

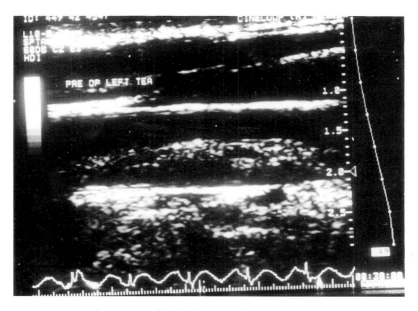

FIGURE 3. *B-mode image of a thick carotid plaque that is heterogeneous. It contains both echolucent and echogenic regions. (Photograph courtesy of Jean Primozich.)*

Several workers have attempted to correlate the presence of these features as well as smoothness or irregularity of the plaque surface as seen on preoperative scanning to pathological findings in the endarterectomy specimen; results have been mixed. The only feature that can be reliably detected is plaque calcification. Some workers have reported high degrees of accuracy for detecting intraplaque hemorrhage or fibrous regions,[53–56] but others have had limited success.[57,58] Plaques with significant areas of hemorrhage often have a heterogeneous pattern with significant anechoic regions. Unfortunately, regions with significant accumulations of lipid have a similar appearance on ultrasound. Detection of plaque ulceration by B-mode imaging is also very difficult. The ultrasound beam should be orthogonal to the surface for optimum imaging, but this is often technically difficult or impossible. Furthermore, imaging of the entire surface of the plaque is difficult because of physical constraints imposed by the neck anatomy and the ultrasound probe and the fact that some surfaces may be in the acoustic shadow of calcified regions on the opposite wall (Figure 4).

Sampling error has been a significant problem in previous studies correlating ultrasound features with plaque histology. Some studies have relied on gross findings of the surgeon and

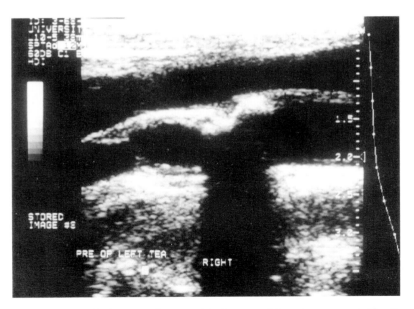

FIGURE 4. *B-mode image of a carotid plaque with extensive calcification of the anterior wall. The resulting acoustic shadowing prevents imaging of the posterior wall. (Photograph courtesy of Jean Primozich.)*

pathologist while others have studied a limited number of pathological sections from the plaque. None have attempted to correlate ultrasound and histologic features in specific regions of the plaque. This is a much more significant undertaking because it is difficult to define precise anatomical locations in the plaque and the morphology is altered by surgical manipulation and histologic preparation. Another problem with previous studies is the lack of consistent set up of the ultrasound instruments. Plaque appearance changes dramatically with different instruments and probes as well as alterations in the various settings such as gain, dynamic range, and time-gain control. Significant advances in this field will depend on careful correlation of discrete regions of carotid plaques with corresponding histologic findings. In this manner plaque features can be compared between symptomatic and asymptomatic patients and longitudinal studies can be undertaken to determine if ultrasound features can be used to predict clinical outcome.

Investigators at the University of Washington in Seattle, Washington have undertaken a prospective study to systematically and precisely correlate ultrasound findings with histologic features of carotid plaque morphology. Three-dimensional histologic reconstructions are being correlated with sonographic findings using standardized ultrasound protocols. The first study concentrated on echolucent regions from plaques of 24 patients (14 asymptomatic, 10 symptomatic).[59] An ATL Ultramark 8 scanner with a 7.5-mHz mechanical sector transducer (Advanced Technology Laboratories, Bothell, WA) was set up with maximal dynamic range (60 dB) to display the most levels of gray. The time-gain compensation was set flat through the lumen of the artery, and the gain was adjusted so blood appeared at the lowest level. Images were taken from multiple angles in both longitudinal and cross-sectional views. Multiple cross-sectional images were taken at 1-mm intervals throughout the plaque. Echolucent regions were defined as distinct zones at least 4 mm^2 in area within the plaque with echogenicity similar to luminal blood (56 to 60 dB). Histologic sections were made at 0.5-mm intervals through the plaque. Each section was then mapped by planimetry into six regions of interest: 1) fibrous tissue, rich in collagen bundles and cells; 2) loose necrosis, with loosely aggregated necrotic debris without viable nuclei or collagen bundles; 3) calcified areas; 4) regions of thrombus/hemorrhage; 5) regions with foam cells; and 6) cholesterol clefts.

Plaques were subdivided into four quadrants with the bifurcation and origin of the external carotid artery serving as reference points. The 33 quadrants with echolucent areas had a significantly higher percentage of hemorrhage, foam cells, necrotic regions, and calcification than did the 63 quadrants without echolucent areas (Table 1). A significant number of quadrants with echolucent areas contained hemorrhage (25%). This is consistent with previous studies that have found an association between the ultrasound finding of heterogeneity and histologic features of intraplaque hemorrhage, lipid, and necrosis. This method of analyzing plaques by quadrants is an improvement over previous studies, but still lumps together large regions that contain many different histologic features.

Efforts are underway to quantitate plaque features more thoroughly both by ultrasound and pathologically. Careful histologic assessment of carotid plaques in symptomatic and asymptomatic patients will help determine if there are features of the plaque that correspond with development of neurological events. If there are such features then noninvasive methods to detect them can be tested. For example, the ability to measure the thickness of the fibrous cap may be emphasized if the presence of a continuous, thick fibrous cap with no underlying large areas of lipid, hemorrhage, or necrosis is predictive of plaque stability. Workers at the University of Washington are currently performing systematic evaluation of carotid plaques from symptomatic and asymptomatic patients to determine the location, distribution, orientation, and volume of plaque components and their relationship to the fibrous cap.[60] Three-dimensional histologic reconstructions are made using three sciatic nerve fibers along the sides of the embedded specimens as fiducial markers for orientation (Figure 5). It is hoped that this

TABLE 1

Distribution of Intraplaque Hemorrhage, Foam Cells, Necrotic Cores, Speckled Calcification, Cholesterol Clefts, and Dense Calcification in Plaque Quadrants with an Echolucent Zone (ELZ) Compared with Quadrants without an Echolucent Zone

Histologic Finding	% of quadrants with an ELZ with histologic finding	% of quadrants without an ELZ with histologic finding	P value
Hemorrhage	55% (18/33)	25% (16/63)	<.01
Foam cells	70% (23/33)	37% (23/63)	<.01
Necrotic core	79% (26/33)	54% (34/63)	<.05
Speckled calcium	67% (22/33)	33% (21/63)	<.01
Cholesterol clefts	52% (17/33)	40% (25/63)	NS
Dense calcification	76% (25/33)	62% (39/63)	NS

Reprinted with permission from Reference 59.

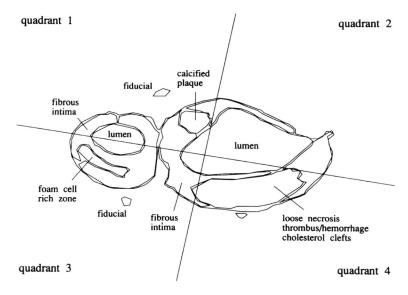

quadrant 1

quadrant 2

fiducial

calcified
plaque

fibrous
intima

lumen

lumen

foam cell
rich zone

fiducial

fibrous
intima

loose necrosis
thrombus/hemorrhage
cholesterol clefts

quadrant 3

quadrant 4

FIGURE 5. *Diagram of histologic features from cross section of a carotid plaque. Fiducial markers are sciatic nerves embedded with the specimen. Similar diagrams from sections taken serially along the length of the plaque are reconstructed in three dimensions to determine the location, distribution, orientation, and volume of the various elements. Reprinted with permission from Reference 60.*

analysis will yield insight into the causes of plaque rupture and thrombosis. It is likely that findings in carotid plaques will be applicable to the coronary circulation. It is much easier to obtain carotid specimens than coronary lesions for assessment of plaque morphology and correlation with noninvasive testing.

The Role of Magnetic Resonance Imaging

Many centers have recently reported promising results using magnetic resonance angiography for diagnosis of carotid artery disease.[61–70] Several small, retrospective studies have suggested that this method can eliminate the need for arteriography in selected patients prior to carotid endarterectomy.[71–75] Magnetic resonance angiography of the cerebral vascular system can be obtained at the time of magnetic resonance imaging of the brain with 15 to 20 minutes of additional scan time. This technique makes it possible to obtain detailed anatomic information concerning the extracranial and intracranial circulation in addition to detection of brain parenchymal disease in patients who are suspected of having symptoms of cerebral ischemia. The combination of magnetic resonance imaging of the brain and magnetic resonance angiography is attractive as a complete study of patients with possible cerebrovascular disease. High-resolution MRI has promise as another method to evaluate atherosclerotic plaque morphology (Figure 6). Studies are underway at the University of Washington using a 1.5-

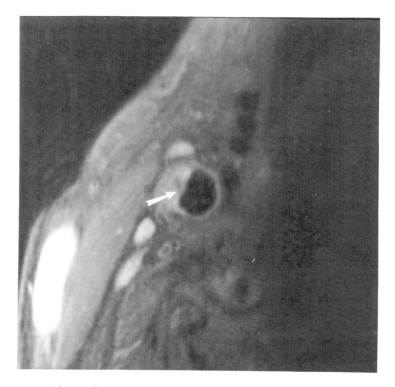

FIGURE 6. *High-resolution magnetic resonance image of a diseased common carotid artery characterized by histology. The hyperintense signal surrounding the entire vessel circumference corresponds to fibrous plaque . The arrow indicates an ulcerated area. The region of the dark band contains foam cells and thrombus. The rest of the plaque consists of a pool of loose necrosis, foam cells, organized thrombus, and cholesterol. (Proton density weighted image, TR 3956 msec, TE 24 msec, field-of-view 9 cm, slice thickness 3 mm, 256×256 matrix, 2 excitations, cardiac gated. Photo courtesy of C. Yuan, K. Beach, and D.E. Strandness, Jr, University of Washington Departments of Radiology and Surgery.)*

T whole-body imager with a custom-built surface coil for characterizing the composition and morphology of plaque removed at carotid endarterectomy. Preliminary data suggest that good correlation between MRI and histologic features can be achieved.[76]

Conclusion

Carotid plaques usually are present for decades before they become unstable and produce symptoms. The transition from a stable to unstable state is likely to involve disruption of the fibrous plaque and to depend on certain plaque characteristics such as the thickness and integrity of the fibrous cap, intraplaque hemorrhage, the extent of central necrosis, and the composition of the matrix. Noninvasive determination of plaque composition with modalities like ultrasound or magnetic resonance imaging may enhance our ability to predict which lesions will produce symptoms. Unfortunately, it has been difficult to associate characteristics noted on imaging studies with histologic features, such as intraplaque hemorrhage, and correlation of these features with the clinical course is lacking. Detailed studies of the histology of plaques from symptomatic and asymptomatic patients are underway and may yield important insight. An accurate, reliable method for identifying plaque characteristics in vivo would be invaluable for prospectively studying the relationship between plaque composition and clinical events. Longitudinal studies could then be performed to determine which factors are important in the development of specific plaque features, and to evaluate the response to therapeutic intervention.

References

1. *Statistical Abstract of the United States.* 111st Ed. Washington, DC: US Bureau of the Census, 1991:80.
2. Bogousslavsky J, van Melle G, Regli F. The Lausanne Stroke Registry: Analysis of 1,000 consecutive patients with first stroke. *Stroke* 1988;19: 1083–1092.
3. Bogousslavsky J, Cachin C, Regli F, et al. Cardiac sources of embolism and cerebral infarction—Clinical consequences and vascular concomitants: The Lausanne Stroke Registry. *Neurology* 1991;41:855–859.
4. Fisher CM. Occlusion of the internal carotid artery. *Arch Neurol Psych* 1951;65:346–377.
5. Hollenhorst RW. Significance of bright plaques in the retinal arterioles. *JAMA* 1961;178(1):123–129.
6. Zukowski AJ, Nicolaides AN, Lewis RT, et al. The correlation between carotid plaque ulceration and cerebral infarction seen on CT scan. *J Vasc Surg* 1984;1:782–786.

7. Julian OC, Dye WS, Javid H, et al. Ulcerative lesions of the carotid artery bifurcation. *Arch Surg* 1963;86:803–809.
8. Drake WEJ, Drake MAL. Clinical and angiographic correlates of cerebrovascular insufficiency. *Am J Med* 1968;45:253–270.
9. Sterpetti AV, Hunter WJ, Schultz RD. Importance of ulceration of carotid plaque in determining symptoms of cerebral ischemia. *J Cardiovasc Surg* 1991;32:154–158.
10. Moore WS, Hall AD. Importance of emboli from carotid bifurcation in pathogenesis of cerebral ischemic attacks. *Arch Surg* 1970;101:708–716.
11. Moore WS, Hall AD. Ulcerated atheroma of the carotid artery. *Am J Surg* 1968;237:242.
12. Steed DL, Peitzman AB, Grundy BL, et al. Causes of stroke in carotid endarterectomy. *Surgery* 1982;92:634–641.
13. Hafner CD. Minimizing the risks of carotid endarterectomy. *J Vasc Surg* 1984;1:392–397.
14. Davies MJ, Richardson PD, Woolf N, et al. Risk of thrombosis in human atherosclerotic plaques: Role of extracellular lipid, macrophage, and smooth muscle cell content. *Br Heart J* 1993;69:377–381.
15. Lendon CL, Davies MJ, Born GV, et al. Atherosclerotic plaque caps are locally weakened when macrophages density is increased. *Atherosclerosis* 1991;87:87–90.
16. Richardson PD, Davies MJ, Born GV. Influence of plaque configuration and stress distribution on fissuring of coronary atherosclerotic plaques [see comments]. *Lancet* 1989;2:941–944.
17. Fuster V, Badimon L, Badimon JJ, et al. The pathogenesis of coronary artery disease and the acute coronary syndromes. *N Engl J Med* 1992;326:242–250.
18. Haudenschild CC. Pathogenesis of atherosclerosis: State of the art. *Cardiovasc Drugs Ther* 1990;4(suppl 5):993–1004.
19. Martin MJ, Whisnant JP, Sayre GP. Occlusive vascular disease in the extracranial cerebral circulation. *Arch Neurol* 1960;3:530–538.
20. Fuster V, Stein B, Ambrose JA, et al. Atherosclerotic plaque rupture and thrombosis: Evolving concepts. *Circulation* 1990;82:II47–II59.
21. Fisher M, Blumenfeld AM, Smith TW. The importance of carotid artery plaque disruption and hemorrhage. *Arch Neurol* 1987;44:1086–1089.
22. Imparato AM, Riles TS, Mintzer R, et al. The importance of hemorrhage in the relationship between gross morphologic characteristics and cerebral symptoms in 376 carotid artery plaques. *Ann Surg* 1983;197:195–203.
23. Beach KW, Hatsukami T, Detmer PR, et al. Carotid artery intraplaque hemorrhage and stenotic velocity. *Stroke* 1993;24:314–319.
24. Pokras R, Dyken ML. Dramatic changes in the performance of endarterectomy for diseases of the extracranial arteries of the head. *Stroke* 1988;19:1289–1290.
25. Chambers BR, Norris JW. The case against surgery for asymptomatic carotid stenosis. *Stroke* 1984;15:964–967.
26. Barnett HJ, Plum F, Walton JN. Carotid endarterectomy—An expression of concern. *Stroke* 1984;15:941–943.
27. North American Symptomatic Carotid Endarterectomy Trial Collaborators. Beneficial effect of carotid endarterectomy in symptomatic patients with high-grade carotid stenosis. *N Engl J Med* 1991;325:445–453.
28. European Carotid Surgery Trialists' Collaborative Group. European carotid surgery trial: Interim results for symptomatic patients with se-

vere (70–99%) or with mild (0–29%) carotid stenosis. *Lancet* 1991;337: 1235–1243.

29. Mayberg MR, Wilson SE, Yatsu F, et al. Carotid endarterectomy and prevention of cerebral ischemia in symptomatic carotid stenosis. Veterans Affairs Cooperative Studies Program 309 Trialist Group. *JAMA* 1991;266:3289–3294.

30. Roederer GO, Langlois YE, Jager KA, et al. The natural history of carotid arterial disease in asymptomtic patients with cervical bruit. *Stroke* 1984;15:603–613.

31. Moneta GL, Taylor DC, Zierler RE, et al. Asymptomatic high-grade internal carotid artery stenosis: Is stratification according to risk factors or duplex spectral analysis possible? *J Vasc Surg* 1989;10:475–483.

32. Moneta GL, Taylor DC, Nicholls SC. Operative versus nonoperative management of asymptomatic high-grade carotid stenosis: Improved results with endarterectomy. *Stroke* 1987;18:1005–1010.

33. Hobson RW, Weiss DG, Fields WS, et al. Efficacy of carotid endarterectomy for asymptomatic carotid stenosis. *N Engl J Med* 1993; 328:221–227.

34. Ricotta JJ, Holen J, Schenk E, et al. Is routine angiography necessary prior to carotid endarterectomy. *J Vasc Surg* 1984;1:96–102.

35. Dawson DL, Zierler RE, Kohler TR. Role of arteriography in the preoperative evaluation of carotid artery disease. *Am J Surg* 1991;161: 619–624.

36. Blackshear WM Jr, Connar RG. Carotid endarterectomy without angiography. *J Cardiovasc Surg* 1982;23:477–482.

37. Crew JR, Dean M, Johnson JM. Carotid surgery without angiography. *Am J Surg* 1984;148:217–220.

38. Flanigan DP, Schuler JJ, Vogel M, et al. The role of carotid duplex scanning in surgical decision making. *J Vasc Surg* 1985;2:15–25.

39. Walsh J, Markowitz I, Kerstein MD. Carotid endarterectomy for amaurosis fugax without angiography. *Am J Surg* 1986;152:172–174.

40. Moore WS, Ziomek S, Quiñones-Baldrich WJ, et al. Can clinical evaluation and noninvasive testing substitute for arteriography in the evaluation of carotid artery disease. *Ann Surg* 1988;208:91–94.

41. Geuder JW, Lamparello PJ, Riles TS, et al. Is duplex scanning sufficient evaluation before carotid endarterectomy? *J Vasc Surg* 1989;9:193–201.

42. Knox RA, Breslau PJ, Strandness DE Jr: A simple parameter for accurate detection of severe carotid disease. *Br J Surg* 1982;69:230–233.

43. Blackshear WM Jr, Phillips DJ, Thiele BL, et al. Detection of carotid occlusive disease by ultrasonic imaging and pulsed Doppler spectrum analysis. *Surgery* 1979;86:698–706.

44. Langlois Y, Roederer GO, Chan A, et al. Evaluating carotid artery disease. The concordance between pulsed Doppler/spectrum analysis and angiography. *Ultrasound Med Biol* 1983;9:51–63.

45. Roederer GO, Langlois YE, Jager KA, et al. A simple spectral parameter for accurate classification of severe carotid disease. *Bruit* 1984;Vol. VII:174–178.

46. Blackshear WM Jr, Phillips DJ, Chikos PM, et al. Carotid artery velocity patterns in normal and stenotic vessels. *Stroke* 1980;11:67–71.

47. Langlois YE, Roederer GO, Chan A, et al. The use of common carotid waveform analysis in the diagnosis of carotid occlusive disease. *Angiology* 1983;34:679–687.

48. Breslau PJ, Fell G, Phillips DJ, et al. Evaluation of carotid bifurcation

disease—The role of common carotid artery velocity patterns. *Arch Surg* 1982;117:58–60.

49. Thomas GI, Jones TW, Stavney LS, et al. Carotid endarterectomy after doppler ultrasonographic examination without angiography. *Am J Surg* 1986;151:616–619.

50. Goodson SF, Flanigan DP, Bishara RA, et al. Can carotid duplex scanning supplant arteriography in patients with focal carotid territory symptoms? *J Vasc Surg* 1987;5:551–557.

51. Dawson DL, Zierler RE, Strandness DE Jr, et al. The role of duplex scanning and arteriography before carotid endarterectomy. A prospective study. *J Vasc Surg* 1993;18:673–683.

52. Belcaro G, Laurora G, Cesarone MR, et al. Ultrasonic classification of carotid plaques causing less than 60% stenosis according to ultrasound morphology and events. *J Cardiovasc Surg (Torino)* 1993;34:287–294.

53. Reilly LM, Lusby RJ, Hughes L, et al. Carotid plaque histology using real-time ultrasonography. Clinical and therapeutic implications. *Am J Surg* 1983;146:188–193.

54. O'Donnell TF, Erdoes L, Mackey WC, et al. Correlation of B-mode ultrasound imaging and arteriography with pathological findings at carotid endarterectomy. *Arch Surg* 1985;120:443–449.

55. Weinberger J, Marks SJ, Gaul JJ, et al. Atherosclerotic plaque at the carotid artery bifurcation. Correlation of ultrasonographic imaging with morphology. *J Ultrasound Med* 1987;6:363–366.

56. Bluth EI, Kay D, Merritt CR, et al. Sonographic characterization of carotid plaque: Detection of hemorrhage. *AJR* 1986;146:1061–1065.

57. Widder B, Paulat K, Hackspacher J, et al. Morphological characterization of carotid artery stenoses by ultrasound duplex scanning. *Ultrasound Med Biol* 1990;16:349–354.

58. Ratliff DA, Gallagher PJ, Hames TK, et al. Characterisation of carotid artery disease: Comparison of duplex scanning with histology. *Ultrasound Med Biol* 1985;11:835–840.

59. Hatsukami TS, Thackray BD, Primozich JF, et al. Echolucent regions in carotid plaque: Preliminary analysis comparing three-dimensional histologic reconstructions to sonographic findings. *Ultrasound Med Biol* 1994;20:743–749.

60. Thackray BD, Burns DH, Ferguson MS, et al. A new method for studying plaque morphology. *Am J Cardiac Imaging* 1995;9:149–156.

61. Grevers G, Balzer JO, Vogl TJ. [Magnetic resonance angiography—A new procedure for vascular imaging in the area of the head-neck]. *Laryngorhinootologie* 1993;72:116–124.

62. Kramer J, Wimberger D, Haimberger K, et al. [Stenosis of the extracranial carotid artery]. *Wien Klin Wochenschr* 1993;105:194–199.

63. Furuya Y, Isoda H, Hasegawa S, et al. Magnetic resonance angiography of extracranial carotid and vertebral arteries, including their origins: Comparison with digital subtraction angiography. *Neuroradiology* 1992;35:42–45.

64. Pan XM, Anderson CM, Reilly LM, et al. Magnetic resonance angiography of the carotid artery combining two- and three-dimensional acquisitions. *J Vasc Surg* 1992;16:609–615.

65. Anderson CM, Saloner D, Lee RE, et al. Assessment of carotid artery stenosis by MR angiography: Comparison with x-ray angiography and color-coded Doppler ultrasound. *Am J Neuroradiol* 1992;13:989–1003.

66. Carriero A, Salute L, Toppetti A, et al. [Comparison of magnetic reso-

nance angiography and digital angiography of the epiaortic vessels]. *Radiol Med (Torino)* 1991;81:781–786.

67. Mattle HP, Kent KC, Edelman RR, et al. Evaluation of the extracranial carotid arteries: Correlation of magnetic resonance angiography, duplex ultrasonography, and conventional angiography. *J Vasc Surg* 1991;13:838–844.

68. Kido DK, Barsotti JB, Rice LZ, et al. Evaluation of the carotid artery bifurcation: Comparison of magnetic resonance angiography and digital subtraction arch aortography. *Neuroradiology* 1991;33:48–51.

69. Kido DK, Panzer RJ, Szumowski J, et al. Clinical evaluation of stenosis of the carotid bifurcation with magnetic resonance angiographic techniques. *Arch Neurol* 1991;48:484–489.

70. Manning WJ, Li W, Edelman RR. A preliminary report comparing magnetic resonance coronary angiography with conventional angiography. *N Engl J Med* 1993;328:828–832.

71. Turnipseed WD, Kennell TW, Turski PA, et al. Combined use of duplex imaging and magnetic resonance angiography for evaluation of patients with symptomatic ipsilateral high-grade carotid stenosis. *J Vasc Surg* 1993;17:832–839.

72. Chiesa R, Melissano G, Castellano R, et al. Three dimensional time-of-flight magnetic resonance angiography in carotid artery surgery: A comparison with digital subtraction angiography. *Eur J Vasc Surg* 1993;7:171–176.

73. Anson JA, Heiserman JE, Drayer BP, et al. Surgical decisions on the basis of magnetic resonance angiography of the carotid arteries. *Neurosurgery* 1993;32:335–343.

74. Freeman J, Free T, Payne H, et al. Assessing extracranial carotid stenosis: Magnetic resonance angiography, duplex scanning, and digital angiography. *S D J Med* 1993;46:53–56.

75. Wesbey GE, Bergan JJ, Moreland SI, et al. Cerebrovascular magnetic resonance angiography: A critical verification. *J Vasc Surg* 1992;16:619–628.

76. Yuan C, Tsuruda JS, Beach KN, et al. Techniques for high-resolution MR imaging of atherosclerotic plaque. *J Magn Reson Imaging* 1994;4:43–49.

Chapter 12

The Natural History of Atherosclerosis in the Aorta in the First Forty Years of Life

Herbert C. Stary, MD, James D. Stoll, MD, Jianfang Yin, MD, Kenneth B. Fallon, MD, and Zhongxin Yu, MD

Introduction

This chapter summarizes the findings in the aortas in our recent autopsy studies of the intima and the atherosclerotic lesions of infants, children, and young to middle-aged adults. Data from the coronary arteries of these cases are summarized in the companion chapter in this volume, Chapter 4. The aortas were examined both with the unaided eye and with various histologic techniques. Studies with the unaided eye included the following determinations:

- The extent of the aortic intimal surface involved with the three types of grossly distinguishable lesions;
- The locations in the aorta at which raised (and presumably histologically advanced) types of lesions are predictably found and at which they are most severe.

The histological studies included light and electron microscopic and immunohistochemical methods and consisted of the following determinations:

- Comparisons of the thickness, composition, and structure of the intima in lesion-prone and in lesion-resistant parts of the aorta;
- The composition, structure, and thickness of advanced le-

From: Fuster V, (ed.) *Syndromes of Atherosclerosis: Correlations of Clinical Imaging and Pathology.* Armonk, NY: Futura Publishing Company, Inc.: © 1996.

sions, the frequency of different types of histologically advanced lesions, and the frequency of thrombosis.

Human aortic atherosclerosis has been studied at autopsy by many investigators. The frequency, extent, and location of changes of the intima were most often measured or estimated by examining the aortic surface with the unaided eye.[1-6] In other autopsy studies of aortas, sections of lesions were examined with the light or electron microscope, after various histochemical or other histologic techniques had been applied.[1,2,7-11] Even when examined with a microscope, the same three types of lesion were described that were also visible with the unaided eye: fatty streaks, fibrous plaques, and complicated lesions, although some authors[12] have suggested that the histologic range of lesions was wider than these three types.

The new findings in the present study were obtained mainly because some new techniques were used, because particular attention was paid to the advanced lesion-prone locations of the aorta, and because the composition and the structure of the intima in the lesion-prone locations (and the evolution of lesions in these locations) was studied from birth. The aortas (and the coronary arteries) used were obtained between 1980 and 1989 from 1286 human subjects. Most of these subjects, who were up to 39 years of age, had either died in accidents or as a result of violence.[13,14] The data in this chapter are mostly from the aortas of the 691 cases in which the coronary arteries were perfused under pressure with glutaraldehyde (see also Chapter 4). However, of the 691 cases with pressure-perfused coronary arteries, the aortas were only available in 648 cases.

In most cases, whole aortas were available. The remaining aortas consisted of only the left longitudinal half, because the right half had been used up for chemical analysis in the belief (based on earlier observations but not on measurements) that lesions were similarly present and distributed in the two opposing halves. The specific methods used in each substudy and the findings that have been obtained are summarized and discussed in the following sections.

Frequency, Extent, and Locations of Lesion Types Visible with the Unaided Eye

To date, we have evaluated the lesions that are grossly visible on the intimal surface of these aortas in three separate studies. The methods of evaluation differed in each study, but the initial processing of the aortas was the same and as follows.

All aortas were opened longitudinally along their dorsal aspect by cutting between the paired origins of the intercostal and lumbar arteries. The portion of the aorta that was proximal to the first pair of intercostal orifices (the arch of the aorta) was detached and not used in these studies. The aortas were then flattened, fixed in formalin, stained with Sudan IV, and preserved in individual transparent plastic bags.

In the first of these studies, data were obtained on the grossly visible lesions of all of the 648 aortas that were available from cases in which the coronary arteries had been fixed by pressure perfusion. The percentage of the intimal surface covered with lesions was estimated by examining the surface with the unaided eye. Only when some doubt about the presence or the identity of a lesion existed was a magnifying glass used. Although we could distinguish eight types of lesion when we subsequently studied 1-μm thick sections with the microscope, with the unaided eye we distinguished the usual three types:

- Fatty streaks, ie, lesions that are flat or raised $<$ 1 mm and stain red with a Sudan dye. Such lesions are equivalent to histologic type II, sometimes to type I or type III.
- Raised lesions, ie, circumscribed lesions elevated 1 mm or more with an apparently intact surface. Such lesions are generally considered as advanced atherosclerosis. Histologically, they are equivalent mostly to types IV, V, VII, and VIII.
- Raised lesions with a disrupted surface, and/or hematoma, and/or thrombus. Such lesions are equivalent to histologic type VI.

The results of the gross frequency estimates of raised lesions are summarized in Figures 1 and 2.

When we later studied the compositions of the grossly raised lesions by microscopy of the 1-μm thick sections, we found that the gross interpretations were incorrect in some cases. Thus, many of the smaller raised "lesions" were not lesions, but localized adaptive intimal thickenings. Adaptive intimal thickening is defined in the companion chapter on the coronary arteries (Chapter 4). The misinterpretations of the gross are explained by the fact that as an aorta without pressure collapses, and as elastic fibers further shorten when the aorta is disengaged from its attachments at autopsy, circumscribed parts of the intima that are thick protrude above the surface of adjacent thinner intima. This artifact of collapsed aortas facilitates the identification of advanced lesions with the unaided eye, but as we now show, it is also misleading because

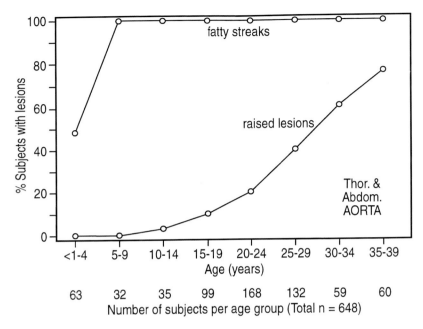

FIGURE 1. *The percentage of the population having fatty streak lesions and the percentage also having localized intimal elevations (raised lesions) is shown for successive 5-year age groups. The data were obtained by examining the thoracic and abdominal aortic intimal surface with the naked eye as described in the text.*

many of the smallest protrusions are not lesions. Detailed postmortem measurements of the elasticity and size of human aortas were made by Wilens[15] and confirmed by our own observations. When freed from their attachments at autopsy, the aortas of subjects 20 to 39 years old contract in length from 25% to 35%, both longitudinally and around the circumference. In an older population than the one studied here, the force of the postmortem elastic recoil of the aorta would not be as strong. Postmortem aortas continue to increase in surface area as adults become older.[1] In an unrelated study of a population 30 to 59 years old, the thickness of the raised aortic lesions did not appear to increase much in the older persons, possibly for this reason (Yin and Stary, unpublished data). The degree of our overestimate of the frequency of raised lesions in the present study of young people is given in the subsequent section of this chapter on the histologic compositions of the raised lesions.

In an additional study of the gross aortas we determined the

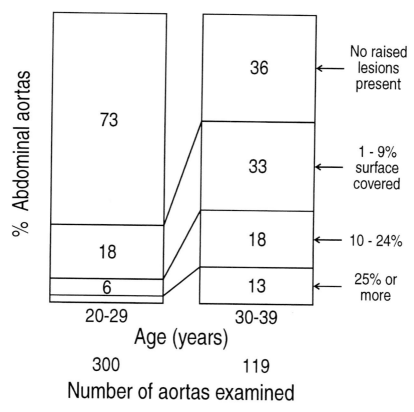

FIGURE 2. *Different degrees of involvement of the intimal surface of the abdominal aorta with raised lesions for the two successive 10-year age groups ranging from 20 to 39 years. Of subjects 20–29 years old, 27% had raised lesions in the abdominal aorta; in 3% the lesions covered 25% or more of the intimal surface. Of those subjects aged 30 to 39 years, 64% had raised lesions in the abdominal aorta; in 13% they covered 25% or more of the surface.*

frequency and the locations of only the sudanophilic (ie, the red-staining) lesions by image analysis. Sites on the aortic surface that become red when stained with a Sudan dye are predominantly type II (fatty streak) lesions, particularly in children and young adults. Whole aortas from 109 male subjects aged 15 to 29 years were selected for this substudy. The intimal surface of the aortas was photographed, the images were digitized from the 35-mm color slides, and the data were transformed spatially to standard templates of the opened aorta. The methods were devised and the analyses were performed at the Biomedical Engineering Center of Ohio State University.[16,17] The resulting probability of occurrence maps demonstrated that in the thoracic aorta, the highest probability of fatty streaks was associated with the dorsal surface while the ventral surface was virtually spared. The dorsal 50% of the circumference of the aorta had a probability of fatty streaks >20% while the dorsal 25% had a probability >40%. The probability of fatty streaks increased as one proceeded circumferentially towards the axial lines defined by the origin of the intercostal ostia. The mean percentage surface area covered with sudanophilic lesions was 20%. The dorsal distribution of fatty streaks continued into the abdominal aorta, but here the ventral intimal surface was another region of high probability. The regions of highest probability of sudanophilia were associated with the inflow tracts of the celiac, superior mesenteric, right and left renal, and inferior mesenteric ostia. The mean intimal surface of the abdominal aorta covered with sudanophilic lesions was 25%.

In another gross study, we determined the locations of raised lesions rather than the locations of fatty streaks. In this study, 211 whole aortas that had raised lesions and were from male and female subjects 20 to 39 years old were analyzed.[18] As already stated, the term raised lesion refers to any localized elevation of 1 mm or more and some of the smaller elevations were found to be adaptive intimal thickening rather than atherosclerotic lesions in subsequent histologic studies. The grading form that was developed for this study included a sketched standard outline (a map or template) of the inner aortic surface on which the four circumferential quadrants of the aorta (left posterior, left anterior, right posterior, right anterior) were indicated by vertical lines. The map also subdivided the descending thoracic and the abdominal aortas into longitudinal quadrants by means of horizontal lines and indicated the orifices of major branch vessels. Thus, when the raised lesions were recorded on the maps both their circumferential and longitudinal locations were recorded. The percentage area of each location covered with raised lesions was estimated and recorded on the form. When 61% or more of the raised lesion area was located in one of the two opposing longitudinal halves (posterior half vs. anterior half, left half vs. right half, separately for the descending thoracic aorta, and the abdominal aorta) we considered raised lesions to be dominant in that half. When each of the opposing halves contained 40% to 60% of the raised lesions the two halves were considered balanced. Only 38% of the 211 aortas had raised lesions in the descending thoracic segment and the mean intimal area covered was 5.1%. Conversely, 95% of the 211 aortas had raised lesions in the abdominal aorta and the mean intimal area they covered was 9.3%. The locations of the raised lesions around the circumference of the two aortic segments are shown in Figure 3. In the thoracic segment there was no significant difference between the left and right sides or between the anterior and posterior halves. In the abdominal aorta, raised lesions predominated on the left side, in the posterior half, and in the most distal quadrant. Thus, raised lesions were most frequent, most extensive, and most advanced (ie, most often complicated) in the left posterolateral part between the level of the inferior mesenteric artery orifice and the aortoiliac bifurcation. Between 20 and 29 years of age, most raised lesions were oval, extending longitudi-

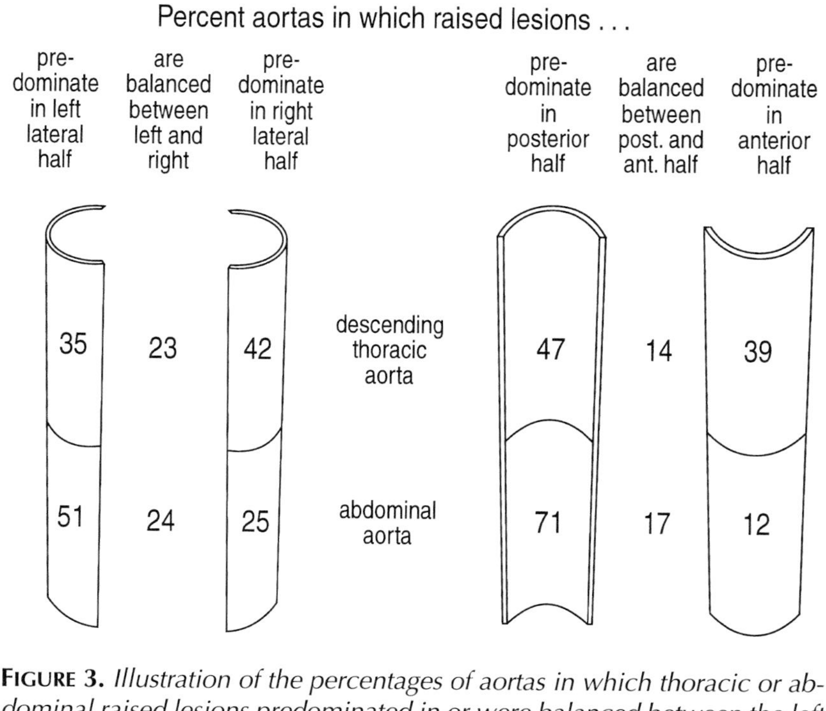

Percent aortas in which raised lesions . . .

pre-dominate in left lateral half	are balanced between left and right	pre-dominate in right lateral half		pre-dominate in posterior half	are balanced between post. and ant. half	pre-dominate in anterior half
35	23	42	descending thoracic aorta	47	14	39
51	24	25	abdominal aorta	71	17	12

FIGURE 3. *Illustration of the percentages of aortas in which thoracic or abdominal raised lesions predominated in or were balanced between the left and the right half and the posterior or anterior half. In thoracic aortas, lesions predominated about equally often in the left and right half and the posterior and anterior half; less often were they balanced. In most abdominal aortas, raised lesions predominated most often in the left lateral half and the posterior half. Furthermore, raised lesions predominated most often in the distal quarter of the abdominal aorta. Therefore, the most frequent location of raised lesions in the aorta is the left posterolateral segment between the inferior mesenteric artery and the aortoiliac bifurcation.*

nally along the left or right side, or the left and right side of the posterior abdominal aorta. Between ages 30 and 39, increase in lesion size and evolution of new raised lesions sometimes caused the confluence of left- and right-sided raised lesions, particularly in the posterior half of the aorta. Subsequent histologic studies confirmed that advanced atherosclerotic lesions usually emerge first, and are usually most advanced, in the posterolateral parts of the distal abdominal aorta.

Composition and Thickness of the Intima in Lesion-Prone and in Lesion-Resistant Locations

To distinguish lesions from normal aortic intima and media, both in pathological studies and by clinical imaging, we must know the range of thickness and the composition of undiseased intima and media, particularly in locations of the aorta that are predisposed to the development of advanced atherosclerosis. We therefore took sections from 72 aortas that were without grossly visible raised lesions and without or with only the most minimal fatty streaks (aortas completely without fatty streaks are not available in adults). Thirty-nine of the aortas were from the 5-year age group from birth to 4 years and 33 were from the 5-year age group from 20 to 24 years, about equally from males and females. Two regions of the aorta were studied, the distal thoracic and the distal abdominal segment. One aim of this sampling was to compare the histology and thickness of the intima of a part of the aorta that is not very susceptible to the development of advanced lesions (distal thoracic) with a part that is highly susceptible (distal abdominal). The distal abdominal aorta was sampled in more (in 72 cases) than the thoracic (27 of these cases) because our main objective was to discover the components and features of the intima that might explain why advanced disease favors the distal abdominal aorta.

The distal abdominal aorta was examined at up to five equally spaced levels between the inferior mesenteric artery and the aortoiliac bifurcation. At each level, a 2-mm thick slice of the left half of the circumference was removed. Each slice was then divided into the quarter from the posterior aorta and the quarter from the anterior aorta. The samples were embedded in Maraglas and cut into 1-μm thick sections. Sections from the anterior and posterior aorta were put on separate slides and stained with toluidine blue and basic fuchsin. Thus for each distal abdominal aorta up to 10 slides were evaluated with the light microscope. On each slide the intima and the media were measured at three equidistant points along the quarter (anterior or posterior) of the circumference. When a branch vessel was present at a standard point that was to be measured that point was omitted. Thus, variations in thickness caused by the shoulders of branch vessels are not part of these data. The measurements of up to 15 points from the posterior aorta were averaged and the same was done for the anterior aorta measurements. The distal thoracic aorta was sectioned at four equally spaced levels and the same determinations were made as described for the distal abdominal aorta.

The results of the measurements are summarized in Figure 4. Between individuals of the same age, the thickness of the intima was more variable than the thickness of the media in every location. Posterior intima was thicker than anterior intima in both thoracic and abdominal aorta at every age although this difference was significant only in adults. The distal abdominal aortic intima was thicker (both posteriorly and anteriorly) than the distal thoracic intima, particularly when compared to the media of which the reverse was true.

Detailed data of the histology will be published elsewhere. Briefly, the basic composition of aortic intima resembled that de-

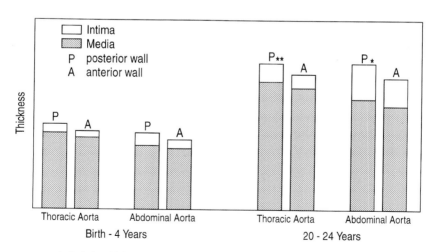

* posterior intima thicker than anterior intima, P < 0.05
** posterior intima thicker than anterior intima, P < 0.01

FIGURE 4. *Thickness of lesion-free intima and media in two locations along the aorta and in two locations around the circumference in infants and in young adults. Intima is thickest in the posterior half of the abdominal aorta of the adults.*

scribed earlier for the coronary arteries.[19] Both an inner and an outer intima layer were present. As in the coronary arteries, the aortic layers differed in the densities and morphologies of intimal smooth muscle cells and in type of intercellular matrix. In some infants, a few isolated macrophages and macrophage foam cells were found about equally in thoracic and abdominal aortic intima. In the aortic intima of young adults intimal macrophages were numerous, even in young adults without type II lesions in the sectioned location (ie, even in those without groups or layers of intimal macrophage foam cells). Macrophages and macrophage foam cells in the distal abdominal aorta were similar in number to those in the thoracic aorta or they outnumbered them.

The internal elastic lamina in the aortas of infants was generally a relatively continuous single lamina. In young adults, there were often several parallel but often discontinuous internal elastic laminas with islands or layers of myofilament-rich smooth muscle cells between them, particularly in the abdominal aorta.

The Composition of Advanced Lesions and the Frequency of Thrombosis

The composition of raised lesions (the concept of "raised" is defined earlier in this chapter) was studied in 166 aortas in which such localized elevations of the intima were grossly visible. The 166 aortas were the aortas that had raised lesions among the 648 aortas available from cases with pressure-perfused coronary arteries.

The aortas varied in the number, thickness, and gross surface characteristics of the raised lesions they contained. In some cases only one was present while in other cases a large part of the aortic intimal surface was covered with confluent raised lesions. We decided to study the one location in every aorta that appeared to contain the most advanced lesion. We considered as most advanced the one that was raised most above the surrounding intimal surface (ie, the thickest elevation). Lesions in which disruptions of the surface, hematoma, or thrombotic deposits could be recognized took precedence. The samples were adjacent 2-mm thick cross sections. One was embedded in Maraglas, cut into 1-μm thick sections, and sections were stained with toluidine blue and basic fuchsin. An adjacent 2-mm thick cross section was embedded in paraffin, cut into 5-μm thick sections, and sections were stained for fibrin-fibrinogen with the avidin-biotin complex immunoperoxidase method and with hematoxylin and eosin. In a subsample of raised lesions a third cross section was frozen, sectioned in a cryostat, and stained for fat with oil-red-O. From a further subsample of raised lesions, sequential cross sections extending from the proximal to the distal ends of the lesions were prepared, the histology was digitized, and three-dimensional reconstructions of the lesions were prepared with the Jandel Scientific PC3D reconstruction software.

The presence of thrombi or thrombotic remnants was based on the positive immunostaining, the mesh-like structure, and the wavy band-like pattern of deposits on the surface and/or among the fibrous tissue or within the lipid core of lesions. This structure and pattern of deposits is considered as characteristic of thrombi and the remnants of thrombi.[11,20,21] Diffuse fibrin-fibrinogen immunostaining without this structure or pattern was not considered thrombus or remnant. Diffuse fibrinogen enters the intima as do many other plasma proteins. Diffuse immunostaining for fibrinogen was found in almost all advanced lesions, in most of their precursors (type II and type III lesions), and occasionally even in localized adaptive intimal thickening.

Lesions were classified according to their histologic characteristics as explained in Chapter 4. Briefly, this classification consists of eight types of lesion. Type I and type II designate relatively minimal, mainly intracellular, accumulation of lipid in the intima. Type III designates lesions that contain, in addition, small, scattered pools of extracellular lipid. Type IV designates atheroma, ie, a large accumulation of extracellular lipid which disrupts normal structure in the deep core of the intima. Type V contains, in addition, layers of newly formed fibrous tissue (collagen). Type VI contains, in addition, disruption of the intimal surface, hematoma, and generally also thrombosis. Type VII designates a lesion in which deposition of mineral predominates. Type VIII designates a mainly fibrotic lesion without or with only minimal lipid. In addition to classifying lesions according to their composition, the thickness was also measured with a micrometer scale mounted in an ocular of the microscope.

As mentioned, some protrusions above the aortic surface (ie, some raised lesions) had, when studied with the microscope, the composition not of lesions but of focal adaptive thickening. As already explained, protrusion of adaptive intimal thickening is the consequence of postmortem collapse of blood vessels. Because aortas are always studied in their collapsed state after death, this problem pervades all autopsy studies. When the localized elevations that were adaptive intimal thickening, or adaptive thickening with only a type I or type II lesion, were measured, they were found to be the least elevated when compared to elevations that were advanced lesions histologically.

With the immunohistochemical technique, thrombi and rem-

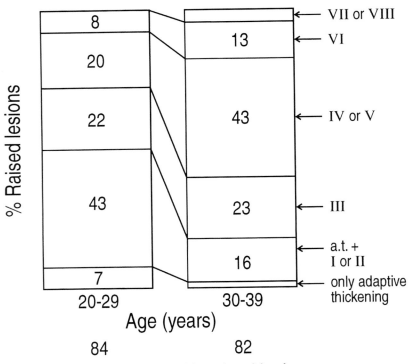

FIGURE 5. *Frequency of the various characteristic histologies of localized elevations in the aortas of the two successive age groups from 20 to 39 years. Between ages 20 to 29, 50% of the localized elevations were caused primarily by adaptive intimal thickening plus (43%) a minimal superimposed foam cell lesion. In the subsequent 10-year age group, only 17% of elevations had this histology whereas 60% had the composition of advanced (type IV to type VIII) lesions.*

nants of thrombi were also found on or within lesion types that were not atheroma or fibroatheroma. For the purpose of presenting the immunohistochemical results we therefore modified our standard histologic classification. In this modification type VI denotes a lesion with any kind of disruption of the surface and/or intimal hematoma. Thrombi or thrombotic remnants associated with type VI and with any other lesion type are noted in addition and separately.

The types of histology of the 166 localized elevations sampled from 166 aortas are illustrated in Figure 5. Seven of the sampled raised locations were only adaptive intimal thickening. None of these contained thrombotic deposits or remnants. An additional 49 of the sampled elevations were adaptive thickening containing only a type I or type II lesion. Four (8%) of these contained thrombotic deposits or remnants. Thirty-seven of the 166 sampled elevations were adaptive thickenings containing a type III (preatheroma) lesion and 8 (24%) of these contained thrombotic deposits or remnants. Fifty-two of the 166 elevations were type IV or type V lesions (atheroma, fibroatheroma) and 33 (64%) contained thrombotic deposits or remnants. Eighteen of the 166 elevations were type VI lesions (lesions with a surface defect or hematoma) and 17 (94%) contained thrombotic deposits or remnants. Only one of the elevations was a completely calcified (type VII) lesion and a thrombotic deposit or remnant was not found. Of two completely fibrotic (type VIII) lesions one contained a thrombotic deposit or remnant. Of the 166 sampled raised locations, 84 were in persons 20 to 29 years old and 24% had thrombotic deposits or remnants; 82 were in persons 30 to 39 years old and 54% had thrombotic deposits or remnants.

The frequency of thrombosis in the present study of a young population is high. Nevertheless, our data may still understate the contribution thrombosis makes to atherosclerosis progression since we only examined one raised lesion per aorta. Our judgement that we had selected the lesion most likely to be thrombotic may not always have been correct.

References

1. Aschoff L. *Lectures on Pathology*. New York: Paul B. Hoeber, Inc.; 1924.
2. Jores L. Arterien. In: Henke F, Lubarsch O, eds. *Handbuch der speziellen pathologischen Anatomie und Histologie, vol. 2: Herz und Gefaesse.* Berlin: Springer Verlag; 1924:608–786.
3. Zinserling WD. Untersuchungen ueber Atherosklerose. 1. Ueber die Aortaverfettung bei Kindern. *Virchows Arch* 1925;225:677–705.
4. Holman RL, McGill HC, Strong JP, et al. The natural history of atherosclerosis. The early aortic lesions as seen in New Orleans in the middle of the 20th century. *Am J Pathol* 1958;34:209–235.

5. Strong JP, McGill HC. The natural history of aortic atherosclerosis: Relationship to race, sex, and coronary lesions in New Orleans. *Exp Molec Pathol* 1963;1(Suppl):15–27.
6. Tanganelli P, Bianciardi G, Simoes C, et al. Distribution of lipid and raised lesions in aortas of young people of different geographic origins (WHO-ISFC PBDAY study). *Arterioscler Thromb* 1993;13:1700–1710.
7. Duguid JB. Thrombosis as a factor in the pathogenesis of aortic atherosclerosis. *J Pathol Bacteriol* 1948;60:57–61.
8. Geer JC. Fine structure of human aortic intimal thickening and fatty streaks. *Lab Invest* 1965;14:1764–1783.
9. Mitchell JRA, Schwartz CJ. *Arterial Disease*. Philadelphia, PA: F.A. Davis; 1965.
10. Haust MD, More RH. Mechanism of fibrosis in white atherosclerotic plaques of human aorta. An electron microscopic study. *Circulation* 1966;34(Supp III):14. Abstract.
11. Woolf N. *Pathology of Atherosclerosis*. London: Butterworth & Company Publishers Ltd.; 1982.
12. McGill, HC. The lesion. In: Schettler G, Weizel A, eds. *Atherosclerosis III*. Berlin: Springer-Verlag; 1974:27–38.
13. Stary HC. Evolution and progression of atherosclerotic lesions in coronary arteries of children and young adults. *Arteriosclerosis* 1989; 9(Suppl I):19–32.
14. Stary HC. The sequence of cell and matrix changes in atherosclerotic lesions of coronary arteries in the first forty years of life. *Eur Heart J* 1990;11(Suppl E):3–19.
15. Wilens SL. The postmortem elasticity of the adult human aorta. Its relation to age and to the distribution of intimal atheromas. *Am J Pathol* 1937;13:811–834.
16. Cornhill JF, Stary HC, Herderick EE, et al. Topographic probability mapping of human aortic atherosclerosis. *Arteriosclerosis* 1984;4:52a.
17. Cornhill JF, Herderick EE, Stary HC. Topography of human aortic sudanophilic lesions. *Monogr Atheroscler* 1990;15:13–19.
18. Stary HC, Fallon KB. Asymmetrical location of advanced atherosclerotic lesions in the aortas of young people. *Arteriosclerosis* 1990;10:791a. Abstract.
19. Stary HC. Macrophages, macrophage foam cells, and eccentric intimal thickening in the coronary arteries of young children. *Atherosclerosis* 1987;64:91–108.
20. Schwartz J, Valente AJ, Kelley JL, et al. Thrombosis and the development of atherosclerosis: Rokitansky revisted. *Sem Thromb Hemostasis* 1988;14:189–195.
21. Woolf N, Davies MJ. Interrelationship between atherosclerosis and thrombosis. In: Fuster V, Verstraete M, eds. *Thrombosis in Cardiovascular Disorders*. Philadelphia, PA: W.B. Saunders Co.; 1992:41.

Chapter 13

A Clinician's View of
Aortic Atherosclerosis

*Steven M. Santilli, MD, PhD and
Jerry Goldstone, MD*

Introduction

Aortic atherosclerosis is a common clinical problem in western societies. This disease process is typically found in populations with other risk factors for atherosclerosis including hypertension, hyperlipidemia, cigarette smoking, and diabetes mellitus. The overall cost in patient suffering as well as actual monetary costs to society are staggering and continuing to rise. Aortic atherosclerosis most commonly presents as one of six clinical syndromes including: 1) aortoiliac occlusive disease; 2) coral reef lesions of the abdominal aorta; 3) splanchnic atherosclerotic occlusive disease; 4) atherosclerotic occlusive disease of the renal arteries; 5) blue toe syndrome and; 6) abdominal aortic aneurysms. Treatment of these clinical syndromes has traditionally required some form of invasive surgical therapy with conservative treatment being reserved for those patients who are minimally symptomatic, with significant medical risk factors for operative intervention or relatively short life expectancies. Although surgical therapy has been effective, new treatment options of a less or minimally invasive form are currently being investigated. These new treatment options include angioplasty, stent placement, atherectomy devices, laser treatment, and endovascular stent-gaft placement. Though the incidence of aortic atherosclerosis and its clinical syndromes continue to rise, these new less invasive forms of therapy may lead to less patient suffering, quicker return to work, and less overall cost to society.

From: Fuster V, (ed.) *Syndromes of Atherosclerosis: Correlations of Clinical Imaging and Pathology.* Armonk, NY: Futura Publishing Company, Inc.: © 1996.

Aortoiliac Occlusive Disease

Aortoiliac occlusive disease is especially common in the western world. The aortoiliac segment of the vascular tree is frequently involved with atherosclerosis. Historically, the series of three articles first describing this syndrome was published by Dr. Rene Leriche between 1923 and 1948.[1-3] His descriptions are still valid today, although diagnostic and treatment options have changed significantly.

Diagnosis

Leriche stated that, as a rule, his patients were young adults and most were males. They usually had no other significant past medical history, but smoking was a common habit. Most complained of "extreme liability to fatigue of both lower limbs". This has been subsequently described as intermittent claudication. Leriche also described a "global atrophy of both lower limbs." This was a subtle but reliable finding present in all patients. The skin had "no trophic changes". Because of the lack of trophic changes in the skin and nails and normal-appearing feet and toes, he found it difficult to believe that circulation was severely impaired. Leriche did note that wound healing was significantly impaired, but there was "power of the legs and feet" present even with standing. In males, most also complained of an inability to maintain a stable erection. By physical examination there were absent or severely diminished pulses in both lower extremities beginning at the groin, and often an iliac pulse could not be felt, but the aortic pulsation was palpable high in the abdomen well above the umbilicus. In addition, most patients had hypertension although no evidence of renal impairment.[1-3]

In addition to the patient's history and physical examination, Doppler-derived segmental pressures are now beneficial in aiding the diagnosis of aortoiliac occlusive disease. This is an easy clinical test to perform, although its major disadvantage is that some forms of infrainguinal occlusive disease can give false-positive test results. Accuracies of 73% to 97% to detect significant aortoiliac occlusive disease are reported if a 30-mm pressure gradient from the brachial to proximal thigh cuff is used.[4,5] Doppler-determined thigh pressure should be considered a useful adjunct to taking a good history and physical examination or, in patients with aortoiliac occlusive disease.

Natural History

The natural history of aortoiliac occlusive disease was also accurately recorded by Leriche.[1-3] Aortoiliac occlusive disease can be well tolerated for a number of years. Patients usually note the onset of intermittent claudication associated with muscle atrophy of the legs and thighs. The claudication is progressive, followed by edematous changes in the lower extremities with a cyanotic or violaceous hue to the skin preceding tissue loss. In Dr. Leriche's descriptions, most untreated patients developed progressive tissue loss and gangrene that was slow, but relentless. The end result was that the patient would usually succumb to some other complication of the occlusive disease, usually cardiac, cerebrovascular or renovascular in origin. The disease progression paralleled the increasing involvement of the vascular tree with occlusive disease both proximal and distal to the aortoiliac segment.

Treatment Options

The initial treatment for aortoiliac occlusive disease was bilateral lumbar sympathectomies with or without aortectomy.[1-3] This is no longer appropriate and treatment of aortoiliac occlusive disease now varies from conservative (noninvasive) management to minimally invasive percutaneous therapy, and finally to invasive surgical procedures for which aortofemoral bypass grafting is the gold standard. Other invasive treatment options include aortoiliac endarterectomy, and extra-anatomic bypass in selected patients.

Conservative Treatment

Claudication may sometimes be considered an indication for intervention in aortoiliac occlusive disease, usually in those good risk patients with severely limiting incapacitating claudication. Intervention need not be considered if the patient does not have disabling claudication or critical ischemia, although the natural history of this disease process suggests relentless progression.[1-3] Invasive treatment is used selectively because operative mortality varies from 5% to 10%,[6,7] and patients with aortoiliac occlusive disease have a rapidly declining late survival, averaging approximately 60% at 5 years, 33% at 10 years, and 14% at 15 years after surgery or diagnosis.[7,8] With this combination of operative mortality and poor long-term survival, a conservative approach to patients with claudication and aortoiliac occlusive disease seems warranted in many cases.

Minimally Invasive Treatment

Dotter and Judkins[9] first reported the performance of percutaneous transluminal angioplasty (PTA) in 1964. The balloon catheter for dilation was introduced by Gruntzig in 1974,[10] and since then PTA has become a widely accepted alternative form of therapy for arterial occlusive disease. Results of iliac angioplasty vary widely in the literature. One of the largest series is that reported by Johnston et al[11] in 1987. This series included 984 angioplasties with 5-year follow-up results by both clinical examination and hemodynamic parameters. They reported a 60% 5-year patency rate for angioplasty of the common iliac artery, and a 48% 5-year patency rate for angioplasty of the external iliac artery. Patency rates were slightly greater if good distal run-off was present, and those patients with iliac occlusion had slightly worse long-term patency rates. Of note, this is one of the few studies in the literature where primary patency rates were reported that included initial failures. In 1989, Wilson et al[12] reported a randomized trial comparing angioplasty with surgery for 263 patients. After a 3-year follow-up, there was no significant difference in results between operation and angioplasty in common iliac artery lesions. The American Heart Association published *Guidelines for Peripheral Percutaneous Transluminal Angioplasty of the Abdominal Aorta and Lower Extremity Vessels*.[13] These guidelines were approved by the Councils of Cardiovascular Radiology, Cardiovascular Surgery, Clinical Cardiology and Epidemiology. They categorized the iliac lesions into varying degrees of suitability including: 1) lesions that were concentric noncalcified stenoses of <3 cm in length; 2) lesions or stenoses 3 to 5 cm in length or calcified or eccentric stenoses <3 cm in length; 3) lesions or stenoses 5 to 10 cm in length or occlusions <5 cm in length after thrombolytic therapy; 4) lesions or stenoses >10 cm in length, occlusions longer than 5 cm, extensive bilateral disease, or iliac stenoses in patients with abdominal aortic aneurysms. Category 1 and 2 patients should anticipate an 80% 5-year patency rate with angioplasty with decreasing rates of patency of 65% to 75% for category 3 patients. It is currently felt that surgical therapy should be performed for all patients in category 4.

More recently vascular stents have been used with increasing frequency for the treatment of aortoiliac occlusive disease after successful angioplasty of various short-segment iliac lesions and even some terminal aortic lesions. The only current prospective randomized trial of iliac stent placement versus angioplasty that was published came from Germany in which the group used a Palmaz stent.[14] In the stent arm of the study, the 5-year clinical success rate was 92.7% and angiographic patency rate was 93.6%. The 5-year angioplasty angiographic patency rate was 64.6% with a clinical success rate of 69.7%. The comparisons between these data were significant at the P=0.001 level and seem to validate the superiority of stents over simple angioplasty of localized short segment aortoiliac occlusive lesions. In conclusion, it seems that angioplasty alone or with stent placement is a durable and effective procedure in the treatment of aortoiliac occlusive disease. The ideal candidates for angioplasty in this segment are patients with intermittent claudication and discrete stenoses. It appears that angioplasty plus stent placement is superior to angioplasty alone. Future treatment of aortoiliac occlusive disease will probably see the more widespread application of stents and angioplasty, however, the role of endovascular grafting as an alternative is currently being evaluated. The advantage of endovascular grafting is that it may be able to be used for more extensive aortoiliac disease than is currently felt applicable to angioplasty and/or stent placement.

Invasive Treatment

The gold standard in the treatment of aortoiliac occlusive disease is aortobifemoral bypass. Aortobifemoral bypass currently enjoys one of the best success rates, between 80% and 90%, of any vascular surgery operation at 5 five years.[6-8] Classically, surgical alternatives to aortobifemoral bypass for aortoiliac occlusive disease have been considered in the following clinical settings: 1) hostile abdominal pathology; 2) high-surgical risk; and 3) occlusive disease of lesser severity or limited extent. Recent studies have suggested that extra-anatomic (axillobifemoral) bypass graft patency rates are better than previously reported, however, their patency rates still do not equal those of aortobifemoral bypass.[15,16] Although there are many controversies surrounding the technical aspects involved in aortobifemoral bypass grafting, its role and status as the gold standard remain unchanged. In the upcoming era in which outcome assessment and cost-benefit analysis will receive greater weight, the role of aortofemoral bypass will need to be reevaluated.

Coral Reef Lesions of the Abdominal Aorta

Coral reef atherosclerosis of the abdominal aorta describes a localized exophytic obstruction that usually involves the suprarenal aorta.

Diagnosis

Patients with coral reef lesions of the abdominal aorta are usually middle-aged women between the ages of 45 and 70, smoke between 1 and 3 packs of cigarettes per day, with a high incidence of hyperlipidemia, and a strong family history of atherosclerotic occlusive disease. These patients rarely have diabetes mellitus, but there is a fair incidence of coronary artery disease and many have previously undergone other vascular surgical procedures. Classic presenting symptoms in these patients are hypertension and varying degrees of lower extremity ischemia ranging from claudication to rest pain. Some patients will have other signs and symptoms of visceral ischemia including intestinal angina. On physical examination, the patients typically have abdominal bruits and absent or diminished femoral pulses. Though renal artery disease is common with resulting hypertension, abnormalities in renal function tests are not usually encountered.[17,18]

Natural History

There are no published reports on the natural history of coral reef lesions of the abdominal aorta, however, it is felt that the natural history of these lesions is to progress to total occlusion with probable catastrophic results due to renal and visceral artery occlusion.[17–19]

Treatment

Currently, all patients presenting with symptomatic coral reef lesions of the abdominal aorta require some form of treatment to relieve their symptoms as well as prevent progression to total occlusion. For this reason, conservative measures are only considered in patients who are prohibitive operative risks or with very shortened life spans. Conservative management consists of risk-factor control of hypertension, hypercholesterolemia, diabetes mellitus, and cessation of smoking.

Minimally Invasive Procedures

At the current time, there are no accepted or proposed methods for minimally invasive management of patients with coral reef lesions of the abdominal aorta.

Invasive Procedures

Transaortic thromboendarterectomy is the procedure of choice in treating patients with coral reef lesions of the abdominal aorta.[17-19] Most series report good success with this procedure, with the majority of patients remaining symptom-free without evidence of recurrence of the lesion at an average of 4 years follow-up. Most patients will require some other form of concomitant aortoiliofemoral revascularization based on the associated atherosclerotic lesions throughout the vascular tree. In some patients, the disease is found to circumferentially involve the aortic wall and extend distally into the visceral vessels. In these very rare patients, endarterectomy is felt to be a less safe procedure and bypass grafting from the thoracic to the abdominal aorta is preferable.

Future Directions in the Treatment of Coral Reef Lesions of the Abdominal Aorta

It is possible that atherectomy or some form of laser treatment could effectively deal with isolated coral reef lesions (without associated atherosclerosis elsewhere in the vascular tree requiring operative intervention). However, there are no known reports of these treatment modalities being used for this type of lesion.

Splanchnic Arteriosclerotic Occlusive Disease

Atherosclerotic disease of the celiac and superior mesenteric arteries is the most common cause of intestinal ischemia.[20] Patients with intestinal angina typically exhibit either total occlusion or stenoses of >90% to 95% in both of these arteries.[20] The natural history of patients who have intestinal angina due to splanchnic atherosclerotic occlusive disease is one of progressive weight loss and emaciation. These patients then may succumb to their debilitating illness and are also at high risk for acute arterial occlusion with extensive intestinal infarction and subsequent death.[21-24] Because of the dismal natural history of symptomatic splanchnic atherosclerotic occlusive disease, treatment is indicated when symptoms become clinically evident.

Diagnosis

The majority of patients with symptomatic splanchnic atherosclerotic occlusive disease are women. The hallmark symptom is weight loss that is usually associated with progressive severe post-prandial midabdominal pain. Classically, this "intestinal angina" begins 30 to 45 minutes after eating, often lasts for several hours, which is associated with the normal transit time of food through the small bowel. These patients develop a real fear of eating, which explains the severe weight loss. On physical examination, patients will appear to be quite thin and frail. Most will exhibit an abdominal bruit in the epigastrium. The remainder of the examination may demonstrate some other sequelae of atherosclerotic vascular occlusive disease including processes in the coronary, carotid, or extremity circulation.[21-23]

Treatment

Decision to Treat

The decision to intervene in a patient with splanchnic atherosclerotic occlusive disease is based on the patient's symptoms. The progressive weight loss and worsening abdominal pain mandate some invasive form of intervention due to the dismal prognosis. The only exceptions are patients who are prohibitive operative risks or with very short life spans due to other pathological processes.

Minimally Invasive Therapy

Atherosclerotic occlusive disease of the celiac and superior mesenteric arteries can be considered as an extension of aortic atherosclerosis, and balloon angioplasty has had about the same results as it has in the treatment of orificial renal artery lesions. Initial success can be expected in the majority of patients, but recurrence rates are high.

Invasive Therapy

Surgical therapy consists of either endarterectomy or bypass grafting. The choice depends on the anatomic distribution of the disease and the experience and expertise of the surgeon; both procedures have good long-term patency rates. Clinical improvement is reported in approximately 90% of cases with an acceptably low operative mortality of approximately 5% to 10%.[25-31] Due to the relatively uncommon nature of this disease process, there have been no prospective randomized studies to compare these two treatment choices, however, both are effective procedures with good long-term results.

Future in the Treatment of Splanchnic Atherosclerotic Occlusive Disease

There is a modest accumulated experience with balloon angioplasty and/or stent placement in the treatment of celiac or superior mesenteric artery atherosclerotic occlusive disease. As noted above, the results with angioplasty of the superior mesenteric and celiac arteries is about as good as for other similar vascular beds with low rates of morbidity. Future technological innovations can be expected to provide a less invasive, but technically successful method to manage these serious clinical problems.

Atherosclerotic Occlusive Disease of the Renal Arteries

Occlusive lesions of the renal arteries are like the superior mesenteric artery and celiac lesions discussed above, an extension of aortic atherosclerosis and most commonly involve the ostium of the left renal artery.[32] The first observation that atherosclerotic occlusive disease in the renal artery may be related to a clinical syndrome was by Richard Bright of Guy's Hospital in London who observed the apparent association between hypertension and renal disease in 1836.[33] Subsequently, a renal pressor substance named renin was discovered in 1887, which led to the understanding of the clinical syndrome related to atherosclerotic occlusive disease of the renal arteries.

Diagnosis

Atherosclerotic occlusive disease of the renal arteries can result in renovascular hypertension, with or without renal failure, mediated by the renin-angiotensin system. Renovascular hypertension is generally felt to account for between 5% and 10% of those patients in the population classified as having "essential hypertension." Numerous epidemiologic studies have found that severe hypertension at the two extremes of life carries the highest probability of being renovascular in origin. Children under the age of 5 and adults over the age of 60 are more likely to have hypertension based on a renovascular cause. Atherosclerotic renovascular hypertension is the usual cause in the elderly and fibromuscular dysplasia is more common in the young. In general, patients with severe diastolic hypertension (>105 mm Hg) are those at highest risk for having renovascular hypertension. Therefore, elderly patients with risk factors for atherosclerosis and severe diastolic hypertension will be those most likely to have atherosclerotic lesions of the renal arteries. Depending on the duration and severity of hypertension and the degree of atherosclerotic renal artery occlusive disease, some patients may present with elevations in their serum renal function tests indicating some degree of renal failure. On physical exam, these patients will classically have severe diastolic hypertension and possibly an abdominal bruit. Many patients will also have other sequelae of atherosclerotic vascular occlusive disease including disease within the coronary, cerebrovascular, and peripheral vascular beds. Laboratory evaluation may reflect the underlying degree of renal dysfunction and the electrocardiogram may show myocardial hypertrophy or ischemic heart disease because of the prolonged hypertension.[35-40]

Treatment

Decision to Treat

Atherosclerotic renal artery stenosis is usually diagnosed in patients being evaluated for hypertension. This hypertension can often be effectively treated with medical therapy. Dean[41] reported the results of serial renal function studies performed on 41 patients with renovascular hypertension secondary to atherosclerotic renal artery disease. These patients all had attempts at blood pressure control with medical management. A significant number with acceptable blood pressure control went on to have progressive renal failure and progression of their renal artery disease, suggesting that the control of hypertension does not change the natural history of renal artery stenosis with regard to the loss of renal function. Therefore, it would seem that the conservative management of atherosclerotic renal artery stenosis is not warranted in patients who are acceptable operative risks.

Minimally Invasive Procedures

PTA has been widely used for the treatment of atherosclerotic lesions of the renal artery. Miller[42] reported that in his series, only 45% of ostial lesions of the renal arteries improved over a 6-month follow-up. Sos[43] reported that only 14% of patients with bilateral ostial lesions treated with percutaneous angioplasty had any significant benefit in follow-up. In reviewing these series, it is apparent that PTA has limited value in the treatment of atherosclerotic lesions affecting the renal artery orifices. The risks of cholesterol embolization or thrombosis of the renal artery with loss of renal function must be weighed against the minimal long-term benefits observed with this form of therapy. The addition of stents to balloon angioplasty has been reported to have better results.

Invasive Procedures

Operative therapy of atherosclerotic renal artery occlusive disease has been well described in the literature. Treatment options include aortorenal bypass, thromboendarterectomy, and ex vivo renal artery reconstruction. Procedure selection is based on the individual patient and the anatomic pattern of renal artery disease. These procedures can all be accomplished with low rates of morbidity and mortality (5% to 10%).[44-46] Most studies report a beneficial hypertension response in 80% to 90% of patients. Although improvement is noted in 90% of cases, cure rates are lower, between 40% and 50%.[44-46] Most studies support the concept that revascularization procedures for renal artery occlusive disease have some beneficial effect on the ischemic nephropathy observed in many of these patients. Long-term follow-up shows that the reconstructions remain patent with good function in 85% to 95% of cases,[46] and long-term life table analysis reveals a definite survival benefit to those patients successfully treated.[46]

Future Treatment Options

The early results with PTA are not encouraging for renal artery occlusive disease. However, further refinement in the technique and construction of catheters and balloons will lead to a more positive outlook. In addition, the role of stents and atherectomy devices in this disease process may have a beneficial effect. Due to the morbidity and mortality rates of 5% to 10% with open operative procedures, the less invasive procedures (angioplasty, stent placement, atherectomy), when further refined, will likely play a major role in the treatment of this disease process.

Blue Toe Syndrome

Aortoiliac occlusive disease resulting in blue toe syndrome is a potentially limb-threatening condition. The concept of some form of atheromatous debris resulting in emboli was first noted by Panum in 1862,[47] who reported on a fatal coronary artery occlusion. Extensive documentation of cholesterol emboli to various parts of the arterial system is noted throughout the literature, and in 1952, Venet and Friedfeld[48] first documented atheromatous embolization of the lower extremity.

Natural History

The natural history of blue toe syndrome can be determined from various reported series in the literature.[49–53] It appears that patients with blue toe syndrome are at significant risk for suffering an adverse outcome. Less than half of untreated patients in most reported series have an uncomplicated course during a follow-up period. Approximately one third of patients will present with initial and subsequent tissue loss, and 20% to 25% will undergo amputations, most of which will involve a toe or foot. There is approximately a 20% 7-year mortality in this group of patients. It is therefore reasonable to conclude that blue toe syndrome is a potentially life- and limb-threatening clinical situation that deserves prompt, aggressive diagnosis and treatment. The majority of patients are males with a mean age of 64 years, who usually have associated atherosclerotic risk factors including cigarette smoking (77%), hypertension (67%), and diabetes (19%). Patients will classically present with the sudden onset of **p**ain and **p**eripheral discoloration of a toe(s) in the presence of a palpable peripheral (pedal) **p**ulse. These are the so-called three p's of the blue toe syndrome. These patients will usually manifest atherosclerotic occlusive disease in other vascular beds including the coronary, cerebral, and peripheral arterial systems. Noninvasive evaluation may reveal normal proximal vessels but significant occlusive disease is present in approximately half of those studied.

Treatment

Decision to Treat

In the past, treatment for patients with blue toe syndrome has been reserved for those with progressing tissue loss or threatened limbs. Because of the poor natural history of this disease process in most patients, surgically correctable lesions probably should be treated operatively and conservative management reserved for those patients who are prohibitive operative risks or have relatively short life spans. Conservative management consists of optimization of risk factors including good control of diabetes, hypertension, and hypercholesterolemia, as well as smoking cessation. Long-term anticoagulant therapy is advisable. The role of aspirin therapy has not been studied, however, it may be of some benefit.

Minimally Invasive Therapy

There are no reports in the literature on the results of angioplasty, stent, or stent-graft placement for blue toe syndrome caused by aortoiliac occlusive disease. This would seem to be a reasonable alternative for some patients, but there is only anecdotal experience available on which to make such a decision.

Invasive Therapy

It would seem logical that blue toe syndrome caused by aortoiliac disease would benefit from surgical intervention to repair that segment of the aortoiliac system responsible for the emboli that lodge distally in the lower limb. There are no prospective randomized data comparing surgical and medical therapy in the treatment of this disease process, but the recommendation of surgical treatment is a natural extension of our current knowledge given the poor natural history of this disease process. Surgical treatment consists of either aortofemoral grafting to exclude and replace the diseased segments or aortoiliac endarterectomy for relatively localized aortoiliac occlusive disease. The operative morbidity and mortality rates[6–8] of each of these procedures is excellent.

Future Directions in Treatment

Blue toe syndrome is uncommon, so it is unlikely that a prospective randomized trial comparing surgical therapy with medical therapy for this condition will ever be conducted. There is great interest in the use of minimally invasive procedures such as PTA with or without stent placement, atherectomy devices, or the use of endoluminal grafting to exclude the atheromatous debris from the circulatory system. Until more data are available, surgical therapy seems to be of greater benefit to these patients than does the conservative or medical approach.

Abdominal Aortic Aneurysms

Abdominal aortic aneurysms are relatively common, and recent studies suggest that their incidence is increasing.[54–57] There is some disagreement as to what constitutes an aneurysm, but the Ad Hoc Committee on Reporting Standards of the Society for Vascular Surgery and the International Society for Cardiovascular Surgery has recently suggested that an aneurysm is a permanent localized dilation of an artery with an increase in diameter of >1.5 times its normal diameter.[58] Aneurysms of the abdominal aorta located between the renal arteries and the iliac bifurcation are by far the most common encountered in clinical practice. Men are affected more often than women in a ratio of 4:1.[59] Aneurysms of other arteries are common in patients with abdominal aortic aneurysms. These include the common and internal iliac (41%) and femoropopliteal aneurysms (15% to 50%). The etiology and pathogenesis of abdominal aortic aneurysms has not been defined, but there are numerous studies that suggest that decreased quantities of elastin and collagen are present in the artery wall of an aneurysm.[60–63] There also is considerable evidence that there is some genetic susceptibility to aortic aneurysm formation.[64] Hemodynamic factors are also thought to have a significant role in this disease process. Once an aneurysm develops (regardless of cause), its enlargement is based on certain physical principles, most notably La Places's law that states that the circumferential wall stress is proportional to the transmural pressure muliplied by the radius of the vessel. Therefore, as the radius of the vessel increases, so does the transmural wall stress and the incidence of rupture. This accounts for the 12-fold increase in wall tension found when an aortic aneurysm increases from 2 to 6 cm in diameter.

Diagnosis

Aneurysms of the aorta occur most often in elderly men, whose average age is about 70 years. Aortic aneurysm disease is found in patients with other risk factors for atherosclerosis including cigarette smoking, hypertension, and hypercholesterolemia.[8] Of those patients with abdominal aortic aneurysms, 70% to 75% are asymptomatic when first diagnosed.[65] Most aortic aneurysms are discovered as a pulsatile abdominal mass during a routine physical examination, more commonly during a radiological study for some other reason. Aneurysms may also cause symptoms as a result of pressure, rupture, or expansion. Symptoms of rupture include severe pain in the back, flank, or abdomen that is also consistent with expansion. Other symptoms may include a sensation of fullness, or nausea or vomiting due to compression of adjacent viscera.

Natural History

The natural history of abdominal aortic aneurysms was originally described by Estes[66] in the early 1950s. In his series, patients with abdominal aortic aneurysms found on physical examination were followed, as at the time, there was no definitive therapy available. Most of these aneurysms were large. During the follow-up period, the mortality was nearly 100%, with the majority of patients dying from aneurysmal rupture. Other investigators have reported similar findings. The natural history of untreated abdominal aortic aneurysms seems to be one of progressive expansion, followed by rupture and death.

Treatment Options

Decision to Treat

Because of the poor prognosis for untreated abdominal aortic aneurysms, most patients should be considered for surgical intervention. The timing of intervention depends primarily on the size of the aneurysm at the time of diagnosis. Using currently available data, almost all aneurysms >5 cm in diameter should be treated. This is based on a rupture risk of approximately 5% to 7.5% per year for untreated aneurysms of this size.[67–70] With rupture, the overall mortality is at least 78%.[54,59] with approximately 50% of patients dying before reaching the hospital. Acceptable surgical candidates with aneurysms ≥5 cm in diameter should not be treated conservatively. The objective of treatment is to prevent rupture and thereby prolong life. Currently, controversy exists regarding the treatment of small aneurysms, ie, aneurysms <5 cm in diameter. There are many anecdotal reports of rupture of these small aneurysms, and although there have been no large series to document the true rupture risk, it is low. Because abdominal aneurysms tend to occur in elderly patients with other sequelae of atherosclerotic vascular disease, and because the morbidity and mortality rates of 1% to 5% for surgical aneurysm repair,[71–76] although low are real, elective aneurysm repair is not recommended for most patients with small abdominal aortic aneurysms (<4.5cm.) At least three randomized prospective studies are currently underway that should define the natural history of these small aneurysms.

Minimally Invasive Therapy

Currently there is an ongoing prospective randomized trial evaluating minimally invasive treatment of abdominal aortic aneurysms by placement of an endovascular graft. Initial results are promising, but long-term follow-up is not yet available.

Surgical Therapy

Surgical therapy for abdominal aortic aneurysms was first performed in 1951 and there have been large numbers of publications documenting the operative and long-term survival after surgical treatment.[71–76] There has been steady improvement in operative results for elective operations. Large contemporary series report current operative mortality rates between 0.9% and 5%.[71–76] The usual form of surgical therapy consists of opening and replacing the aneurysmal segment of aorta with a suitable prosthetic graft. Long-term results show that there is increased patient survival over those treated nonsurgically, however, the rate never quite achieves the normal age and sex match control survival curves.[77–80] All aneurysmal portions of the aorta and iliac arteries are usually replaced. The operations are well tolerated by most patients, including those 80 to 90 years old.

Future Directions

Endovascular treatment of abdominal aortic aneurysms is currently undergoing clinical trials in many centers around the world. Initial results suggest that in anatomically favorable conditions, the endovascular placement of a graft is associated with very low morbidity and mortality rates with good early success and freedom from subsequent aneurysm rupture. Patients tolerate the procedure well with short-term hospitalizations and quickly return to normal activity levels.

New Directions in the Treatment of Atherosclerosis that Affects the Aorta

PTA with or without stent placement for treatment of athero-sclerotic disease of the aorta is currently a valid clinical tool. The indications for and application of these techniques have been increasing since their introduction. With the help of carefully planned prospective randomized studies, the scope of this therapeutic option will increase even more. Atherectomy devices and lasers, although initially felt to be quite effective, have had their use curtailed because of problems with early restenosis secondary to myointimal hyperplasia. Currently, molecular biologists are investigating the cellular mechanisms responsible for this process, which is thought to be an overexuberant healing response of the artery wall. When the pathophysiological mechanisms responsible for myointimal hyperplasia are defined in detail, it will become possible to control the process and then atherectomy and laser therapy for atherosclerosis of the abdominal aorta and its branches should become effective and durable procedures. There is tremendous enthusiasm and interest in the use of endovascular grafting in the treatment of aneurysmal disease. Favorable results were obtained with phase I clinical trials and phase II clinical trials are currently underway. It appears that endovascular grafting will soon become an effective form of therapy for certain anatomic variations of abdominal aortic aneurysmal disease. Its long-term durability will, in great part, depend on the method of attachment as well as the reaction of the artery wall to the graft itself. The role of endovascular grafting in the treatment of occlusive disease may also depend on effective forms of procedures to first open the arteries, followed by placement of grafts or stents. All of these minimally invasive procedures, although attractive in design, have so far been hampered by the same problems of intimal hyperplasia, ie, the reaction of the artery wall to manipulation. Once again, the role of molecular biology in the future of vascular surgery will be in the hands and minds of scientists who hopefully will resolve this problem. Controlling the reaction of the artery wall to manipulation and foreign materials will allow the further development of minimally invasive procedures. Society, government, and insurance companies may force this issue to the forefront with the current and future trends in medicine that are moving toward outcome assessment, cost containment, and early return to work.

References

1. Leriche R, Morel A. The syndrome of thrombotic obliteration of the aortic bifurcation. *Ann Surg* 1948;127:193–206.
2. Leriche R. Des obliterations arterielles hautes (obliteration de la terminaison de l'aorte) comme causes des insuffisances circulatoires des membres inferieurs. *Bull Mem Soc Chir (Paris)* 1923;49:1404–1406.
3. Leriche R. De la resection du carrefour aortico-iliaque avec double sympathectomie lombaire pour thrombose arteritique de l'aorte' le syndrome de l'obliteration termino-aortique par arterite. *Presse Med* 1940;48:601–604.
4. Flanigan DP, Gray B, Schuler JJ, et al. Utility of wide and narrow blood pressure cuffs in the hemodynamic assessment of aortoiliac occlusive disease. *Surgery* 1982;92:16–20.
5. Lynch TG, Hobson RW, Wright CB, et al. Interpretation of Doppler segmental pressures in peripheral vascular occlusive disease. *Arch Surg* 1984;119:465–467.
6. Malone JM, Moore WS, Goldstone J. Life expectancy following aortofemoral arterial grafting. *Surgery* 1977;81:551.
7. Crawford ES, Bomberger RA, Glaeser DH, et al. Aortoiliac occlusive disease: Factors influencing survival and function following reconstructive operation over a twenty-five-year period. *Surgery* 1981;90:1055–1067.
8. Szilagyi DE, Elliott JP, Smith RF, et al. A thirty-year survey of the reconstructive surgical treatment of aortoiliac occlusive disease. *J Vasc Surg* 1986;3:421–436.
9. Dotter CT, Judkins MP. Transluminal treatment of arteriosclerotic obstruction: Description of a new technique and a preliminary report of its application. *Circulation* 1964;30:654–670.
10. Gruntzig A, Hopff H. Perkutane rekanalisation chronischer arterieller verschlusse mit einem neuen dilation-skatheter: Modifikation der dotter-technik. *Dtsch Med Wochenschr* 1974;99:2502–2510.
11. Johnston KW, Rae M, Hoss-Johnston SA, et al. Five-year results of a prospective study of percutaneous transluminal angioplasty. *Ann Surg* 1987;206:404–413.
12. Wilson SE, Wolf GL, Cross AP. Percutaneous transluminal angioplasty versus operation for peripheral arteriosclerosis: Report of a prospective randomized trial in a selected group of patients. *J Vasc Surg* 1989;9:1–9.
13. Pentecost MJ, Criqui KH, Dorros G, et al. Guidelines for peripheral percutaneous transluminal angioplasty of the abdominal aorta and lower extremity vessels. *Circulation* (in press).
14. Richter GM, Roeren T, Brado M, et al. Further update of the randomized trial: Iliac stent placement versus PTA-morphology, clinical success rates, and failure analysis. *JVIR* 1993;4:30.
15. Schneider JR, McDaniel MD, Walsh DB, et al. Axillofemoral bypass: Outcome and hemodynamic results in high-risk patients. *J Vasc Surg* 1992;15:952–963.
16. El-Massry S, Saad E, Sauvage LR, et al. Axillofemoral bypass with externally supported, knitted Dacron grafts: A follow-up through twelve years. *J Vasc Surg* 1993;17:107–115.
17. Qvarfordt PG, Reilly LM, Sedwitz MM, et al. "Coral reef" atheroscle-

rosis of the suprarenal aorta: A unique clinical entity. *J Vasc Surg* 1984; 1:903–909.

18. Sako Y. Arteriosclerotic occlusion of the midabdominal aorta. *Surgery* 1966;59:709–712.

19. Stoney RJ, Wylie EJ. Surgical management of arterial lesions of the thoracoabdominal aorta. *Am J Surg* 1973;126:157–164.

20. Zelenock GB, Graham LM, Whitehouse WM Jr, et al. Splanchnic arteriosclerotic disease and intestinal angina. *Arch Surg* 1980;115:497–501.

21. Baccelli F, cited by Goodman EH. Angina abdominis. *Am J Med Sci* 1918;155:524.

22. Chiene J. Complete obliteration of celiac and mesenteric arteries: Viscera receiving their blood supply through extraperitoneal system of vessels. *J Anat Physiol* 1869;3:65.

23. Conner LA. Discussion of role of arterial thrombosis in visceral diseases of middle life, based upon analogies drawn from coronary thrombosis. *Am J Med Sci* 1933;185:13.

24. Dunphy JE. Abdominal pain of vascular origin. *Am J Med Sci* 1936;192:102.

25. Mikkelson WP. Intestinal angina: Its surgical significance. *Am J Surg* 1957;94:262.

26. Hollier LH, Bernatz PE, Pairolero PC, et al. Surgical management of chronic intestinal ischemia: A reappraisal. *Surgery* 1981;90:940.

27. Rapp JH, Reilly LM, Qvarfordt PG, et al. Durability of endarterectomy and antegrade grafts in the treatment of chronic visceral ischemia. *J Vasc Surg* 1986;3:799.

28. Rheudasil JM, Stewart MT, Schellack JV, et al. Surgical treatment of chronic mesenteric arterial insufficiency. *J Vasc Surg* 1988;8:495.

29. Crawford ES, Morris GC Jr, Myhre HO, Roehm J Jr. Celiac axis, superior mesenteric artery, and inferior mesenteric artery occlusion: Surgical considerations. *Surgery* 1977;82:856–866.

30. Hansen HJB. Abdominal angina: Results of arterial reconstruction in 12 patients. *Acta Chir Scand* 1976;142:319–325.

31. Rapp JH, Reilly LM, Qvarfordt PG, et al. Durability of endarterectomy and antegrade grafts in the treatment of chronic visceral ischemia. *J Vasc Surg* 1986;3:799–806.

32. Stanley JC. Pathologic basis of macrovascular renal artery disease. In: Stanley JC, Ernst CB, Fry WJ, eds. *Renovascular Hypertension.* Philadelphia: WB Saunders; 1984:46–74.

33. Bright R. Cases and observations illustrative of renal disease accompanied with the secretion of albuminous urine. *Guy's Hospital Rep* 1836;1:388.

34. Tigerstedt R, Bergman PG. Niere und Kreislauf. *Scand Arch Physiol* 1898;8:223.

35. Tucker RM, Labarthe DR. Frequency of surgical treatment for hypertension in adults at the Mayo Clinic from 1973 through 1975. *Mayo Clin Proc* 1977;52:549.

36. Shapiro AP, Perez-Stable E, Scheib ET, et al. Renal artery stenosis and hypertension. *Am J Med* 1969;47:175.

37. Davis BA, Crook JE, Vestal RE, et al. Prevalence of renovascular hypertension in patients with Grade III or IV hypertensive retinopathy. *N Engl J Med* 1979;301:1273.

38. Lawson JD, Boerth RK, Foster JH, et al. Diagnosis and management of renovascular hypertension in children. *Arch Surg* 1977;112:1307.

39. Simon N, Franklin SS, Bleifer KH, Maxwell MH. Clinical characteristics of renovascular hypertension. *JAMA* 1972;220:1209.
40. Foster JH, Dean RH, Pinkerton JA, et al. Ten years experience with the surgical management of renovascular hypertension. *Ann Surg* 1973; 177:755.
41. Dean RH, Kieffer RW, Smith BM, et al. Renovascular hypertension. *Arch Surg* 1981;116:1408.
42. Miller GA, Ford KK, Braun SD, et al. Percutaneous transluminal angioplasty vs. surgery for renovascular hypertension. *AJR* 1985;144: 447–450.
43. Sos TA, Pickering TG, Sniderman K, et al. Percutaneous transluminal renal angioplasty in renovascular hypertension due to atheroma of fibromuscular dysplasia. *N Engl J Med* 1983;309:274–279.
44. Wylie EJ, Perloff DL, Stoney RJ. Autogenous tissue revascularization techniques in surgery for renovascular hypertension. *Ann Surg* 1969;170:416.
45. Eggers PW. Effect of transplantation on the medicare endstage renal disease program. *Transplant Medicare ESRD Prog* 1988;318:223.
46. Dean RH, Krueger TC, Whiteneck JM, et al. Operative management of renovascular hypertension: Results after 15–23 years follow-up. *J Vasc Surg* 1984;1:234.
47. Panum PL. Experimentelle beitrage zue hehre von der embolie. *Virchows Arch Pathol Anat* 1862;25:308–310.
48. Venet L, Friedfeld L. Avulsion and embolization of a calcific arterial plaque: Femoral embolectomy. *Surgery* 1952;32:119–122.
49. Richards AM, Eliot RS, Kanjuh VI, et al. Cholesterol embolism. A multiple-system disease masquerading as polyarteritis nodosa. *Am J Cardiol* 1965;15:696–707.
50. Crane C. Atherothrombotic embolism to lower extremities in arteriosclerosis. *Arch Surg* 1967;94:1368–1377.
51. Wagner RB, Martin AS. Peripheral atheroembolism: Confirmation of a clinical concept, with a case report and review of the literature. *Surgery* 1973;73:353–359.
52. Karmody AM, Powers SR, Monaco VJ, et al. "Blue toe" syndrome: An indication for limb salvage surgery. *Arch Surg* 1976;111:1263–1268.
53. Wingo JP, Nix ML, Greenfield LJ, Barnes RW. The blue toe syndrome: Hemodynamics and therapeutic correlates of outcome. *J Vasc Surg* 1986;3:475–480.
54. Bickerstaff LK, Hollier LH, Van Peenen HJ, et al. Abdominal aortic aneurysm: The changing natural history. *J Vasc Surg* 1984;1:6–12.
55. Castelden W, Mercer J. Abdominal aortic aneurysms in western Australia: Descriptive epidemiology and patterns of rupture. *Br J Surg* 1985;72:109–112.
56. Melton L, Bickerstaff L, Hollier LH, et al. Changing incidence of abdominal aortic aneurysms: A population based study. *Am J Epidemiol* 1984;120:379–386.
57. Norman PE, Castleden WM, Hockey RL. Prevalence of abdominal aortic aneurysm in Western Australia. *Br J Surg* 1991;78:1118–1121.
58. Johnston KW, Rutherford RB, Tilson MD, et al. Suggested standards for reporting on arterial aneurysms. *J Vasc Surg* 1991;13:452–458.
59. Taylor LM, Porter JM. Basic data related to clinical decision-making in abdominal aortic aneurysms. *Ann Vasc Surg* 1980;1:502–504.
60. Busuttil RW, Abou-Zamzam AM, Machleder HI. Collagenase activity

of the human aorta: Comparisons of patients with and without abdominal aortic aneurysms. *Arch Surg* 1980;115:1373–1378.
61. Busuttil RW, Heinrich R, Flesher A. Elastase activity: The role of elastase in aortic aneurysm formation. *J Surg Res* 1982;32:214–217.
62. Dobrin PB, Baker WH, Gley WC. Elastolytic and collagenolytic studies of arteries: Implications for the mechanical properties of aneurysms. *Arch Surg* 1984;119:405–409.
63. Dobrin PB, Baker WH, Schwarcz TH. Mechanisms of arterial and aneurysmal tortuosity. *Surgery* 1988;104:568–571.
64. Majumder PP, St. Jean PL, Ferrell RE, et al. On the inheritance of abdominal aortic aneurysm. *Am J Hum Genet* 1991;48:164–170.
65. Szilagyi DE. Clinical diagnosis of intact and ruptured abdominal aortic aneurysms. In: Bergan JJ, Yao JST, eds. *Aneurysms: Diagnosis and Treatment*. New York: Grune & Stratton; 1982:205–215.
66. Estes JE Jr. Abdominal aortic aneurysm: A study of 102 cases. *Circulation* 1950;2:258–264.
67. Darling RC, Messina CR, Brewster DC, et al. Autopsy study of unoperated aortic aneurysms. *Circulation* 1977;56(suppl 2):161–164.
68. Cronenwett JL, Murphy TF, Zelenock GB, et al. Actuarial analysis of variables associated with rupture of small aortic aneurysms. *Surgery* 1985;98:472–483.
69. Bernstein EF, Chan EL. Abdominal aortic aneurysm in high risk patients: Outcome of selective management based on size and expansion rate. *Ann Surg* 1984;200:255–263.
70. Szilagyi DE, Elliott JP, Smith RF. Clinical fate of the patient with asymptomatic abdominal aortic aneurysm and unfit surgical treatment. *Arch Surg* 1972;104:600–606.
71. Thompson JE, Hollier LH, Purment RD, et al. Surgical management of abdominal aortic aneurysms. *Ann Surg* 1975;181:654–660.
72. Baird RJ, Gurry JF, Kellam JF, et al. Abdominal aortic aneurysms: Recent experience with 210 patients. *Can Med Assoc J* 1978;118:1229–1235.
73. Crawford ES, Saleh SA, Babb JW III, et al. Infrarenal abdominal aortic aneurysm: Factors influencing survival after operation performed over a 25 year period. *Ann Surg* 1981;193:699–709.
74. Whittemore AD, Clowes AW, Hechtman HB, et al. Aortic aneurysm repair reduced operative mortality associated with maintenance of optimal cardiac performance. *Ann Surg* 1980;120:414–421.
75. Ramos TK, Goldstone J. Should small abdominal aortic aneurysms by operated on? In: Veith F, ed. *Current Critical Problems in Vascular Surgery*. Volume 4. St. Louis: Quality Medical Publishing; 1992:197–206.
76. Pairolero PC. Repair of abdominal aortic aneurysms in high-risk patients. *Surg Clin North Am* 1989;69:755–763.
77. Burnham SJ, Johnson G Jr, Gurri JA. Mortality risks for survivors of vascular reconstructive procedures. *Surgery* 1982;92:107.
78. Johnson G Jr, Gurri JA, Burnham SJ. Life expectancy after abdominal aortic aneurysm repair. In: Bergan JJ, Yao JST, eds. *Aneurysms: Diagnosis and Treatment*. New York: Grune & Stratton; 1982:279–285.
79. Hollier LH, Plate G, O'Brien PC, et al. Late survival after abdominal aortic repair: Influence of coronary artery disease. *J Vasc Surg* 1984;1:290–299.
80. Hertzer NR. Fatal myocardial infarction following abdominal aortic aneurysm resection: 343 patients followed 6–11 years post-operative. *Ann Surg* 1980;190:667–673.

Chapter 14

Peripheral Vascular Disease:
A Clinician's View

William Insull, Jr, MD

Introduction

Lower extremity arterial disease (LEAD) is a signifcant clinical disease, particularly in patients with diabetes mellitus. The clinician currently addressing LEAD expects that the newer concepts of atherogenesis, the clinical syndromes, and the newer imaging techniques that are successfully being applied to the coronary arteries, aorta, and carotid arteries can also be applied to the arterial disease of the lower extremities leading to improved diagnosis and treatment. However, this expectation has yet to be fulfilled in clinical practice, although significant progress has been achieved in recent years. A major problem is that the correlations of the clinical disease with pathological descriptions of the lesions and their imaging characteristics are limited because of insufficient tissue studies.

This chapter uses the clinician's perspective to evaluate the current status of the correlation of clinical syndromes of peripheral vascular disease with the morphology of the arterial lesions by pathology and by imaging techniques and how this may be used in the diagnosis and management of treatment. This chapter is confined to atherosclerotic LEAD and addresses five topics crucial for successful correlation and clinical application: 1) knowledge of atherosclerosis and its treatment supports expectation for LEAD; 2) clinical characteristics and risk factors for LEAD; 3) clinical uses and requirements for imaging techniques for LEAD; 4) Potential imaging techniques for LEAD; and 5) future research needs for LEAD

From: Fuster V, (ed.) *Syndromes of Atherosclerosis: Correlations of Clinical Imaging and Pathology.* Armonk, NY: Futura Publishing Company, Inc.: © 1996.

Knowledge of Atherosclerosis in LEAD

The recently demonstrated correlation between coronary lesion morphology and clinical disease, the lesions' successful treatment, and the increasing experience with LEAD strongly indicates that for LEAD, the correlation of clinical syndromes with morphology and with the medical treatments will be similarly successful. Four recent developments are pertinent. First, the classification of atherosclerotic lesions and their probable developmental sequence, and the identifcation of the culprit lesion for many clinical coronary events can be applied in principle to lower extremity disease.[1,2] Second, the treatment-induced alteration of coronary lesions of atherosclerosis and the prevention of clinical disease in multiple clinical trials with a variety of cholesterol-lowering agents has clearly demonstrated that atherosclerotic vascular disease can be controlled to a major degree.[2,3] Third, three clinical trials of some of these agents lowering low-density lipoprotein cholesterol (LDL-C) have demonstrated reduction of LEAD.[4–6] Fourth, new more potent agents for monotherapy that lower LDL-C promise to make regression of lesions and prevention of clinical coronary disease more readily achievable in clinical practice.[7]

LEAD Clinical Characteristics and Risk Factors

The major clinical characteristics of LEAD indicate the circumstances where the clinician would use imaging techniques. Most clinical disease is caused by occlusive atherosclerosis, with an incidence that is greater in men than women, 0.3% and 0.1%, respectively, and a fivefold increase when diabetes is present.[8] The anatomic distribution under age 40 is primarily aortoiliac (53%); over age 40 the distribution is primarily femoropopliteal (65%), with multisegmental envolvement in about 20% of patients.[9] The initial presentation is mostly with intermittent claudication (73%), less often with ischemic pain at rest (16%), and ulceration or gangrene (11%).[10] Late complications can include severe ischemia that can lead to surgery in 19% to 27%, with amputation in 3% to 8%.

The risk factors for LEAD are being defined and their relative effects determined. The most prominent risk factor is cigarette smoking. The relative importance of other factors for the clinical syndromes and for the morphology of arterial lesions and how they interact with smoking and with diabetes mellitus has not yet been established. These factors include lipid peroxidation, fibrinogen and inhibition of fibrinolysis as determinants of blood viscosity, endothelial dysfunction centered around the von Willebrand factor, platelet activation by beta thyroglobulin, and plasminogen activator inhibitor.[11]

The diagnosis of LEAD must recognize that the diagnostic accuracy of a modern vascular laboratory is superior to that of traditional clinical assessment, the latter having significant false positives or false negatives, 44% and 19%, respectively.[12] Isolated posterior tibial artery disease and its lack of exercise-induced calf pain is signifcant because it carries increased risks of mortality from all causes and from coronary artery disease.[13]

The recomendations for the primary care assessment for LEAD in diabetes describe the initial diagnostic procedures and the criteria for referral for further study at a vascular laboratory or clinic.[14] These recommendations present the elements of the clinical history, clinical examination, and readily available elective tests: claudication, signs of critical ischemia, palpation of tibialis posterior and dorsalis pedis pulses, femoral bruits, and the ankle brachial index. Arteriography is the definitive diagnostic procedure prior to surgical intervention, but its use must consider associated increased risks with older patients and limited renal function, and also recognize that arteriography does not detect early lesions.

Clinical Uses and Requirements for Imaging Techniques for LEAD

The clinical uses for imaging LEAD set the requirements for the imaging techniques that can also be used to evaluate the correlation between the clinical syndrome and the images. Each imaging technique should be evaluated for its capacity to fulfill these clinical requirements. Eight major clinical uses have been identified: 1) to diagnose the presence of LEAD; 2) to assess the characteristics and severity of LEAD; 3) to assess remaining arterial function; 4) to guide intervention by intravascular techniques and by surgery; 5) to assess postinterventional arterial patency; 6) to assess the complications of angiography; 7) to perform serial examinations in order to monitor disease development and to evaluate treatments; and 8) to aid research on LEAD epidemiology and clinical trial evaluation of interventions.

Further requirements for the imaging techniques include the detailed descriptions of individual arterial lesions. Eight major lesion characteristics have been identified for their clinical usefulness: 1) the lesion's length and the occurrence of segmentation; 2) the degree of stenosis or presence of occlusion; 3) eccentricity; 4) irregularity, 5) calcification; 6) the status of the runoff for the common femoral, superficial, and deep femoral arteries, and for the popliteal artery, the number of patent vessels; 7) the status of the arteries' compensatory enlargement;[15] and 8) the identifcation of pathological types of lesions and especially the potential culprit lesions.[2]

Increased emphasis on diagnostic imaging techniques is resulting from improved treatments. Treatment of LEAD is currently undergoing a revolution based on improvements in percutaneous revascularization and successful clinical trials of medical intervention.[4–6,16] The developing techniques for percutaneous revascularization are redefining alternatives to surgery and are identifying optimal procedures from a broad range of technical procedures including hydrophilic guidewires, clot lysis with perfusion systems, stents, directional atherectomy, rotational atherectomy, and laser angioplasty. Treatment selection is directed in part by arterial anatomy. Occluded arteries may be opened by partially intramural new courses. Restenosis, postgraft or angioplasty, is frequently managed.

Clinical trials are demonstrating that medical treatments with lipid-altering regimens are effective for prevention of LEAD. While three trials of drugs lowering low-density lipoprotein cholesterol have demonstrated significant treatment effects, additional trials in progress should add more data in the near future. Endothelial dysfunction, such as abnormal endothelium dependent vascular relaxation, has not been reported for lower extremity arteries, but may be assumed to occur.

Potential Imaging Techniques for LEAD

The imaging techniques that are potentially useful for the LEAD are all those that can be applied to the coronary and carotid arteries. For some techniques, applications to LEAD may be advantageous because the extremity arteries have greater physical accessibility. The techniques most successfully applied are contrast arteriography, B-mode ultrasound, and duplex scanning by B-mode ultrasound and Doppler. The evolving procedures with intravascular ultrasound appear promising. Other potentially useful techniques that are not yet well developed and that are frequently restricted by limited resolution include magnetic resonance angiography, electron beam computer aided tomography, and radioisotope imaging of atheroma. Details of these techniques are reviewed elsewhere in this book. Each technique needs to be evaluated for its application to LEAD by considering the requirements for imaging and correlation discussed above. Some of these in vivo imaging techniques may be useful for measuring endothelium dysfunction, eg, abnormal vascular relaxation, as part of the clinical syndromes.

Research Needs for Correlations of Clinical Syndromes with Imaging and Pathology

Because of the paucity of LEAD studies correlating clinical syndrome with arterial lesion pathological morphology and imaging, it is appropriate to identify and recommend the types of research studies that are needed. These studies should lead to better understanding of the pathogenesis of the disease, improved diagnosis, and more effective and better focused treatments and preventive measures. Our suggestions are as follows.

For the arterial lesions of LEAD, determine their pathological morphology and the sequence of development guided by the concepts applied to the coronary artery lesions. Emphasis should be placed on the early lesions and the potential culprit lesions predisposed to thrombosis or occlusion and causing a clinical event because these lesions are the targets for primary and secondary prevention of clinical disease. Correlate the pathological morphology of arterial lesions with the lesions' morphology by sensitive imaging techniques. This validates the lesion specificity of the imaging techniques. Correlate the clinical syndromes of LEAD and the clinical tests with the arterial lesions that can be evaluated by pathological morphology and by imaging techniques. This enables clinical treatment to be based on the tissue diagnosis of arterial lesions evaluated by the imaging techniques. An evaluation of the cost effectiveness of the clinical useful imaging procedures should be performed.

Conclusions

Evaluation of the status of the correlation of the clinical syndrome of lower extremity arterial disease with lesion morphology by pathology and imaging techniques can be judged by comparison with similar correlations being obtained for lesions of the coronary and carotid arteries. By these criteria, the LEAD correlations have not been signifcantly developed to the same extent. Although the knowledge base for LEAD is substantial, the elements essential for these correlations are weak or missing. The requirements for LEAD images based on their clinical usefulness have been identified. Several methods of imaging have been refined or are being refined, so that comparative evaluation of the imaging methods for clinical use can be performed. However, the adequate research correlating the lesions' pathology with their morphology by the imaging techniques has not been performed. After this is attained, research can be directed to correlating the imaging morphology with the clinical syndrome of LEAD. Achievement of these latter correlations promises to make possible the improved diagnosis, treatment, and prevention of LEAD.

References

1. Stary HC, Chandler AB, Glagov S, et al. A definition of advanced lesions of atherosclerosis and a classification of lesions: A report from the Committeee on Vascular Lesion of the Council on Arteriosclerosis. *Arterioscler Throm Vasc Biol* 1995;15:1512–1531.
2. Brown BG, Zhao X-Q, Sacco DE, et al. Lipid lowering and plaque regression: New insights into prevention of plaque disruption and clinical event in coronary disease. *Circulation* 1993;87:1781–1791.
3. Scandinavian Simvastatin Survival Study Group. Randomized trial of cholesterol lowering 4444 patients with coronary heart disease: The Scandinavian Simvastatin Survival Study (4S) *Lancet* 1994;344:1383–1389.
4. Blankenhorn DH, Azen SP, Crawford DW, et al. Effects of colestipol-niacin therapy on human femoral atherosclerosis. *Circulation* 1991;83:438–447.
5. Bourdages HR, Campos CT, Nyugen R, et al. Peripheral vascular results on the surgical control of the hyperlipidemias (POSCH). *Circulation* 1994;90:1–585.
6. Salonen R, Nyyssonen K, Porkkala E, et al. KAPS: The effect of pravastatin on atherosclerotic progression in carotid and femoral arteries. *Circulation* 1994;90:I–127.
7. Nawrocki J, Weiss S, Sprecher D, et al. Reduction of LDL-C by more than 60% with the HMGCoA reductase inhibitor atorvastatin. *Atherosclerosis* 1994;109:313.
8. Kannel WB, McGee DL. Diabetes and cardiovascular disease. The Framingham Study. *JAMA* 1979;241:2035–2038.
9. McDaniel MD, Cronenwett JL. Basic data related to the natural history of intermittent claudication. *Ann Vasc Surg* 1989;3:273–277.
10. Juergens IL, Barker NW, Hines EA, Jr. Atheriosclerosis obliterans: Review of 520 cases with special reference to pathogenic and prognostic factors. *Circulation* 1960;21:118–195.
11. Smith FB, Lowe GDO, Fowkes FGR, et al. Smoking, hemostatic factors and lipid peroxides in a popluation case control study of peripheral vascular disease. *Atherosclerosis* 1993;102:155–162.
12. Marinelli MR, Beach KW, Glass MJ, et al. Non-invasive testing vs clin-

ical evaluation of arterial disease: A prospective study. *JAMA* 1979;241: 2031–2034.

13. Criqui MH, Fronek A, Klauber MR, et al. The sensitivity, specifcity, and predictive values of traditional clinical evaluation of peripheral vascular arterial disease, results from noninvasive testing in a defined population. *Circulation* 1985;71:516–522.
14. Orchard TJ, Strandness DE. Assessment of peripheral vascular disease in diabetes. Report and recomendations of an International Workshop. *Circulation* 1993;88:819–828.
15. Glagov S, Zarins CK, Giddens DP, et al. Hemodynamics and atherosclerosis, insights and perspectives gained from studies of human arteries. *Arch Pathol Lab Med* 1988;112:1018–1031.
16. Isner IM, Rosenfield K. Redefining the treatment of peripheral artery disease. *Circulation* 1993;88:1534–1557.

Panel Discussion II

Pathology
Clinical Correlation
of Carotid, Aortic, and
Peripheral Vascular Disease

Dr. Valentin Fuster: I would like to discuss carotid disease first, then aortic disease, and finally peripheral vascular disease. Drs. Weinberger and Kohler, can you begin by clarifying one issue for us? The North American Symptomatic Carotid Endarterectomy Trial (NASCET) indicated that patients with symptomatic carotid disease and >70% stenosis would benefit from surgery. But, Dr. Weinberger tells us that after several months, perhaps 18, after the last carotid or cerebrovascular event, it doesn't make a difference. Then, the Asymptomatic Carotid Arteriosclerosis Study (ACAS) tells us that we should perform the operation in an asymptomatic patient with >60% stenosis. So, how can you reconcile these different approaches?

Dr. Jesse Weinberger: First, we can't make any comments about the ACAS study until we have seen all of the data. The first thing you have to remember is that, as Dr. Kohler shows us, about 75% of these symptomatic patients with severe lesions aren't having any strokes. It's the exception, not the rule, that they are going to have a stroke. That has to do with other things that are going on. For instance, if you have good posterior communicating collateral circulation, you may have transient ischmemic attacks (TIA), but you won't have a stroke no matter the state of the artery. There are data showing that in the presence of normal opthalmic artery pressure, a high-grade stenosis gives you a 2% risk of stroke, whereas if the pressure is reduced, the risk is 20%. So, there are other factors in the brain circulation and brain biochemistry in addition to what's happening at the carotid artery that determine outcome. We use this information clinically, for example, with ocular plethysmography or transcranial Doppler, to determine which are the high-risk patients.

Dr. Ted R. Kohler: I would just like to point out that another deficiency of NASCET and other trials is that they did not correlate

269

the incidence of strokes with disease progression in the medical group, so we don't know if the strokes that occurred were associated with progression. I think that's data that will be very important. In getting at the important question, how long are these patients at risk and how should they be followed, Dr. Strandness' group will soon publish their 10-year follow-up of asymptomatic patients with mild to moderate disease. And, going along with what Dr. Weinberger presented earlier, of the 12 patients who had strokes in that group, 8 patients had progressed, so progression is obviously an important thing to pick up. However, only about 3% of the patients with the 50% to 79% stenosis progressed per year and only about 7% of those patients over 10 years had a stroke. I think that's important to keep in mind.

Dr. Fuster: At this time, would you operate on a completely asymptomatic patient who has an 80% stenotic lesion?

Dr. Kohler: We do operate upon asymptomatic patients, who are good surgical risks, with 80% stenotic lesions.

Dr. Fuster: Dr. Glagov, have you studied the intracerebral circulation in patients who have transient cerebral ischemic attacks and in patients who have a stroke? Let me ask this question. The heart appears to be relatively insensitive to emboli. For example, during angioplasty in an epicardial artery I am sure emboli are common and nothing really happens to the patient. Is the brain more sensitive to microemboli? What is the size of the cerebrovascular artery that is occluded, for example, in a transient cerebral ischemic attack? Is it very tiny?

Dr. Seymou Glagov: This is an area that is very poorly studied because the cerebral circulation is not really very accessible, either to demonstrate micro-occlusions or to compare with what's in the carotid bifurcation. We've been trying to look at carotid bifurcations after carotid endarterectomy to see what the healing process is like and what the recurrence rate is like and so on. This information is very difficult to come by. Looking at small vessels in the brain is much more difficult than in the heart and the peripheral arteries where the channels are anatomically identifiable in a rather simple way. The brain is far more complex. There certainly is going to be a difference between blockage of an ophthalmic artery and the motor cortex and the sensory areas. I think that the clinicians really can better identify the regions that are at risk and the regions that present the symptoms. I think it's much easier to identify which vessels are obstructed that way than by an anatomical study.

Discussant A from the Audience: The brain, in many ways, is not sensitive. Patients who have asymptomatic carotid stenosis have an incidence of silent infarcts of up to 25% on CT scans, so clearly there are lots of things going on that are not clinically apparent.

Dr. Weinberger: Also, if you look sequentially with transcranial Doppler at patients with carotid disease, they have findings that are consistent with microemboli going on all the time.

Dr. Fuster: Dr. Imperato (in the audience), I was very impressed by what you found in your studies of carotid disease in terms of intracarotid hemorrhage as a cause of acute cerebrovascular events. Perhaps you are talking about the same thing we are in the study of coronary plaque rupture? Would you comment.

Dr. Anthony M. Imperato: First, we studied carotid plaques with grossly visible hemorrhage, not the microscopic hemorrhages that Dr. Glagov alluded to. These were huge, thumb-sized collections of hematoma confirmed by histologic examination. So this is grossly visible bleeding into a plaque. Second, it was possible to show in a certain number of instances that the fibrous cap was totally intact, sometimes quite thick. However, there were encysted hematomas. Also, in following a larger series of plaques, and we are now going into hundreds and hundreds, it was possible to show degradation. We could see fresh hemorrhage, hemorrhage that is undergoing degradation, degradation and cholesterol crystals, and finally the eruption of a hemorrhage through the overlying fibrous cap. So, the observation in the carotid surgical specimens, I think is incontrovertible. The next point I would like to make has to do with stenosis. The degree of stenosis that one reports depends on the technique used to estimate this stenosis. In the NASCET study, the narrowest area at the origin of the internal carotid artery was compared with the normal artery distally. In the European Carotid Endarterectomy Trial, the method of measuring the stenosis was entirely different. It was dependent upon a technique originally described to us by Dr. Juan Taveras, in which we found the narrowest area at the carotid bifurcation, and then created an imaginary line, estimating where the arterial wall should be on the angiogram, and used that in estimating stenosis. Most importantly, I believe the major factor is probably not the degree of stenosis, which is simply a marker of the fact that the pathological process has undergone great progression, and that there has been thorough degeneration of the plaque.

Dr. Fuster: Thank you very much. Dr. Glagov, do you have anything to add regarding the frequency of carotid plaque hemorrhage leading to acute cerebrovascular events?

Dr. Glagov: All of our carotid endarterectomy plaques come to me; I section them at 5-mm intervals, and I examine each and every section. The incidence of hemorrhage is very small. I don't see big hematomas. I see footprints indicating that there have been hemorrhages, and occasionally I do see a hemorrhage where a plaque has been broken by immediately subjacent calcification. But that's not a dominant feature in the plaques at the University of Chicago.

Dr. Imperato: With all due respect to Dr. Glagov, we had the same experience with our pathologist who received the plaques without having seen what was going on in the operating room. When we finally gave him a Kodachrome of what that plaque looked like in the operating room before it was removed, he came to an entirely different conclusion as to what was going on in the vessel. At that point, he understood the importance of hemorrhage. I would suspect that anybody who has not seen what the plaque looks like in vivo ought to take a look in order to get a better impression of how to reconstruct the histologic sections.

Dr. Fuster: Thank you. Let's go to another controversial issue. Dr. Stary has described a very high frequency of microscopic thrombotic material on atherosclerotic plaques of the aorta. It is my impression that in the coronary arteries, thrombotic material may be seen principally in acute coronary syndromes and sometimes in people at high risk with small plaque ruptures. What's the difference? Is it the size of the vessel or is the pathogenesis of the disease more thrombogenic in the large vessel than in the small vessel?

Dr. Herbert C. Stary: I cannot answer reliably whether or not aortic lesions are thrombotic more often than coronary lesions. We did not use quite the same methods to study the two vessels. The aortic lesions were larger in every dimension and lesion composition was not quite the same. These factors may influence susceptibility to thrombosis. But evidence of thrombi was by no means rare in the coronary arteries. One must also remember that in this population of young and middle-aged adults thrombotic deposits and remnants in both coronary and aortic lesions, though frequent, were in fact quite small.

Dr. Fuster: I also have the impression from talking to surgeons who deal with coronary disease and peripheral vascular disease that there is more thrombosis in peripheral than in coronary disease, at least grossly.

Dr. Jerry Goldstone: I don't think that they are more frequent, but I think that there are larger and more extensive thrombi in peripheral vascular diseases because of the nonbranching longer segments of arteries.

Dr. Stary: Many years ago I collected amputated legs from diabetics and nondiabetics and I cross-sectioned the arteries from beginning to end and looked at them under the microscope. I was impressed by frequency and extent of thrombosis. I thought at the time there was more extensive thrombosis in the legs than in coronary arteries of hearts with myocardial infarcts I was seeing at autopsy.

Dr. Fuster: Let me ask about calcification. Dr. Stary, you indicated that calcification appears late, in advanced lesions. But I haven't had the impression from studies of the coronary arteries with ultrafast computed tomography that the presence of calcification necessarily means advanced lesions.

Dr. Stary: Calcification appears early in life because lesions I include and label as advanced by histology (type IV) appear early. Type IV lesions may not obstruct the lumen much. Although there was calcium in all such advanced lesions, the amount was extremely variable for lesions that were otherwise quite similar. Often the amount of calcium was so small that I am convinced it cannot be detected with any of the available clinical techniques.

Dr. J. Frederick Cornhill: If I could make a comment based on studies of young people. Less than 20% of lesions in the abdominal aorta that are advanced by Dr. Stary's classification had calcium recognized by soft x-ray, and <10% of advanced lesions in the right coronary arteries had significant calcium.

Discussant B from the Audience: Diffuse calcification of the lower limb arteries is a very common clinical observation. This is especially frequent in conditions of aging, diabetes, and chronic renal insufficiency. I want to ask what it corresponds to—is it something like the type VIII of Dr. Stary?

Dr. John T. Fallon: I think what you are referring to is the disease called Mönckeberg's sclerosis. This is a fibrotic lesion, with very little or no lipid.

Discussant B from the Audience: Yes, but don't you think that it interferes with the circulation in the lower limbs and adds something to atherosclerosis?

Dr. Fallon: It may have an effect on the capability of the vessel to dilatate and increase flow, but Mönckeberg's sclerosis is not an obstructive process.

Dr. Fuster: Dr. Insull, when I was resident in cardiology and cardiovascular diseases 25 years ago, peripheral vascular disease at Mayo Clinic was a surgical disease. Today, you were talking about it as a medical or interventional disease, but not necessarily surgical. Do you think things have changed over the years? What do you think is happening?

Dr. William Insull, Jr: My impression is that there is a discourse in the literature regarding whom the specialty belongs to, interventional cardiologists or radiologists, surgeons, or less frequently internists. But I think that as therapeutic efforts shift it more into prevention and vigorous medical treatment, it will become more the domain of the general practitioner, and he/she will refer more advanced cases to the specialists.

Dr. Fuster: Dr. Goldstone, you are a surgeon, and it was mentioned this morning that exercise is good for the legs because it improves collateral circulation. Why are we so successful with the legs and less with the heart?

Dr. Goldstone: I don't have the answer to that question, but I have a comment on what Dr. Insull said about the primary care physicians of the future. I think the challenge is that there are few, if any, internal medicine or family practice training programs that teach anything about peripheral vascular disease. So, either all those educational programs are going to have to change or patients aren't going to properly be cared for. I think there will be a new generation of physicians who are likely to be a hybrid between what we now look at as vascular surgery and either interventional radiology or cardiology.

Dr. Fuster: Dr. McGill, you have a lot to offer on these discussions, and you have been rather silent.

Dr. Henry C. McGill: Throughout the day there have been many references to the similarity between atherosclerosis in carotids, coronaries, and aorta, and also many references to differences in behavior. My question to the panel is, with regard to the dogma that most of us subscribe to, that it's the same process modified perhaps by anatomy—is it time to reexamine that dogma systematically in light of what we know now about the pathogenesis of it in various places?

Dr. Colin J. Schwartz: I just wanted to say that I think Henry McGill's comment is extremely important. We tend to gloss over this, but if you look at some of the potential differences, they are quite perplexing. For example, the effect of hypertension in an experimental model system in nonhuman primates is primarily evidenced in the survival vessels to the brain and has much less measurable effect in other vascular beds. So there are differences in the way different parts of our arterial tree respond to at least some of the risk factors, and I think Dr. McGill's point is very well taken.

Dr. Fuster: You don't think that an anatomical component, such as topography and size, plays a role? Why don't we have atherosclerotic disease in our brachial arteries or internal mammary arteries, for example?

Dr. Schwartz: There is a sequence in which lesions develop in the different arterial beds. They don't occur at the same time in all beds. Even if disease advances in one bed, it doesn't necessarily have to be advanced in another bed. And because there's a difference in that sequence, the developmental ages of the lesions can be quite different in different places. That sometimes creates the impression that there are different processes going on. That isn't necessarily true, though it may be true, and is worth investigating. We know that people with carotid disease almost always have coronary disease, but people with coronary disease don't always have carotid disease. There are different sequences depending on geometry, on artery size, and different reactions to different risk factors.

Dr. Cornhill: From our studies it would appear that different risk factors operate at different locations. And I think what that really suggests is we really do need to understand which risk factors work in the lesions we see, such as smoking in one and high-density lipoproteins (HDL) or age in another. We really do need to reevaluate this, based on topography and localization.

Dr. Insull: It would be very useful to know if the lesions in the different artery beds are equivalent, particularly because peripheral arteries could be used as surrogates for more central arteries. That issue has come up repeatedly in the past and we have never had an adequate answer as to what can be a surrogate for what. A careful comparison might enable us to answer that question and have a useful surrogate for coronary arteries.

Dr. Fuster: We have started a collaborative study with nuclear magnetic resonance (NMR) in the carotid arteries, and one of the first things that became obvious is that rupture occurs in much more complex lesions than in the coronary arteries. Accordingly, it is unclear whether imaging the carotid artery is really going to help us to better understand the coronary arteries.

Discussant C from the Audience: I would like to comment, as someone who has practiced the medical side of peripheral vascular disease for many years, that the term "peripheral vascular disease" refers to arterial, venous, and lymphatic diseases. We ought to use the term "atherosclerosis obliterans" when referring to arterial disease. It would save some confusion.

Dr. Fuster: Perhaps it would be nice to have a final comment from Dr. Wissler about the importance of thrombosis and its organization by connective tissue in the progression of atherosclerosis in all vascular beds.

Dr. Robert W. Wissler: I just want to say one brief word about immunochemistry and fibrin and fibrinogen. I think we probably published the first evidence, around 1970, that there is an antigenic component of fibrin and fibrinogen in practically every lesion of atherosclerosis at no matter how young an age, and there is a good deal of evidence the fibrin and fibrinogen may be very important components of the lesion as it develops. But, these are not thrombi. These are fibrin and fibrinogen incorporated into the lesion as a part of the pathogenesis of the lesion. We know from many studies that these molecules do make their way into the intima and they do get deposited. So, I think in order to really be more certain about the role of thrombosis and organization, we probably have to take another look with another set of tools. So far, we don't see very much in coronaries or the aorta below the age of 35, so it's still an open question, at least in the young.

Dr. Schwartz: I just want to add a point here, which I think is quite important. Dr. Wissler is, of course, perfectly correct in pointing out that fibrinogen enters the vessel wall. It does so readily and specifically in lesion-prone areas, and so this is almost a physiological phenomenon. But the point that I think is important is it's not the presence of fibrin, it's the pattern in which the antigen is distributed in the vessel wall that really is critical. This is true also in antiplatelet antigen distribution. The point is that you get a very distinct banded pattern as distinct from flecks and little spots. The banded pattern is the one that is regarded as reflecting the footprints of past thrombi in the vessel that I feel, as do other observants, play a critical role in the progression of atherosclerosis in all vascular beds.

Dr. Stary: We too have found that most lesions, and sometimes even nonatherosclerotic intima, stain positively for fibrinogen. This fibrinogen gets into the intima from the plasma as do many other proteins. But the morphology of this ubiquitous fibrinogen differs from that of the fibrinogen-positive thrombotic remnants that we show to be present in many lesions. We regard as thrombotic remnants only the fibrinogen-positive bands of matrix material that have a morphology similar to that of proven thrombi.

Dr. Fuster: This issue is obviously quite important. If indeed mural thrombi are critical in the progression of atherosclerosis in all vascular beds, the question for future investigators is this: Can we develop antithrombotic agents that prevent mural thrombi without causing bleeding? Certainly today, aspirin and oral anticoagulants are of benefit for the prevention of occlusive thrombus, but are of no benefit at all for the prevention of mural thrombi, the most active part of the clots, or those closer to the vessel wall.

Chapter 15

Imaging Techniques in Carotid and Peripheral Vascular Disease

Robert E. Dinsmore, MD and S. Mitchell Rivitz, MD

Introduction

Most imaging studies of the carotid and peripheral vessels are done for clinical indications, usually the signs and symptoms of ischemia. The pathophysiology of carotid and iliofemoral atherosclerosis is similar; both are associated with obstructive vascular lesions or thromboembolism. Although the clinical objectives in imaging of the two vascular beds are not identical, in each the approach to imaging has traditionally focused on evaluation of the vascular lumen for stenosis severity, and more recently, for stenosis morphology.

Another important indication for carotid or peripheral vascular studies is as a component of clinical trials correlating the effect of risk-factor modification on atherosclerosis progression or regression. These studies may be a part of an evaluation of the general nature of arteriosclerosis, or the carotid and peripheral arteries may be used as surrogates for atherosclerosis of the coronary arteries because of their greater accessibility to low-risk noninvasive imaging methods. The results of these studies extend our understanding of vascular disease and offer the possibility of identifying and following persons with risk factors for atherosclerosis before the onset of symptoms in order to prevent or ameliorate the clinical sequelae.

From: Fuster V, (ed.) *Syndromes of Atherosclerosis: Correlations of Clinical Imaging and Pathology.* Armonk, NY: Futura Publishing Company, Inc.: © 1996.

Imaging Objectives and Selection of Imaging Techniques

The choice of imaging technique depends on the questions being asked, and on the specific capabilities of the available methods for display of the characteristics of the vascular lesions that are of clinical or research interest, including stenosis severity, morphology, distribution, and extent. A large number of imaging techniques are now available for these studies. Among the techniques, conventional angiography, intra-arterial digital subtraction angiography (DSA), and ultrasonography have well-defined roles. Magnetic resonance angiography (MRA) is now widely used, but its specific indications with respect to other noninvasive methods remain to be determined. Intravascular ultrasonography (IVUS) and spiral, or helical computed tomography (CT) are promising for selected applications, but need further evaluation.

Clinical Imaging Objectives

The clinical objectives in the management of patients with carotid vascular disease are preventive, to identify patients at a high risk for stroke, and therapeutic, to determine the cause of and appropriate treatment for stroke or transient ischemic attacks that have already occurred. Because cerebral ischemia may result from either severe arterial stenosis or from cerebral emboli, the usefulness of the various imaging techniques depends on their ability to elucidate these phenomena.

In the case of peripheral vascular disease, the clinical objectives of arterial imaging of the abdominal aorta through the lower extremities are primarily for the management of signs and symptoms already present. Thus, the indications for vascular imaging are, first, intermittent claudication in patients who are candidates for intervention for symptom relief, and second, limb salvage in patients with severe ischemia. In addition to atherosclerosis, rarer causes of occlusive disease such as Burger's disease, fibromuscular dysplasia, and vasculitities must be considered. The goal of the imaging examination is to confirm the diagnosis and to plan the appropriate treatment, usually angioplasty or vascular surgery. In many patients, there will be an intermediate step consisting of non-imaging tests such as pulse volume recordings or segmental limb arterial pressure measurement.

Selection of the best treatment for the individual patient, whether an interventional radiological procedure, an open surgical procedure, or noninterventional management depends on accurate characterization of arterial lesions. Attributes which should be addressed include stenosis severity and length, lesion morphology (eccentricity, presence of thrombus, ulceration, calcification, or aneurysm), distribution and extent of lesions, and presence of collateral vessels. Each of these characteristics can be assessed better with certain imaging modalities than with others, and a combined approach is often useful.

Imaging Method Selection: Characteristics of Lesions

The lesion characteristic that historically has been considered of greatest clinical importance, and that has received the most attention, is *stenosis severity*. However, although available methods can accurately demonstrate stenosis diameter, the hemodynamic significance of a given stenosis is often uncertain. The traditional clinical index of stenosis has been percent diameter reduction, with reference to the diameter of adjacent normal artery.[1] The North American Symptomatic Carotid Endarterectomy Trial (NASCET) showed that for carotid stenosis in the presence of symptomatic cerebral vascular disease, >70% stenosis predicts an increasing risk of major stroke due to compromised blood flow.[2] Roederer et al[3] found that >80% diameter stenosis correlated with the likelihood of progression to total occlusion or development of new symptoms. The kidney is estimated to become ischemic at rest distal to an 80% diameter stenosis.[4] Stenoses of <50% are generally not flow limiting; pressure gradient measurements may be helpful in determining the physiologic significance of stenoses between 50% and 70%.[5,6] However, one must be cautious in interpretation of a "pullback" pressure in which a single measuring catheter is pulled across a stenosis to determine a pressure gradient because the catheter itself can falsely elevate the true gradient by its presence. The best method is simultaneous pressure measurement on both sides of a lesion, but this requires two arterial punctures and is usually not practical in peripheral vascular disease.

Similar to the experience with coronary angiography, percent diameter reduction has limitations as a measurement of carotid and peripheral artery stenosis severity. It does not account for other factors affecting the physiologic effect of the stenosis, such as lesion length and geometry, tandem lesions,[7] or collateral vessels. Its accuracy depends on an assumption that the "normal" reference diameter is in fact normal, whereas an arterial segment used for a reference diameter may be narrowed by diffuse disease,[8] increased slightly by the compensatory response to early atheroma[9,10] or more severely by ectasia associated with medial atrophy.[11]

Because of these problems, some investigators have felt that the use of residual luminal diameter is more meaningful physiologically than percent stenosis,[12] although this also has limitations. The stenosis diameter indicating critical stenosis varies depending on the artery in question, and the method does not account for variations due to patient size, anatomic variations in the amount of tissue supplied, lesion length, the presence of tandem lesions, or the adequacy of collateral supply. In the case of the carotid artery, 1.5-mm residual luminal diameter causes the ipsilateral anterior cerebral artery to fill from the opposite carotid artery, assuming a normal circle of Willis,[13] and stroke is uncommon when minimum luminal diameter is 1.0–1.5 mm or greater.[14] Ackerman et al[13] have concluded that 1.0 mm may be the most useful indicator of potential stroke.

Transfemoral angiography remains the standard with which other methods are compared for the evaluation of lumen stenosis. It has generally been considered to be the technique that most reliably discriminates between virtual and complete occlusion, a distinction that, in patients with carotid disease, may mean the difference between surgical and medical management. Intra-arterial DSA is used with increasing frequency as an alternative to conventional arteriography for cerebral and peripheral vascular disease, allowing a more rapid examination and a lower dose of contrast medium.[15] However, resolution is less than that of film-based arteriography and the lack of gray scale from the subtraction technique makes edge differentiation more difficult. In general, catheter-based angiography has the disadvantages that it is invasive, uses contrast medium and x-radiation, and is expensive. Intravenous DSA is less invasive than intra-arterial DSA, but although initial reports were enthusiastic, sensitivity and specificity were poor and the method is now rarely used.

Noninvasive methods are used increasingly for assessment of stenosis either for screening prior to angiography or as an alternative to catheter studies. Duplex ultrasonography, combining B-mode imaging with pulsed Doppler, and color flow Doppler are now the most widely used noninvasive methods for initial examination for suspected extracranial carotid disease[16,17] and for asymptomatic bruits, or before major vascular surgery. Whereas ultrasound is more commonly used in the evaluation of carotid rather than peripheral disease, in many centers it is used for the assessment of lower extremity arteries as well.

The advantages of ultrasound include absence of radiation,

provision of both anatomic and physiologic information, and patient comfort. In addition, the equipment is mobile and the examination is less expensive than angiography. Disadvantages include a considerable degree of operator dependence and a large time requirement. It is difficult to distinguish near-occlusion from occlusion with ultrasound. It can only be used for vessels that are accessible to the ultrasound transducer. For example, the proximal common carotid artery and abdominal and pelvic vessels can be difficult to examine by ultrasound, and random lesions may be difficult to demonstrate. Calcified plaque can obscure the demonstration of residual lumen.

Pulsed Doppler ultrasound provides a noninvasive measurement of flow velocity, which is related to stenosis severity, and correlates well with angiography for measurement of lumen stenosis. In comparison with angiography, sensitivity and specificity of 84% and 99% for identification of stenosis >50% has been reported for the carotid arteries,[16] and between 80% and 93% for the lower extremity arteries.[17] B-mode ultrasound is an excellent method for demonstrating the vascular wall and lumen, but is less accurate than Doppler ultrasound for evaluation of stenosis severity, particularly because hypoechoic plaques may not be distinguishable from the vascular lumen.[13]

Data obtained via Doppler can help to plan the performance of catheter arteriography for possible angioplasty. In conjunction with a baseline study, it is particularly useful for following patients for possible progression of either carotid or peripheral disease, for postoperative assessment of arterial grafts, or for evaluation of complications of angiography such as pseudo-aneurysm or arteriovenous fistula.[18]

MRA, which is discussed elsewhere in this book, is becoming widely used, often in conjunction with ultrasound, but is not universally available.[19,20] Similar to angiography, MRA shows the entire vascular tree but is completely noninvasive. Presently, MRA appears to be less accurate for stenosis measurement than either contrast angiography or Doppler ultrasound.[21]

Intravascular ultrasound has been shown to be highly accurate for measurement of stenosis area,[22] which unlike stenosis diameter determined by projectional angiographic studies, is independent of cross-sectional luminal shape. However, it is expensive and invasive, and its benefit for stenosis severity determination in clinical practice is unproven.[23]

Helical or spiral CT is the most recent addition to the list of noninvasive methods applied to vascular imaging.[24,25] Iodinated contrast medium is given intravenously and a series of tomographic images of the area of interest is taken at the time of peak contrast intensity, with three-dimensional reconstruction. Theoretically, this method is able to show the vessel wall, but resolution has not been good enough for plaque characterization. Disadvantages include the need for precise timing and for a relatively large contrast medium volume. Helical CT has been used for the carotid bifurcation and major abdominal aortic branches, but has not been useful for peripheral arteries because of dilution of contrast material. Further evaluation is needed before its role is known.

In comparison with stenosis severity, the presence of *ulceration* can be difficult to determine by any of the usual clinical methods. Whereas the classic angiographic "collar stud" appearance is indicative of ulceration, fissures may be microscopic and not identifiable by any available clinical imaging technique. Even large ulcerations may be difficult to identify. They may be mimicked by residual lumen between plaques, or by irregular plaque borders without erosion. An ulceration may be evident, but reendothelialized and no longer a source of emboli. The correlation between either angiography or ultrasound and pathologic examination in identification of ulceration is poor,[26] however, angiography is probably the best available method.[14] MRA has had poorer success than ultrasound. Angioscopy is probably more sensitive than angiography for detection of complex plaques in general, including ulcerated lesions.[27]

Recent tissue characterization studies using B-mode ultrasound have suggested the possibility of identification of unstable lesions with *plaque hemorrhage,*[28] and of *vulnerable, "soft" lesions* at greater risk for becoming unstable.[29] Because of the possibility of determining the composition of plaques by IVUS, it may be possible to identify soft lipid plaques that are vulnerable to rupture by this method as well.[30–32] However, because IVUS is even more invasive than contrast angiography in that it requires passage of the transducer wire through the region to be studied, the potential clinical significance of this application is uncertain. B-mode ultrasonography, helical CT, and IVUS are also highly sensitive for identification of *calcification,*[24,32] which along with lesion *eccentricity* is clinically important primarily for its influence on selection of treatment method.

The determination that ischemia in an individual patient is caused by *thromboemboli* is often difficult. In patients with adequate collateral pathways, the most common cause of carotid-related stroke is cerebral embolus rather than carotid artery stenosis per se.[13] In these patients the importance of the stenotic carotid lesion is in its predisposition to thromboembolus formation due to stasis distal to severe stenosis, or to a ruptured and thrombosed lesion. Cerebral emboli may also arise in the heart or from the aorta,[33] and in the individual case, the cause of embolus commonly remains unexplained. Angioscopy appears to be more sensitive than either angiography or intravascular ultrasound for detection of thrombus.[34] However, angioscopy is invasive, has only a limited range of view, and is presently an investigational method. Currently, contrast angiography is probably the best clinical method for detection of thrombus.

Characterization of the *distribution* and *extent* of disease and the presence of *collateral blood supply* is also important. Demonstration of the circulation of the entire carotid or peripheral vascular tree may be clinically important for demonstration of collateral circulation, retrograde flow, identification of emboli, or recognition of the presence of diffuse or multifocal disease. For example, decreased flow in the carotid system will cause ischemic events only in the 10% to 15% of patients with inadequate collateral paths. The quality of the runoff vascular bed is an important consideration in the management of stenotic lesions. This can best be shown by an angiographic method, whether conventional angiography, DSA, or possibly MRA. In the case of carotid disease, indirect noninvasive tests, including oculoplethysmography and transcranial Doppler are increasingly used as an adjunct to duplex ultrasound to exclude possible internal cerebral disease. Some have predicted that a combination of ultrasound and MRA may ultimately supplant invasive angiography.[16]

Lesion Characteristics and Selection of Treatment

The presence and severity of each of the lesion characteristics bears on management decisions. For example, the criteria for peripheral angioplasty depend on lesion morphology.[35] Relative contraindications include eccentricity, heavy calcification, particularly in an eccentric lesion, ulcerative disease in the presence of evidence of distal embolization, and extensive disease in a long segment.

The performance of endovascular intervention is primarily guided by DSA because of its rapid production of images. However, IVUS may have advantages in guiding certain interventional procedures such as the placement of stents, and in identifying complications of angioplasty such as deep or spiral dissection. Because IVUS can demonstrate plaque thickness and eccentricity, and the presence of calcium, it may be useful in determining the relative merit of different interventional devices for individual lesions.[36] These applications will need further investigation.

Although many of the characteristics of vascular lesions can be imaged by more than one method, and practice patterns are changing to greater use of noninvasive tests, the mainstay of diagnostic and interventional work is still intra-arterial catheter arteriography. Arteriography can delineate stenosis severity, length, eccentricity, thrombus, ulceration, emboli, distribution, and collateral vessels, all during a single examination.

Studies of the Effect of Risk Factors and Their Modification on Progression of Atherosclerosis

Study Objectives and Significance of Lesion Characteristics

Serial angiographic studies have contributed important information about the natural history, influence of risk factors, and the effect of interventions on atherosclerosis of the coronary arteries, allowing smaller sample sizes and shorter study durations than are required if clinical end-points are used. However, the use of angiography is limited by its invasive nature, which for ethical reasons limits studies to symptomatic patients and relatively advanced disease. The traditional angiographic luminal images are most useful if the object of these studies is to relate disease severity to clinical outcome. For studies of atherosclerosis progression, early detection and accurate estimation of the extent of the disease and of change are critical. Because atherosclerosis is a disease of the vascular wall that encroaches on the lumen only in a relatively late stage,[9] an increase in wall thickness is an earlier marker of atherosclerosis than luminal narrowing and is a more sensitive indicator of change. Compared to B-mode ultrasound or IVUS images of the vascular wall, angiograms are not sensitive for detection of early lesions[37] and are inherently less accurate for quantitation of change in lesion size because of their dependence on the indirect effect of lesions on the vascular lumen.

Duplex ultrasound is in many ways a potentially ideal research method for study of atherosclerosis. Stenosis severity of accessible lesions is accurately measured by the Doppler technique. High-resolution B-mode imaging accurately measures wall thickness and is sensitive in detection of early atherosclerosis.[26,38-40] It appears to be reproducible and therefore capable of precise noninvasive assessment of change in plaque size.[41,42] The development of noninvasive methods for study of the carotid and peripheral arteries also opens the possibility of using these vascular beds as surrogate for the less accessible coronary arteries.[43,44] However, Ricotta et al[26] have emphasized the importance of establishing standards for measurement criteria and quality control.

Margitic et al[45] summarized the issues yet to be resolved in epidemiologic and clinical trial studies of carotid atherosclerosis. These include defining the point at which adaptive wall thickening evolves into an atherosclerotic plaque and what risk factors are associated with this transition; determining which risk factors cause destabilization of plaques; establishing standard end-point definitions; and determining the value of ultrasound assessment of carotid atherosclerosis in predicting overall cardiovascular morbidity/mortality.

Relationship of Atherosclerosis Severity and Risk Factors in Carotid, Peripheral, and Coronary Arteries

In order to evaluate the significance of carotid or peripheral artery studies relative to studies of other vascular beds it is important to know the relationship between atherosclerosis severity in each of these vascular beds with the others, as well as the relative effects of the various risk factors on the different vascular beds. Solberg et al[46] reviewed multiple autopsy studies correlating the degree of atherosclerosis of carotid and coronary arteries and the aorta, and concluded that on a group basis, the amount of lesion involvement in one of these vascular regions is correlated with the average amount of lesion involvement in each of the others. In another autopsy study, Young et al[47] found that at any particular age, coronary atherosclerosis was on average more advanced than atherosclerosis of the carotid artery. In the individual subject, the severity of atherosclerosis in one arterial bed does not, however, predict the severity in another.[46,48] The correlation of severity between cerebral and coronary arteries has been found to be less strong than that of the relationship of severity within each of these vascular beds;[48] there is a strong correlation between the severity of lesions in one of a pair of cerebral arteries and the severity in the other artery.[46] In a study of 510 patients, 343 of whom had at least 50% stenosis in one or more coronary arteries, Craven et al[43] found that the severity of carotid disease on B-mode ultrasound study was comparable to the severity of coronary artery disease on angiography.

The effect of any particular risk factor with respect to different vascular beds does not appear to be uniform. For example, Solberg et al[49] and Holme et al[50] found hypertension to be a stronger risk factor for cerebral atherosclerosis than for coronary atherosclerosis. Smoking is a significant risk factor for atherosclerosis of the aorta and coronary arteries,[51] but appears to be a stronger risk factor for aortic, cerebral, and femoral than for coronary artery disease.[50]

Conclusion

Carotid and peripheral vascular imaging studies are performed for a variety of reasons in patients with atherosclerosis, including the evaluation of clinical signs and symptoms, the selection and monitoring of therapy, and investigation of the effect of drugs and other interventions on the progression of atherosclerosis. The purpose of the imaging studies is to determine the presence of lesions, define their characteristics, and assess change. An increasing variety of imaging methods are available, each with known or potential advantages and disadvantages. The selection of optimum imaging methods ultimately depends on their ability to define those lesion characteristics that best relate to the clinical or research questions being asked.

The diagnosis of the presence of ischemia and the determination of when to treat is based primarily on stenosis severity, and the selection of appropriate treatment on lesion morphology and distribution. For risk factor studies, accurate noninvasive detection and measurement of change in vascular lesions is optimum. At the present time, ultrasound appears to be an ideal method for this purpose. However, it is important that examinations and endpoints be standardized.

References

1. Feldman E, Ackerman RH, Rosner B, et al. Progression of carotid disease and onset of ischemic symptoms: A study based on noninvasive/clinical correlations. *Ann Neurol* 1983;14:132.
2. Barnett HJM and the North American Symptomatic Carotid Endareterectomy Trial Collaborators. Beneficial effects of carotid endarectomy in symptomatic patients with high-grade carotid stenosis. *N Engl J Med* 1991;325:445–453.
3. Roederer GO, Langlois YE, Jager KA, et al. The natural history of carotid arterial disease in asymptomatic patients with cervical bruits. *Stroke* 1984;15:605–613.
4. May AG, Deweese JA, Rob CG. Hemodynamic effects of arterial stenosis. *Surgery* 1963;54:250.

5. Brewster DC, Waltman AC, O'Hara PJ. Femoral artery pressure measurements during aortography. *Circulation* 1979(suppl);60:120.
6. Udoff EJ, Barth KH, Harrington DP, et al. Hemodynamic significance of iliac artery stenosis: Pressure measurements during angiography. *Radiology* 1979;132:289.
7. Goldstein RA, Kirkeeide RL, Demer LL, et al. Relation between geometric dimensions of coronary artery stenoses and myocardial perfusion reserve in man. *J Clin Invest* 1987;79:1473–1478.
8. Arnett EN, Isner JM, Redwood DR, et al. Coronary artery narrowing in coronary heart disease: Comparison of cineangiographic and necropsy findings. *Ann Intern Med* 1979;91:350–356.
9. Glagov S, Weisenberg E, Zarins CK, et al. Compensatory enlargement of human atheroosclerotic coronary arteries. *N Engl J Med* 1987;316: 1371–1375.
10. Steinke W, Els T, Hemmerice M. Compensatory carotid artery dilatation in early atherosclerosis. *Circulation* 1994;89:2578–2581.
11. Markis JE, Joffe CD, Cohn PF, et al. Clinical significance of coronary arterial ectasia. *Am J Cardiol* 1976;37:217–222.
12. Ackerman RH, Candia MR. Identifying clinically relevant carotid disease. *Stroke* 1994;25:1–3.
13. Ackerman RH. Cerebrovascular non-invasive evaluation. In: Taveras JT, Ferrucci J, eds. *Radiology/Diagnosis/Imaging/Interventional*. Volume 3. Philadelphia: Lippincott; 1995:1–28.
14. Ackerman RH. Estimation of residual internal carotid artery lumen diameter using arteriographic evidence of intracranial hemodynamic change. *AJNR* 1987;8:950.
15. Carroll BA, Graif M, Orron DE. Vascular ultrasound. In: Kim D, Orron DE. *Peripheral Vascular Imaging and Intervention*. St. Louis, MO: Mosby-Year Book; 1992:211–225.
16. Carroll BA. Carotid sonography. *Radiology* 1991;178:303–313.
17. Taylor DC, Strandness DE Jr. Carotid artery duplex scanning. *J Clin Ultrasound* 1987;15:635–644.
18. Kohler TR, Nance DR, Cramer MM, et al. Duplex scanning for diagnosis of aortoiliac and femoropopliteal disease: A prospective study. *Circulation* 1987;76:1074.
19. Yucel EK, Kaufman JA, Geller SC, et al. Atherosclerotic occlusive disease of the lower extremity: Prospective evaluation with two-dimensional time-of-flight MR angiography. *Radiology* 1993;187:637–641.
20. Edelman RR. MR angiography: Present and future. *AJR* 1993;161:1–11.
21. Atlas SW. MR angiography in neurologic disease. *Radiology* 1994;193: 1–16.
22. Nishimura RA, Edwards WD, Warnes CA, et al. Intravascular ultrasound imaging: In vitro validation and pathologic correlation. *J Am Coll Cardiol* 1990;16:145–154.
23. Nishimura RA, Reeder GS. Intravascular ultrasound. Research technique or clinical tool? *Circulation* 1992;86:322–324.
24. Cumming MJ, Morrow IM. Carotid artery stenosis: A prospective comparison of CT angiography and conventional angiography. *AJR* 1994;163:517–523.
25. Stehling MK, Lawrence JA, Weintraub JL, et al. CT angiography: Expanded clinical applications. *AJR* 1994;163:947–955.
26. Ricotta JJ, Bryan FA, Bond MG, et al. Multicenter validation study of

real-time (B-mode) ultrasound, arteriography, and pathologic examination. *J Vasc Surg* 1987;6:512–520.

27. Sherman CT, Litvack F, Grundfest W, et al. Coronary angioscopy in patients with unstable angina pectoris. *N Engl J Med* 1986;315:913–919.

28. Bluth EL, Kay D, Merritt CRB, et al. Sonographic characterization of carotid plaque detection of hemorrhages. *AJR* 1986;146:1061–1065.

29. Johnson JM, Kennelly MM, Descesane D, et al. Natural history of asymptomatic carotid plaque. *Arch Surg* 1985;120:1010–1012.

30. Tobis JM, Mallery J, Mahon D, et al. Intravascular ultrasound imaging of human coronary arteries in vivo. Analysis of tissue characterizations with comparison to in vitro histological specimens. *Circulation* 1991;83:913–926.

31. Potkin BN, Bartorelli AL, Gessert JM, et al. Coronary artery imaging with intravascular high-frequency ultrasound. *Circulation* 1990;81:1575–1585.

32. Gussenhoven EJ, Essed CE, Lancee CT, et al. Arterial wall characteristics determined by intravascular ultrasound imaging: An in vitro study. *J Am Coll Cardiol* 1989;14:947–952.

33. Amarenco P, Cohen A, Tzourico C, et al. Atherosclerostic disease of the aortic arch and the risk of ischemic stroke. *N Engl J Med* 1994;331:1474–1479.

34. Siegel RJ, Ariani M, Fishbein MC, et al. Histopathologic validation of angioscopy and intravascular ultrasound. *Circulation* 1991;84:109–117.

35. Standards of Practice Committee of the Society of Cardiovascular Interventional Radiology. Guidelines for percutaneous transluminal angioplasty. *Radiology* 1990;177:619–626.

36. Yock PG, Fitzgerald PJ, Linker DT. Intravascular ultrasound guidance for catheter-based coronary interventions. *J Am Coll Cardiol* 1991;17:39B-45B.

37. St. Goar FG, Pinto FJ, Alderman EL, et al. Intracoronary ultrasound in cardiac transplant recipients. In vivo evidence of "angiographically silent" intimal thickening. *Circulation* 1992;85:979–987.

38. Pignoli P. Ultrasound B-mode imaging for arterial wall thickness measurement. *Atheroscler Rev* 1984;12:177–184.

39. Pignoli P, Tremoli, E, Poli A, et al. Intimal plus medial thickness of the arterial wall: A direct measurement with ultrasound imaging. *Circulation* 1986;74:1399–1406.

40. O'Leary DH, Bryan FA, Goodison MW, et al. Measurement variability of carotid atherosclerosis: Real-time (B-mode) ultrasonography and angiography. *Stroke* 1987;18:1011–1017.

41. Salonen R, Salonen JT. Progression of carotid atherosclerosis and its determinants: A population-based ultrasonography study. *Atherosclerosis* 1990;81:33–36.

42. Bond MG, Wilmoth SK, Enevold GL, et al. Detection and monitoring of asymptomatic atherosclerosis in clinical trials. *Am J Med* 1989;86(suppl 4A):33–36.

43. Craven TE, Ryu JE, Espeland MA, et al. Evaluation of the associations between carotid artery atherosclerosis and coronary artery stenosis. *Circulation* 1990;82:1230–1242.

44. Salonen JT, Salonen R. Ultrasonically assessed carotid morphology and the risk of coronary heart disease. *Arterioscler Thromb* 1991;11:1245–1249.

45. Margitic SE, Bond MG, Crouse JR, et al. Progression and regression of carotid atherosclerosis in clinical trials. *Arteriosclerosis* 1991;11:443–451.
46. Sollberg LA, McGarry PA, Moossy J, et al. Severity of atherosclerosis in cerebral arteries, coronary arteries, and aortas. *Ann NY Acad Sci* 1968;149(2):956–973.
47. Young W, Gofman JW, Malamud N, et al. The interrelationship between cerebral and coronary atherosclerosis. *Geriatrics* 1956;11:413.
48. Young W, Gofman JW, Tandy R, et al. The quantitation of atherosclerosis. III. The extent of correlation of degrees of atherosclerosis within and between the coronary and cerebral vascular beds. *Am J Cardiol* 1960;6:300–308.
49. Sollberg LA, Strong JP. Risk factors and atherosclerotic lesions. A review of autopsy studies. *Arteriosclerosis* 1983;3:187–198.
50. Holme I, Enger SC, Helegeland A, et al. Risk factors and raised atherosclerotic lesions in coronary and cerebral arteries. Statistical analysis from the Oslo study. *Arteriosclerosis* 1981;1:250–256.
51. Strong JP, Richards ML. Cigarette smoking and atherosclerosis in autopsied men. *Atherosclerosis* 1976;23:451–476.

Chapter 16

Detection and Quantification of Atherosclerosis:
The Emerging Role For Intravascular Ultrasound

Steven E. Nissen MD, E. Murat Tuzcu MD, and Anthony C. DeFranco MD

Introduction

Accurate detection and precise quantification of coronary atherosclerosis in vivo represents an important, although daunting, challenge for cardiovascular research and clinical practice. Until recently, atherosclerotic coronary lesions could not be directly visualized by any available imaging modality. Accordingly, detection of coronary artery disease has relied principally on indirect methods that either depict the vessel lumen (angiography) or unmask the ischemic effect of coronary obstructions (nuclear or stress echocardiography). However, both methods are insensitive to the early, minimally obstructive disease associated with the dramatic and often lethal consequences of coronary atherosclerosis—acute coronary syndromes.

After its introduction by Sones et al in 1958, and in the absence of a direct method for visualizing atherosclerotic plaques, angiography has constituted the principal modality used by clinicians and investigators to determine the anatomic severity of coronary artery disease. For more than 35 years, coronary angiography has represented the "gold standard" for the diagnosis of coronary disease, growing in frequency to more than 1 million procedures annually in the United States. The diagnos-

From: Fuster V, (ed.) *Syndromes of Atherosclerosis: Correlations of Clinical Imaging and Pathology.* Armonk, NY: Futura Publishing Company, Inc.: © 1996.

tic preeminence of coronary angiography remained unchallenged during the development of balloon angioplasty and other per-cutaneous coronary revascularization techniques in the 1980s. This practice has resulted in a particularly singled-minded, non-critical acceptance by clinicians of the "luminogram" as the principal determinant of the indications and success of coronary interventions.

Presently, an alternative imaging modality, ie, intravascular ultrasound, is challenging the dominance of coronary angiography in the diagnosis and therapy of coronary disease. Catheter-based ultrasound represents a radically different approach to the imaging of vascular anatomy. The incremental value of coronary ultrasound originates principally from two key features: the cross-sectional, tomographic perspective of the images and the ability to image atheromata directly. Whereas angiography depicts the complex cross-sectional anatomy of a human coronary as a planar silhouette, ultrasound directly examines the anatomy within the vessel wall, allowing the operator to measure atheroma size, distribution, and composition precisely (Figure 1). Accordingly, coronary ultrasound is yielding important insights into diverse phenomena, ranging from the pathophysiology of coronary syndromes to the mechanical effects of interventional devices.

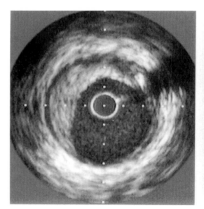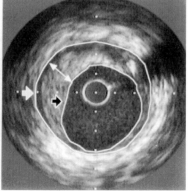

FIGURE 1. *Intravascular ultrasound of typical coronary atheroma. In the right panel, the white arrow indicates planimetry of the media-adventi-tial border and the black arrow shows the tracing of the intimal leading edge. The double-headed arrow shows the maximal thickness of the atherosclerotic plaque.*

Limitations of Angiography

The rationale for intracoronary ultrasound arises from well-established limitations of coronary angiography. In the 1960s and 1970s, investigators first began questioning the accuracy and reproducibility of the coronary angiogram.[1,2] Studies established that visual interpretation of angiograms exhibit significant observer variability.[1] Other investigations reported major discrepancies between the apparent lesion severity and postmortem examination.[2] More recently, investigators have documented major differences between the apparent severity of lesions and measurements of the physiologic effects of stenoses.[3] Although quantitative coronary angiography has improved the reproducibility of coronary luminal measurements, this technique is limited by magnification errors, inability to detect disease at the reference segment, and by the limited number of the projections available.[4]

In percutaneous intervention, the theoretical limitations of angiography are particularly relevant. Radiographic imaging depicts complex coronary cross-sectional anatomy from a planar silhouette of the contrast-filled lumen. Most mechanical interventions exaggerate the extent of luminal eccentricity by fracturing or dissecting the atheroma.[5] This disruption of the atherosclerotic plaque permits extravasation of contrast media into (or beneath) the atheroma. The silhouette (angiographic appearance) of the complex postintervention vessel often consists of an enlarged, although frequently "hazy" lumen. When extensive plaque fracture occurs, the hazy, broadened angiographic silhouette may overestimate the vessel cross section and misrepresent the actual gain in lumen size.

Angiography represents an indirect and relative measure of luminal narrowing. To evaluate the severity of any specific lesion, the angiographer must identify and measure the diameter of an adjacent "reference site," which is presumed free of disease. However, postmortem studies have consistently demonstrated that coronary atherosclerosis is typically a diffuse, rather than focal process. Accordingly, no truly normal reference segment exists from which to calculate percent. In this setting, the calculated percent diameter stenosis will underestimate the true lesion severity by comparing the lesion diameter with a narrowed reference segment. Atherosclerotic involvement of the reference segment also has important implications for interventional practice because reference segment disease will affect assessment of the target vessel, influencing device selection, sizing, and assessment of results.

Coronary Intravascular Ultrasound

Theoretical Advantages

Atherosclerotic plaque morphology constitutes a critical determinant of the prognosis and natural history of coronary disease. Intravascular ultrasound represents the first and only diagnostic technique that provides direct visualization of atherosclerotic coronary plaques in vivo. The tomographic orientation of ultrasound enables visualization of the full 360⁻-circumference of the vessel wall, not merely a silhouette of the lumen. This capability permits direct measurements of lumen dimensions, including minimum and maximum diameter and cross-sectional area. The constant velocity of sound in soft tissue permits ultrasound scanners to overlay a highly accurate, electronically-generated distance scale within the image. This capability obviates the need to correct for radiographic magnification, a troublesome requisite of angiographic methods.[4]

Devices and Techniques

Catheter Designs

The equipment required for intracoronary ultrasound examination consists of two major components, a catheter incorporating a miniaturized transducer and a console containing the necessary electronics to reconstruct an ultrasound image. The current generation of catheters range in size from 2.9F to 3.5F (0.96 to 1.17 mm). The most advanced devices yield remarkably high image quality, primarily as a consequence of the high operating frequency (20 to 30 MHz) and close proximity to the target. Axial resolution typically approaches 80 μm, while lateral resolution is depth-dependent, averaging about 200 μm.

There are two approaches to the design of intracoronary ultrasound devices—mechanical transducers and multielement electronic designs. Mechanical devices use an external motor drive to rotate a single piezoelectric transducer mounted near the distal end of the catheter. Mechanical transducers typically operate at 1800 revolutions per minute to yield 30 frames per second. Rotating mechanical devices provide greater acoustic power than multielement systems because acoustic energy is directed to a single ultrasound element. The higher power yields greater dynamic range and tissue penetration than do electronic probes, resulting in better image quality, although this gap appears to be narrowing.

Some recent catheter designs use a different approach in which sheath-type covering is advanced distally into the vessel, the guidewire removed, and the ultrasound transducer is passed freely within the sheath to image the vessel. Recent sheath-type devices incorporate a distal lumen that is shared by the transducer and guidewire, a feature that allows maximum transducer size with minimum sheath size. The electronic approach to ultrasound catheter design uses 32 elements mounted in an annular array near the distal catheter tip.[6] Precise, sequential timing of various groups of these elements results in a sweep of the ultrasound signal through the 360° vessel arc. The main advantages of this approach include excellent shaft flexibility and optimal guidewire tracking. However, an image quality disadvantage stems from a lower frequency (20 MHz), reduced acoustic power, and a smaller aperture, which limits lateral resolution.

A unique version of the multielement catheter recently approved by the Food and Drug Admionistration, the Oracle-Micro™ (Endosonics Corp, Pleasanton, Ca), uses an imaging transducer mounted a few millimeters proximal to a standard angioplasty balloon. This device allows examination of the vessel before and after angioplasty without requiring a catheter exchange.

Laboratory Technique

Catheter handling procedures are similar to standard interventional techniques. The operator subselective cannulates the vessel using a steerable guidewire and interrogates the vessel by carefully advancing or retracting the imaging catheter over the wire.[7] As the transducer is moved to various points along the vessel, the operator examines the vessel in real time, recording images on videotape for subsequent quantitative analysis. Although currently available ultrasound devices are quite flexible and allow a traumatic coronary examination, these probes have handling characteristics distinctly inferior to modern angioplasty balloons. While typical ultrasound catheters are small and flexible enough for routine imaging, interrogation of heavily diseased or distally located coronary segments remains challenging. Monorail designs facilitate rapid catheter exchanges and allow a guidewire to remain safely in position well beyond critical coronary stenoses.

Safety of Coronary Ultrasound

Although intravascular ultrasound requires intracoronary instrumentation, studies have demonstrated few serious untoward effects.[8] Transient coronary spasm occurs in about 5% of patients, but usually responds rapidly to administration of intracoronary nitroglycerin. The imaging transducer may temporarily obstruct or severely reduce coronary flow when advanced into tight stenoses or small distal vessels, but patients generally do not experience chest pain if the catheter is promptly withdrawn. In both the diagnostic and interventional catheterization, most experienced practitioners administer heparin (5,000 to 10,000 units) prior to intracoronary imaging. Despite the relative safety of coronary ultrasound, any intracoronary instrumentation carries the potential risk of intimal injury or vessel dissection. Although many centers use ultrasound during diagnostic catheterization, most laboratories limit credentialing for intravascular imaging procedures to personnel with interventional training.

Artifacts and Limitations

Mechanical transducers may exhibit cyclical oscillations in rotational speed, nonuniform rotational distortion (NURD), which arises from mechanical drag on the catheter drive shaft producing visible distortion. NURD is most evident when the drive shaft is bent into a small radius of curvature by a tortuous vessel and is recognized as circumferential "stretching" of a portion of the image with compression of the contralateral vessel wall. An additional artifact, transducer ring-down, appears in virtually all medical ultrasound devices. This artifact arises from acoustic oscillations in the piezoelectric transducer material, resulting in high-amplitude signals that obscure the near-field imaging. The resultant inability to image structures immediately adjacent to the transducer yields a device with an "acoustic" size larger than its physical size.

Interpretation of Coronary Ultrasound

Normal Anatomy

A series of investigations have characterized the appearance of normal coronary anatomy by intravascular ultrasound.[8–10] At higher frequencies (25 MHz and above), the vessel lumen is characterized by faint, finely textured specular echoes that move and swirl during active blood flow. The echogenicity within the lumen presumably arises the reflection of acoustic energy by circulating blood elements. In many situations, blood "speckle" assists image interpretation by providing a means to confirm the communication between tissue planes and the lumen.

Morphology in normal arteries consists of two basic patterns: a trilaminar appearance with three discrete layers or monolayered vessel wall. (Figure 2). Although there is still some controversy regarding the genesis of the three ultrasonic layers in normal subjects, most authorities agree that the innermost band represents reflections from the internal elastic lamina, while the middle sonolucent layer is principally composed of the vessel media. In normal segments without a trilaminar appearance, the internal elastic lamina is thin and reflects the ultrasound signal poorly, resulting in a monolayered appearance. In normal subjects, the intimal thickness averages 0.15 ± 0.07 mm with many investigators using 0.25 to 0.30 mm as an upper limit (2 SD >normal). The deepest layer of the arterial wall represents the adventitia and periadventitial tissues, exhibiting a characteristic "onionskin" pattern.

Abnormal Morphology

Arteries with coronary atherosclerosis exhibit a diversity of abnormal features that reflect the distribution, severity, and com-

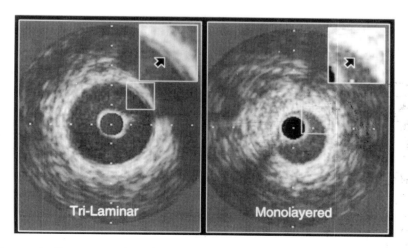

FIGURE 2. *Two examples of normal coronary morphology by intravascular ultrasound. In the left panel, a distinct trilaminar structure is evident. In the right panel, a monolayered artery is apparent.*

position of the atheroma.[8,11] Sites with minimal disease show generalized or focal thickening of the intimal leading edge, whereas advanced lesions appear as large echogenic masses encroaching on the lumen. Most classification schemes differentiate coronary atheromata into one of three categories (soft, fibrous, or calcified) according to plaque echogenicity. (Figure 3–5). Plaques are termed *soft* if they are less echogenic than the adventitia because in vitro studies demonstrate a high lipid content. Plaques with an echodensity similar to the adventitia are described as *fibrous* because studies demonstrate that increasing echogenicity correlates with increasing fibrous tissue content. *Calcified* lesions are recognized as highly echogenic plaques that attenuate transmission of the ultrasound signal thereby obscuring deeper layers.

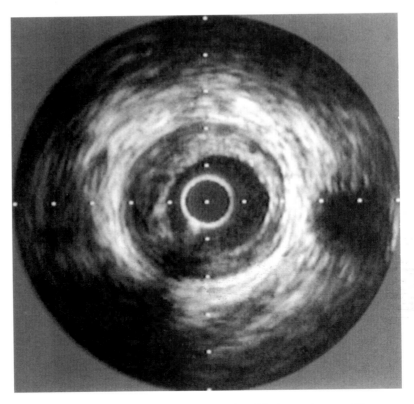

FIGURE 3. *Example of a sonolucent lipid-laden plaque. The mean echogenicity of the atheroma is substantially less than the surrounding adventitia, classifying the lesion as a soft (sonolucent) plaque.*

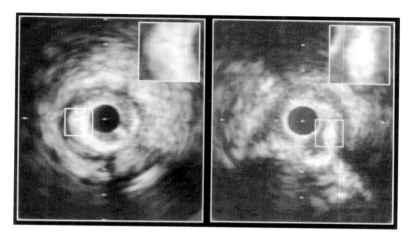

FIGURE 4. *Two examples of "hard" echogenic atherosclerotic plaque. In both examples, the average echogenicity of the plaque is equal or greater than that of the surrounding adventitia. The insets show magnified views of these plaques.*

Caution is warranted in interpretation of intravascular ultrasound images. Methods do not yet exist for automated classification of atheromatous lesions. Although currently available devices produce remarkably detailed views of the vessel wall, interpretation uses visual inspection of acoustic reflections to determine morphology. The echogenicity and texture of different histologic features may exhibit comparable acoustic properties, and therefore appear quite similar by intravascular ultrasound. For example, sonolucent plaque may represent intracoronary thrombus, whereas another nearly identical atheroma may result from a plaque with a high lipid content. Thus, intravascular ultrasound can delineate the thickness and echogenicity of vessel wall structures, but does not provide actual histology.

Despite these limitations, the general classification of coronary plaques into the categories of soft, fibrous, or calcified has significant clinical implications for the interventional practitioner. Initial experience suggests that the three different categories often respond differently to interventional devices. For example, densely fibrotic or calcified plaques resist removal with the current genration of directional atherectomy devices. Armed with this information, the prudent practitioner may choose an alternative revascularization device such as rotational atherectomy for such lesions.

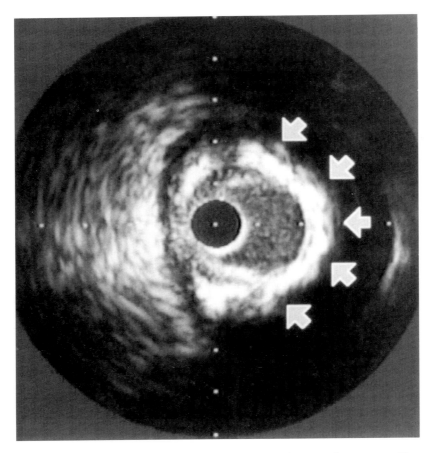

FIGURE 5. *Example of calcified atheromatous plaque. The arrows illustrate a portion of the circumference of the artery in which the plaque obstructs the penetration of ultrasound, thereby concealing the deeper layers. This finding is indicative of lesional calcification.*

Diagnostic Applications

Angiographically Unrecognized Disease

In patients with clinical symptoms of coronary disease, intravascular ultrasound commonly detects atherosclerotic abnormalities at angiographically normal sites.[9,12] There are four principle mechanisms by which angiography may underestimate the amount of atherosclerosis or completely fail to diagnose coronary disease. First, angiography relies on comparison one segment of the vessel to another to detect disease, whereas atherosclerosis is typically a diffuse process. A diffusely diseased vessel may be reduced in caliber along its entire length and contain no truly normal segment for comparison (Figure 6). In the absence of a focal stenosis, the angiographer could erroneously conclude that the vessel is simply "small in caliber."

 ˡᵉsions, plaques that occupy only a portion of the
 ᵖresent ᵃ ᶜond important source of false-
 tions to obtaining optimal an-
 example, at certain angles,
 ᵗcent vessels often obscure seg-
 s in mechanical positioning of
 potentially useful views. There-
 e visualized by angiography be-
 tain an appropriate projection

 n underlying false-negative an-
 nenon of coronary remodeling.[13]
 tory enlargement ("remodeling")
 ᵗque often preserves lumen diam-
 lumen size identical to adjacent,
 Finally, vessel foreshortening can
 ᵗs (usually <1–2 mm).
 of false-negative angiography, ul-
 ᵗresence and estimate the severity
 ᵗinical implications for the higher
 nd in detecting coronary athero-
 ᵗn symptoms suggestive of coro-

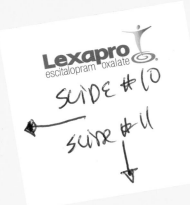

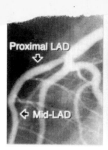

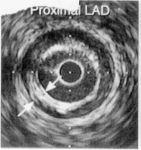

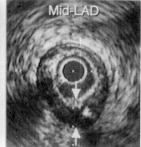

FIGURE 6. *Example of diffuse concentric atherosclerosis resulting in a false-negative angiogram. At both the proximal and mid-left anterior descending (LAD) sites, diffuse concentric atherosclerosis results in a narrowed vessel, but in the absence of a focal stenosis, the angiogram is nearly normal.*

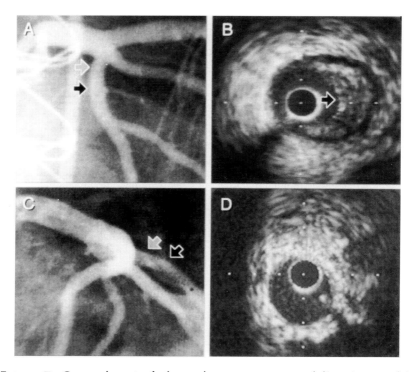

FIGURE 7. *Concealment of plaque by coronary remodeling. In panel **A** and **C**, two angiographic projections are shown. The site indicated by the gray arrow is panel **B**, whereas the site indicated by the black arrow is panel **D**. Note that there is a large atheroma present in panel B, but because the lumen size is similar to the adjacent uninvolved segment (panel **D**), the angiogram is false-negative.*

nary disease, but who have normal angiograms represent a common and perplexing group. In our experience, ultrasound will demonstrate coronary atherosclerosis in the majority of such patients, a finding that impacts on the choice of therapy. Indeed, by the time angiography detects the first luminal irregularity, nearly all of the coronary system will have abnormal intimal thickening by ultrasound.

Lesions of Uncertain Severity

Despite thorough radiographic examination using multiple projections, angiographers commonly encounter lesions that elude accurate characterization. Lesions of uncertain severity often include ostial lesions and moderate stenoses (angiographic severity ranging from 40% to 75%) in patients whose symptomatic status is difficult to evaluate. For these ambiguous lesions, ultrasound provides a precise tomographic measurement, enabling quantitation of the stenosis independent of the radiographic projection.[14] Bifurcation lesions are particularly difficult to assess by angiography (Figure 8). Examination of bifurcation lesions by ultrasound involves specialized techniques, requiring subselective placement of the transducer in the main trunk and each of the daughter branches.

Identification of atherosclerotic lesions in cardiac allograft recipients represents a particularly important and challenging task for diagnostic intravascular ultrasound.[15] These patients may have diffuse vessel involvement that, for reasons already enumerated, conceals the atherosclerosis from the angiographer. Many centers now routinely perform intravascular ultrasound at the time of annual catheterization in all cardiac transplant recipients. Recent studies in our laboratory have revealed dual pathways to transplant atherosclerosis, with some patients receiving atherosclerotic plaques from the donor heart, while others develop immune-mediated vasculopathy.

Risk Stratification of Atherosclerotic Lesions

In the early 1980s, Little et al[15a] confirmed that plaques of minimal to moderate angiographic severity were the most likely to rupture and cause acute myocardial infarction. When intracoronary ultrasound interrogates lesions associated with acute coronary syn-

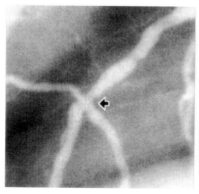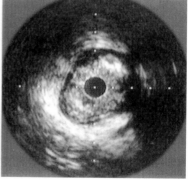

FIGURE 8. *Concealment of severe athersclerosis within a coronary bifurcation. The black arrow indicates the site of intravascular ultrasound imaging. In the ultrasound image, the catheter occupies the entire lumen, illustrating the severity of the atherosclerotic lesion. Because this lesion is most severe near the coronary bifurcation, the the overlapping vessels conceal the disease from the angiographer.*

dromes, most of these plaques contain a relatively echolucent material, consistent with a high lipid content. If a fibrous cap is present, this thick layer is most often ruptured and overlies a large, echolucent, lipid-laden area. Recent research indicates that lipids are the most thrombogenic component of atherosclerotic plaque. The ability of intravascular ultrasound to differentiate predominantly fibrous or calcified plaques from atheromata with a high lipid content offers the potential to determine which plaques are most susceptible to progression to acute coronary syndromes.

Interventional Applications

Quantitative Luminal Measurements

In interventional practice, the precise measurement of vascular dimensions from a tomographic perspective constitutes an important application of intravascular ultrasound. Most investigators report a relatively poor correlation between ultrasonic and angiographic dimensions after intervention. This discrepancy reflects the inability of angiography to accurately portray the complex, irregular cross-sectional profiles of atherosclerotic vessels after mechanical intervention. Careful comparisons of ultrasound and angiographic findings after balloon angioplasty have confirmed that angiography often overestimates the actual gain in luminal cross-sectional area.[16]

Two factors influence the overly optimistic tendency of angiographic imaging. At the reference site, angiography tends to underestimate the true vessel diameter because of the frequent presence of unrecognized atherosclerosis. At the target site, angiography tends to overestimate the actual gain in luminal diameter because contrast material penetrates into complex cracks and fissures produced by the balloon, giving the appearance of a more enlarged lumen. To calculate a postprocedure percent diameter stenosis, the diameter at the target site (an overestimate) is divided by the reference diameter (an underestimate), resulting in a more favorable impression of the actual gain in luminal dimensions. Accordingly, when quantitative angiography reports a residual stenosis of 10% to 15%, ultrasound not uncommonly reports that 60% to 80% of the vessel is still occupied by plaque.

Intravascular Ultrasound and Restenosis

It seems likely that the morphology of the vessel wall after interventions will provide valuable insights into phenomena such as elastic recoil, pathological dissection, abrupt occlusion, and restenosis. The relatively poor correlation between angiographic and ultrasonic dimensions after angioplasty raises provocative clinical and scientific issues. In certain patients, does "restenosis" represent a failure to adequately augment luminal area, rather than the subsequent overexuberant proliferation of cellular elements? Can ultrasound assessment of the residual lumen predict acute postinterventional complications or identify patients with a high likelihood of poor long-term results? Several multicenter clinical trials currently underway are examining whether ultrasound can reliably predict restenosis after intervention. These include a multicenter trial in which the interventional practitioner is blinded to the ultrasound findings. The INSPIRE trial (*In*travascular Ultrasound *P*redictors of *Re*stenosis) will include 500 patients and is expected to complete enrollment in 1996.

Wall Morphology Following Angioplasty

Necropsy studies in patients who have died shortly after balloon angioplasty describe plaque fracturing or disruption as the most common mechanism of successful balloon dilatation.[5] Ultrasound studies have confirmed that plaque fissuring is the most common mechanism of luminal enlargement, occurring in 40% to 80% of patients (Figure 9). Ultrasound often shows other mecha-

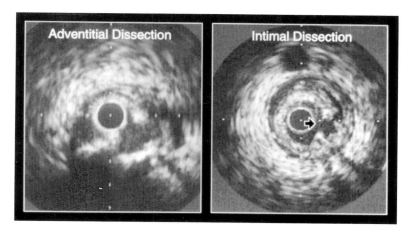

FIGURE 9. *Examples of two types of dissection after coronary balloon angioplasty. In the **left panel**, the dissection (3 o'clock position) extends into the adventitia. In the **right panel**, the black arrow points to a single split within the atheroma that does not extend to the level of the media.*

nisms of luminal enlargement after balloon angioplasty that cannot be discerned in postmortem analyses.[7] Careful imaging before and after percutaneous transluminal coronary angioplasty reveals that stretching of the vessel wall occurs in at least 20% of patients, whereas apparent compression of the atheromatous material occurs in at least 10%. More recent studies using automatic pullback devices (that withdraws the ultrasound catheter at a constant rate through the target site) have shown that compression may represents redistribution of plaque along the long axis of the vessel.

Guidance of Directional Atherectomy

Intravascular ultrasound has proven particularly valuable in guiding directional coronary atherectomy.[17,18] By determining the location and composition of the target atheroma, ultrasound enables optimal preprocedural planning and improved intraprocedural decision making (Figure 10). Lesions that appear concentric by angiography are often eccentric by ultrasound, and conversely, angiographically eccentric lesions are often concentric by ultrasound. The spatial improved perspective provided by ultrasound can assist in the proper orientation of atherectomy cuts. However, successful application of this approach requires experience, patience, and careful planning because precise orientation of the in-

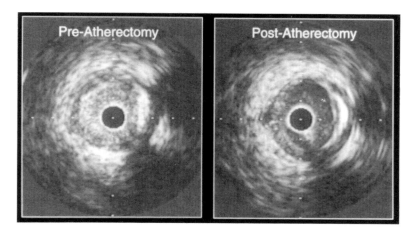

FIGURE 10. *Atherosclerotic lesion pre- and postdirectional atherectomy. Because the ultrasound indicated plaque concentrically distributed in the artery, the operator performed atherectomy cuts throughout the full 360° circumference of the vessel. This results in excellent debulking of plaque, as shown in the right panel.*

travascular image remains a difficult challenge. Experienced operators will carefully examine the target vessel prior to atherectomy to locate anatomic landmarks, especially side branches, and will use these landmarks to orient the ultrasound image. With this information, the operator can then direct atherectomy cuts toward the appropriate side of the vessel. Some operators use repeat ultrasound examinations between passes of the atherectomy device to determine the extent of plaque removal and assess the need for additional cuts.

With currently available directional atherectomy devices, the presence and extent of vessel calcification can dramatically affect the efficiency of plaque removal. For detection of calcification, ultrasound is more sensitive than angiography, permitting identification of extensively calcified atheromata despite the absence of any apparent calcification on fluoroscopy. In our experience, calcification at the luminal surface usually precludes successful tissue removal. However, ultrasound can determine not only the presence of calcification, but also its depth in relation to the lumen. Ultrasound studies have demonstrated that target lesions with extensive calcification deep within the atheroma can undergo successful atherectomy.

In striking contrast to balloon angioplasty, ultrasound studies before and after directional atherectomy confirm that plaque removal is the primary mechanism of luminal enlargement. Nevertheless, ultrasound also reveals that despite a successful angiographic result (<15% residual stenosis), 40% to 60% or more of the target site is still occupied by plaque.[18] Some investigators have proposed that a larger lumen after atherectomy would result in a lower restenosis rate (compared with balloon angioplasty). However, it remains untested whether a larger postprocedure lumen can be achieved using angiographic guidance without a concomitant increase in dissection, perforation, or other complications. In our experience, more aggressive plaque removal is most safely accomplished with the use of ultrasound guidance. Development of a combined atherectomy-ultrasound device represents a major focus of current commercial ventures.

Guidance of Rotational Atherectomy

Rotational ablation (Rotablator™, Heart Technology, Bellevue, WA) uses a high-speed diamond-coated burr to debulk atheromata within coronary stenoses. This approach has been proven particularly effective at removing superficial calcium from stenotic vessels. Interestingly, this morphological subset represents precisely the type of vessel least suitable for directional atherectomy. As previously discussed, there is a poor correlation between ultrasound and fluoroscopy in assessment of the presence and amount of calcification.[19] Accordingly, in our laboratory, practitioners not uncommonly abandon an intended directional atherectomy in favor of rotational ablation because preinterventional ultrasound revealed extensive calcification.

Vessels revascularized using rotational ablation are frequently diffusely diseased and the "normal" dimension can be difficult to determine angiographically. Ultrasound-guided vessel sizing can facilitate the selection of the largest burr. Observational ultrasound studies to date have confirmed that ablation of plaque constitutes the primary mechanism of rotational atherectomy, particularly the more fibrotic or calcified components of the lesion.[20] The residual lumen is usually round or ellipsoid, and may result in a lumen with a 15% to 20% greater area than the largest burr used, presumably due to

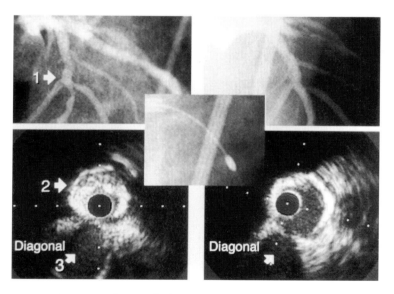

FIGURE 11. *Angiographic and ultrasound appearance after rotational ablation. In the **upper left panel,** the worst lesion in the left anterior descending is near the bifurcation into septal and diagonal branches. The ultrasound image preintervention is shown at the lower left. The lesion is marked by the number 2 and the diagonal branch by the number 3. In the central image, the Rotoblator™ is shown in situ. In the **upper right panel,** the angiographic result of intervention is shown. In the **lower right panel,** the post-Rotoblator™ lumen is enlarged (principally by the cutting of the calcified plaque).*

lateral movement of the burr during the procedure. In certain lesions, rotational atherectomy may be the only device capable of removing a hard, superficial layer of calcium, yet even after this layer is removed, a large volume of plaque may remain. Post-Rotablator™ ultrasound can quantitate the size of the neolumen, characterize the morphology of the remaining plaque, and guide the technique and size of device used for further luminal enlargement (Figure 11). In other target vessels, ultrasound may document restoration of luminal size, obviating the need for an adjunctive device.

Coronary Stent Deployment

Recent studies demonstrating a reduced restenosis rate have stimulated renewed interest in coronary stenting. However, the requirement for vigorous postdeployment anticoagulation have limited more widespread application of this technique. Ultrasound studies have demonstrated that angiography is often inadequate to guide stent deployment. Some stents may appear successfully deployed by angiography, but are actually incompletely apposed to the vessel wall (Figure 12). In such cases, angiographic contrast presumably penetrates the porous stent, giving the false appearance of a large lumen. In other cases, although the stent is well apposed to the wall, the lumen cross-sectional area is considerably reduced in comparison to a proximal or distal reference site.

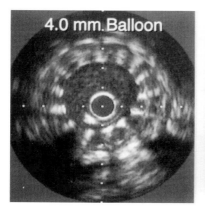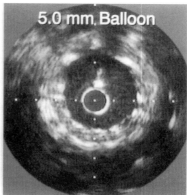

FIGURE 12. *Intravascular ultrasound guidance of stent deployment. After the image in the left panel was obtained, it was evident that several stent struts were not well opposed to the vessel wall (3-o'clock to 6-o'clock position). In the right panel, ultrasound was repeated after several inflations with a larger 5.0-mm balloon, which had a more satisfactory result.*

Ultrasound examination can easily diagnose both of these circumstances. The metallic structure of current coronary stents produces a distinct appearance. Individual struts appear as echo-dense objects with acoustic shadowing similar to vessel wall calcification. A single-center, retrospective analysis has documented that the level of systemic anticoagulation may be safely reduced if ultrasound confirms both adequate stent apposition and restoration of near-normal lumen dimensions, defined as 60% or more of the area of the lumen in a normal or near-normal adjacent segment.[21] However, prospective trials will be required before any widespread application of the practice of reduced anticoagulation.

Intravascular ultrasound is occasionally useful in determining the true longitudinal extent of a dissection before placement of a stent for vessel salvage. Thus, intracoronary imaging is more sensitive in detecting the presence of a dissection, and more accurate in determining the true length of a dissection. In questionable cases, ultrasound examination before stenting can define the limits of the dissection and determine where (and how many) stents should be placed. Although ultrasound is unquestionably useful after stenting, questions of safety in passing any monorail-type catheter through a fine wire, coil design, such as the Gianturco-Roubin™ (Cook) stent remain. It is theoretically possible to dislodge the stent by "snagging" a loop of the struts between the monorail catheter and the guidewire.

Future Directions of Intravascular Ultrasound

Over the next several years, technological advances in intravascular imaging will undoubtedly expand the utility of this procedure. Industry engineers anticipate further reductions in the size of imaging catheters, and animal testing of a guidewire-sized device (<0.025 inches) has already begun. This guidewire-sized ultrasound probe will improve the ease and safety of the examination and may also enable simultaneous imaging during the revascularization procedure. Very small devices would also enable imaging of virtually any coronary stenosis prior to treatment. Combination devices will likely undergo refinement, permitting online guidance during revascularization procedures. An angioplasty balloon with an ultrasound transducer (Endosonics Oracle™) is FDA approved, and a transducer combined with an atherectomy device is also under development. As a consequence of refinements in equipment and knowlege derived from clinical investigations, we anticipate a major role for intravascular ultrasound in the diagnosis and therapy of coronary disease well into the next century.

References

1. Zir LM, Miller SW, Dinsmore RE, et al. Interobserver variability in coronary angiography. *Circulation* 1976;53:627–632.
2. Vlodaver Z, Frech R, van Tassel RA, et al. Correlation of the antemortem coronary angiogram and the postmortem specimen. *Circulation* 1973;47:162–168.
3. White CW, Wright CB, Doty DB, et al. Does visual interpretation of the coronary arteriogram predict the physiologic importance of a coronary stenosis? *N Engl J Med* 1984;310:819–824.
4. Topol EJ, Nissen SE. Our preoccupation with coronary luminology. The Dissociation between clinical and angiographic findings in ischemic heart disease. *Circulation* 1995;92:2333–2342.
5. Waller BF. "Crackers, breakers, stretchers, drillers, scrapers, shavers, burners, welders, and melters": The future treatment of atherosclerotic coronary artery disease? A clinical-morphologic assessment. *J Am Coll Cardiol* 1989;13:969–987.
6. Nissen SE, Grines CL, Gurley JC, et al. Application of a new phased-array ultrasound imaging catheter in the assessment of vascular dimensions: In vivo comparison to cineangiography. *Circulation* 1990;81:660–666.
7. Nissen SE, Tuzcu EM, De Franco AC. Coronary intravascular ultrasound: Diagnostic and interventional applications. In: Topol EJ, ed. *Update to Textbook of Interventional Cardiology*. Philadelphia: WB Saunders; 1994:207–222.
8. Nissen SE, Gurley JC, Grines CL, et al. Intravascular ultrasound assessment of lumen size and wall morphology in normal subjects and coronary artery disease patients. *Circulation* 1991;84:1087–1099.
9. St. Goar FG, Pinto FJ, Alderman EL, et al. Detection of coronary atherosclerosis in young adult hearts using intravascular ultrasound. *Circulation* 1992;86:756–763.
10. Fitzgerald PJ, St. Goar FG, Connolly AJ, et al. Intravascular ultrasound imaging of coronary arteries. Is three layers the norm? *Circulation* 1992;86:154–158.
11. Tobis JM, Mallery J, Mahon D, et al. Intravascular ultrasound imaging of human coronary arteries in vivo. Analysis of tissue characterizations with comparison to in vitro histological specimens. *Circulation* 1991;83:913–926.
12. Nissen SE, De Franco AC, Raymond RE, et al. Angiographically unrecognized disease at "normal" reference sites: A risk factor for suboptimal results after coronary interventions. *Circulation* 1993; 88:412A.
13. Glagov S, Weisenberg E, Zarins CK, et al: Compensatory Enlargement of Human Coronary Arteries. *N Engl J Med* 1987;316:1371–1375.
14. White CJ, Ramee SR, Collin TJ, et al. Ambiguous coronary angiography: Clinical utility of intravascular ultrasound. *Catheterization Cardiovasc Diagn* 1992;26:200–203.
15. Tuzcu EM, Hobbs H, Rincon G, et al. Occult and Frequent transmission of atherosclerosis coronary disease with cardiac transplantation. *Circulation* 1995;91:1706–1713.
15a. Little WC, Constantinescu M, Applegate RJ, et al. Can arteriography predict the site of a subsequent myocardial infarction in patients with

mild-to-moderate coronary artery disease? *Circulation* 1988;78:1157–1166.

16. DeFranco AC, Tuzcu E, Abdelmeguid A, et al. Intravascular ultrasound assessment of PTCA results: Insights into the mechanisms of balloon angioplasty. *J Am Coll Cardiol* 1993;21:485A.

17. Popma JJ, Mintz GS, et al. Clinical and angiographic outcome after directional coronary atherectomy. A qualitative and quantitative analysis using angiography and intravascular ultrasound. *Am J Cardiol* 1993;72:55E-64E.

18. DeFranco AC, Tuzcu EM, Moliterno DJ, et al. "Directional" coronary atherectomy removes atheroma more effectively from concentric than eccentric lesions: Intravascular ultrasound predictors of lesional success. *J Am Coll Cardiol* 1995;137A:730–733.

19. Tuzcu EM, Berkalp B, De Franco AC, et al. The dilemma of diagnosing coronary calcification: Angiography vs. intravascular ultrasound. *J Am Coll Cardiol* In press.

20. Kovach JA, Mintz GS, Pichard AD, et al. Sequential intravascular ultrasound characterization of the mechanism of rotational atherectomy and adjunct balloon angioplasty. *J Am Coll Cardiol* 1993;22:1024–1032.

21. Columbo A, Hall P, Martini G, et al. Results of intravascular ultrasound guided coronary stenting without subsequent anticoagulation. *J Am Coll Cardiol* 1994:335A.

Chapter 17

Magnetic Resonance Coronary Artery Imaging

Mark Doyle, PhD and Gerald M. Pohost, MD

Introduction

Magnetic resonance uses two main imaging approaches to generate images: gradient-echo (bright blood pool) and spin-echo (dark blood pool) imaging. Presently, the coronary arteries are predominantly imaged using gradient-echo methods because gradient-echo techniques produce a bright blood signal in the presence of blood motion. There are several distinct gradient-echo imaging methods, and each is used in a different manner when applied to imaging the coronary arteries. This chapter begins by describing the basic gradient-echo pulse sequence. The other gradient-echo methods will then be described. Then, other more general issues applicable to any magnetic resononance coronary artery imaging technique are discussed, eg, respiratory and cardiac motion compensation methods and image display formats. Finally, other relevant considerations will be discussed, including the information that can be extracted from magnetic resonance images and vessel contrast enhancement approaches.

In the greater context of cardiac magnetic resonance examinations, a coronary artery imaging procedure must be fast enough to be completed without substantially prolonging the examination time. At present, cardiac magnetic resonance imaging can routinely provide information on anatomy, morphology, and function. Magnetic resonance perfusion imaging is under development at a number of sites and shows great promise of becoming more widely available (possibly within the next 2 years). Coronary artery imag-

From: Fuster V, (ed.) *Syndromes of Atherosclerosis: Correlations of Clinical Imaging and Pathology.* Armonk, NY: Futura Publishing Company, Inc.: © 1996.

ing by magnetic resonance angiography will probably become a routine procedure within the next 5 years.

Imaging Techniques

Gradient-Echo Imaging

The basic gradient-echo imaging sequence is shown in Figure 1. The sequence contains two basic components: a slice selection section where the signal for an arbitrarily oriented slice is stimulated (upper two lines), and the image encoding section, where the

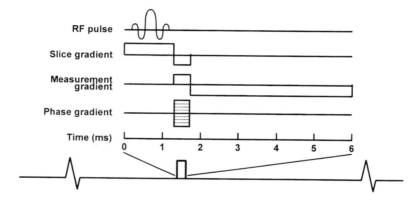

FIGURE 1. *The basic gradient-echo sequence has two distinct sections: slice selection and image encoding. Slice selection is performed by applying a magnetic field gradient perpendicular to the desired slice orientation. The gradient imposes a range of different resonances on the tissue, which vary linearly along the gradient axis. In conjunction with this gradient, a radiofrequency (RF) pulse is applied, such that it is only on resonance for a thin band of tissue (due to the resonance frequency spread caused by the gradient). In this way only a thin band of tissue is stimulated to give off a magnetic resonance detectible signal. Image encoding is performed by application of two orthogonal gradients, the measurement gradient (so called since the signal is detected, or measured, while this gradient is on), and the phase gradient (so called since it changes the phase of the measured signal on repeated applications of the basic sequence). Many applications of the basic sequence are required to encode a complete image, and during each application the amplitude of the phase encoding gradient is stepped to a new value (indicated by the ladder of values). Each application of the sequence takes about 6 msec, depending on scanner capabilities.*

encoded signal is acquired (lower two lines). Images are generally acquired as two-dimensional matrices (planes or slices), and image encoding is accomplished by application of two orthogonal magnetic field gradients, termed the measurement and phase gradients. The phase gradient is drawn schematically as a series of lines with various amplitudes, but only a single amplitude is used for a given application of the basic sequence. Consequently, to acquire sufficient information to encode a complete image, the basic sequence must be repeatedly applied, and on each application the phase encoding gradient is moved to a new amplitude. For instance, to generate a 256^2 image, the phase gradient must be stepped through 256 amplitudes, and thus the basic sequence needs to be repeated 256 times. Each phase step generates a line within the image data set. When applied to coronary artery imaging, the sequence must be synchronized within the cardiac cycle to allow each phase to be acquired at the same time within the cardiac cycle (see ECG tracing, lower portion of Figure 1). Thus, even though the basic gradient-echo sequence requires about 6 msec for each phase step, it must be repeated for each image line in a cardiac synchronized manner, resulting in a minimum imaging time on the order of 5 minutes (depending on heart rate).

Turbo Gradient-Echo Imaging

To encode a single slice using the basic gradient-echo sequence can take an impractically long time (256 cycles per slice), especially when considering that many slices (100 or more) may be required to provide enough resolution to image the coronary arteries in a clinically relevant fashion. Therefore, the turbo gradient-echo technique was devised (Figure 2).[1,2] The turbo gradient-echo approach uses the basic gradient-echo sequence applied many times in rapid succession during each cardiac cycle. For each application of the basic sequence a new phase encoding step is performed, reducing the number of cardiac cycles required to acquire the sequence of images by a factor that depends on the number of phase steps performed during each cycle. Typically, 16 phase steps may be acquired during each cardiac cycle, reducing the imaging time to about 20 seconds. To be effective, cardiac motion must be minimal (relative to the image pixel dimensions) during the application of each burst of turbo gradient-echo sequences. For a train of 16, each burst of gradient-echo sequences could last about 100 msec. If such a burst is applied during mid- to end diastole, the heart is usually in a relatively stationary position. Turbo gradient-echo is some-

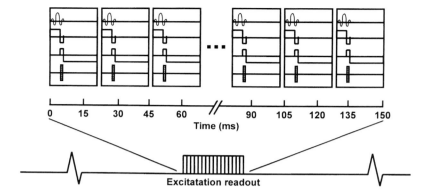

FIGURE 2. *The turbo gradient-echo sequence is similar to the basic sequence except that the basic sequence is applied multiple times during individual cardiac cycles. Thus, turbo methods speed up a cardiac-triggered acquisition by a factor related to the number of basic sequences performed during each cycle.*

times referred to as segmented gradient-echo because a number of data lines (ie, a segment of the complete data matrix) are acquired during each cardiac cycle. Disadvantages of this method include reduction in signal and some blurring due to the prolonged time of acquisition during each cardiac cycle.

Spiral Gradient-Echo Imaging

One disadvantage of the turbo gradient-echo method is that it uses multiple excitations of a given slice during each cardiac cycle. This reduces the maximum signal that can be obtained (the shorter the interval between successive slice selection pulses, the lower the magnetic resonance signal). One technique that can encode a similar amount of data to one turbo burst, but with only one application of the slice selection procedure, is the spiral gradient-echo technique (Figure 3).[3] The sequence encodes data in a spiral manner (top portion of Figure 3) rather than as a series of straight lines as in the basic and turbo gradient-echo sequences. The spiral data trajectory is achieved using sinusoidal and cosinusoidal type waveforms applied in the two orthogonal imaging gradient directions. However, similar to gradient and turbo gradient-echo imaging, a complete image cannot be acquired during a single application of the spiral encoding method. Thus, a number of spirals are interleaved, each acquired during the same point in successive heart cy-

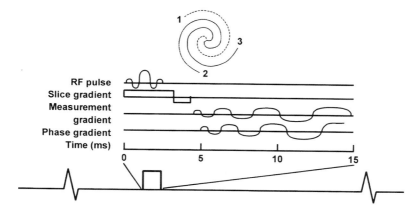

FIGURE 3. *The spiral gradient-echo approach uses sinusoidal and cosi-nusoidal type image encoding gradients (with the gradients increasing in amplitude as the sequence proceeds). As indicated in the top panel, the gradients cause the acquired data to traverse a spiral trajectory in the data matrix with 1, 2, and 3 indicating successive applications of the basic sequence. Typically, 16 interleaved spiral scans are required to produce a complete image, and these are obtained from successive heart cycles.*

cles (Figure 3). Each individual spiral acquisition takes about 15–20 ms to acquire, and about 16 spiral segments are required for each image, resulting in a total scan time of about 20 seconds per plane. A disadvantage of this approach is its greater sensitivity to interference from lipids. Such lipid interference is relatively easily eliminated as described later.

Echo Planar Imaging

A particularly fast imaging method is echo planar imaging (EPI) (Figure 4).[4,5] With a single-slice selection, it is possible to generate a 64x256 image in about 50 msec. To obtain higher resolution images, the basic imaging sequence can be applied multiple times, as in spiral and turbo gradient-echo imaging. However, due to EPIs superior image encoding speed, fewer applications are required compared with the techniques discussed above; for instance to obtain a 256^2 image, as few as four EPI applications are required, which would require four cardiac cycles. The main feature of the EPI sequence that makes it so fast, is the rapidly oscillating measurement gradient. Each oscillation is equivalent to a basic

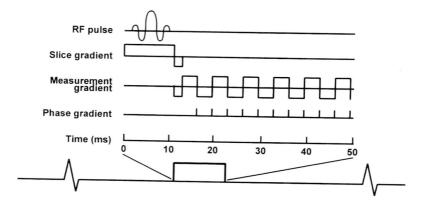

FIGURE 4. *Echo-planar imaging is very similar to the basic gradient-echo sequence with the major exception being that the measurement gradient is rapidly oscillated. The result is that image data are encoded at a very fast rate, and indeed image matrices up to about 64×256 can be acquired in a single application of the basic sequence.*

gradient-echo sequence (compare the measurement gradient of the EPI acquisition with the basic gradient-echo sequence, Figure 1). Unfortunately, EPI gradients place great demands on the scanner hardware, and at present, relatively few scanners are capable of performing EPI. However, scanner performance improves with each new commercial product release. EPI is becoming more widely available and is expected to be a standard feature in the future.

Multiple Slice Gradient-Echo Imaging

Because the basic gradient-echo sequence only lasts about 6 msec, it is possible to image a large number of slices (50–100) during the period of diastole (when coronary artery blood flow is maximal) (Figure 5).[6,7] The multiple-slice acquisition scheme results in a long acquisition train within each cardiac cycle. However, this does not result in slice blurring because the duration of the acquisition per slice remains at 6 msec. Thus, beating motion that occurs during each cardiac cycle merely alters the spatial relationship between each imaged slice, rather than blurring each slice. Just as in the case of the basic gradient-echo sequence, 256 heart cycles are required for a 256^2 matrix image, but during the same imaging time many slices are acquired, making this approach time efficient. By acquiring the slices in a contiguous manner, imaging of the en-

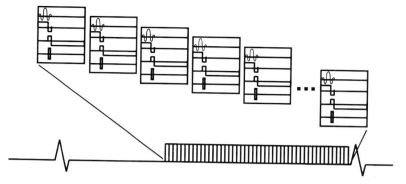

FIGURE 5. *The basic gradient-echo sequence can be applied in a multiple slice mode. Applied in this way, many slices through the heart can be encoded for the entire diastolic period of several hundred milliseconds. It is most convenient to apply this mode to acquire image slices in a contiguous manner and attempt to obtain global coverage of the heart (or at least complete coverage of a portion of the heart).*

tire heart is possible by the end of the acquisition (a minimum of 256 cardiac cycles). Additionally, because the slices are selected in rapid succession, motion occurring between adjacent slice selections is minimal, thus providing reasonable continuity of coronary sections between slices.

Essential Components

Respiratory Compensation

Because multiple heart phases are required to generate a magnetic resonance image, synchronization with the cardiac cycle is essential. However, during these multiple cardiac cycles, the heart undergoes global motion because of respiration. Thus, some form of respiratory motion compensation is required. A number of strategies have been used. Some are more suited for one imaging technique over another, although in general the respiratory compensation techniques can be used in a "mix-and-match" manner with the imaging strategy of choice. Two techniques are used: 1) respiratory gating and 2) breath-holding.

In terms of patient comfort and compliance, synchronizing each acquisition with the patient's respiratory and cardiac cycle is desirable (gating). In this case, the patient must lie still while image acquisition occurs. Various devices are available to monitor the patient's breathing motion, with the most common device being a belt incorporating a bellows that is secured around the patient's abdomen. As the bellows expands and contracts with respiratory motion, the information is transmitted via an air-filled tube to the scanner electronics where it is converted to an electrical signal and digitized for analysis. Typically, the scanner will image during the same phase of the respiration cycle. The typical ratio of the expiration duration to inspiration is 4:1, and the time of least motion occurs during end expiration, potentially allowing imaging for about 80% of the respiratory cycle.[8] An alternative to the belt-and-bellows device for monitoring respiratory induced motion is the use of navigator signals. A navigator signal is derived from a rapid magnetic resonance imaging sequence performed prior to starting the image encoding sequence, and is used to determine whether the correct position in the respiratory cycle has been reached. The navigator sequence selects, with a single excitation procedure, a one-dimensional projection through the abdomen that is quickly processed and analyzed.[9]

In the event that the patient is reasonably fit, some form of breath-holding could be considered. One strategy is to repetitively briefly suspend breathing at end expiration. The scanner is then synchronized to perform a measurement for one cardiac cycle during end expiration.[6] This method of respiratory suspension is nonstrenuous in terms of length of each breath-hold period. Another more strenuous approach is to require that the patient hold their breath continuously for approximately 20 seconds while an acquisition is performed.[1-3,10] The patient is allowed to recover for about a minute, and the procedure is repeated as required. Each 20-second breath-hold generally allows acquisition of a single plane (but multiple-slice acquisitions are feasible). With either breath-hold strategy, reproducibility of the breath-hold position is essential, either for composite acquisitions or comparing slices from different acquisitions. To facilitate consistency in the patient's breath-hold position, some form of feedback (typically auditory or visual) is useful to inform the patient that they are in the correct position of the respiratory cycle.

Cardiac Motion Reduction

For a high-speed imaging technique that can encode an image during a single heartbeat, only a single heartbeat would be required per image plane. However, no such technique currently exists, but EPI comes close. Thus, numerous heartbeats are required to obtain sufficient data to generate each tomographic image. Accordingly, a stable cardiac rhythm and position are essential for good image quality. Some form of arrhythmia rejection is necessary for optimal results.

Image Display Formats

All the magnetic resonace imaging techniques discussed here are two dimensional in that a two-dimensional tomographic image or set of tomographic images are generated. These images can either be viewed individually (Figures 6 and 7), or if there is an anatomic relationship between tomographs, they can be combined

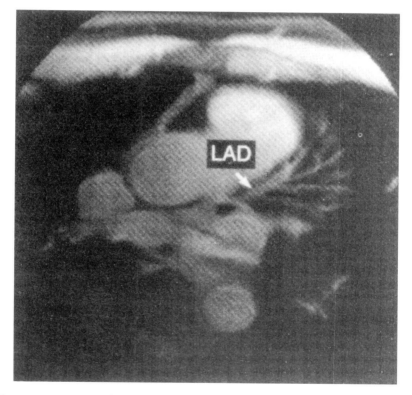

FIGURE 6. *An in-plane view of the left anterior descending coronary artery branch produced by a spiral gradient-echo imaging approach (Figure 3), in 20 heartbeats, with continuous breath-holding, and fat signal suppression was incorporated in the slice selection sequence. Reprinted with permission from Meyer CH, Hu B, Nishimura DG, Macovski A.* Magnetic Resonance in Medicine Fast Spiral Coronary Artery Imaging. *Volume 28. Williams & Wilkins; 1992:202–213.*

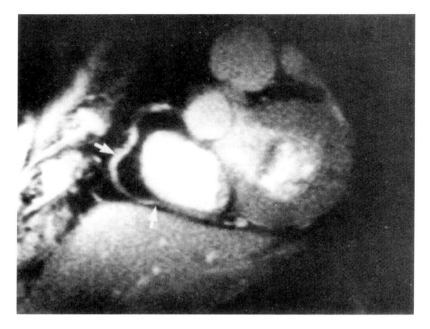

FIGURE 7. *An in-plane view of the right coronary artery branch produced by turbo gradient-echo (Figure 2), in 16–20 heartbeats, with continuous breath-holding, and fat signal suppression applied prior to each turbo burst of acquisitions Reprinted with permission from Manning WJ, Li W, Edelman RR. A preliminary report comparing magnetic resonance coronary angiography with conventional angiography. N Engl J Med 1993;328:828–832.*

to produce a global view of the coronary arteries. The simplest relationship between a series of image slices is that they are parallel to each other and contiguous. With these criteria, four main viewing modes are feasible.

Movie Mode

The series of slices could be reviewed in a movie loop, where contiguous slices are displayed in succession. This mode requires the least computing power, and even small coronary branches can generally be seen because of the continuity between slices. However, particularly tortuous or curved branches are more difficult to appreciate because (depending on slice orientation) a single artery could divide and appear as two diverging dots in the movie sequence.

Multiplanar Reformatting

With a suitably fast computer, reformatted image planes can be generated virtually in real time from the original image set.[8] The reformatted images are composites of the contiguous tomographs that were directly acquired. In this way, it is possible to view coronary vessel segments in single planes (Figure 8). By moving and rotating the imaging plane, various coronary branches can be brought into view, and in particular, the arteries can be traced back to their origin to help distinguish between arteries and veins. For multiplanar reformatting to work optimumly the slice thickness should be the same as the in-plane pixel dimensions.

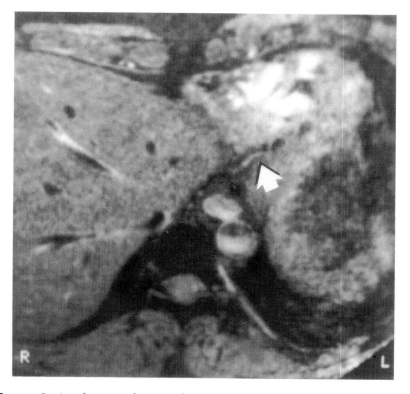

FIGURE 8. *A reformatted image featuring the posterior descending coronary artery, reformatted from a set of 85 parallel thin (1.5 mm) slices, produced with the multiple slice gradient-echo sequence (Figure 5), and acquired with respiratory synchronization (using a belt-and-bellows apparatus). The total acquisition time was about 15 minutes for all 85 slices.*

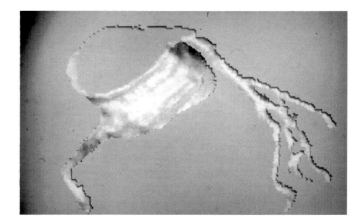

FIGURE 9. *A three-dimensional solid surface rendition of the aortic root, right, and left circumflex coronary branches produced by multiple slice gradient-echo, with multiple short breath-holds at end diastole. The total acquisition time was about 10 minutes to acquire all 30 slices. Reprinted with permission from Doyle M, Scheidegger MB, Graaf RG, et al. Coronary artery imaging in multiple one second breath holds.* Magn Reson Imaging *1993;10:3–6.*

Three-Dimensional Rendition

To visualize the coronary arteries globally (as opposed to the isolated segments of the above described methods) a solid three-dimensional representation can be constructed and viewed on the computer screen (Figure 9).[6] However, prior to rendering as a three-dimensional object, each individual segment of each coronary artery branch must be isolated and identified within each slice. This is time consuming and prone to operator error.

FIGURE 10. *A limited region projection image (a projection of two slices), generated with turbo gradient-echo (Figure 2), magnetization transfer contrast (MTC) enhancement, and breath-holding for about 20 heartbeats. Auditory feedback was used to ensure that the patient held their breath during the correct phase of the respiratory cycle. In the figure, respiratory feedback monitoring (RFM) refers to the feedback system, and the images on the right were acquired with RFM, while those on the left did not use feedback monitoring. Reprinted with permission from Wang Y, Christy PS, Korosec FK, et al. Coronary magnetic resonancel with a respiratory feedback monitor: The 2D imaging case.* Magn Reson Med *1995;33:116–121.*

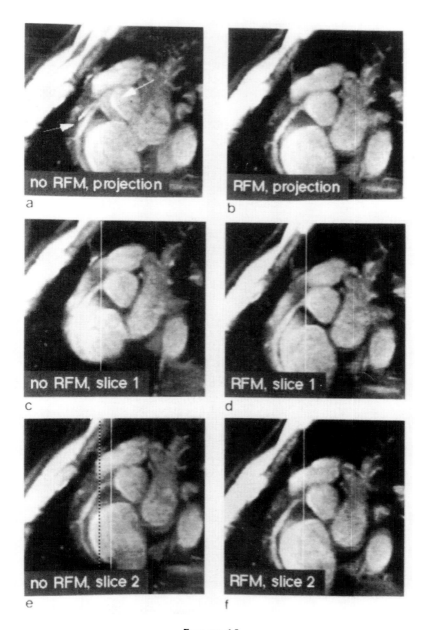

FIGURE 10

Projection

Vasculature, such as the carotid arteries, has been displayed from a series of slices using a projection display. Moving blood appears as a bright signal whereas static tissue appears as a dark signal. A projection (or series of projections) is then retrospectively generated by a mathematical procedure known as maximum intensity projection (MIP).[11,12] In MIPs, the blood is usually the maximum signal in any given projection direction, consequently, MIPS strongly resemble x-ray angiograms. However, for coronary artery imaging, the moving heart tissue and associated large cardiac chamber blood pools usually appear as relatively high signal intensities. Thus, global coronary artery MIPs are generally not feasible. Nevertheless, limited region-of-interest MIPS can be generated to yield local views of coronary segments (Figure 10).[10]

Additional Considerations

Detection Coils

The magnetic resonance radiofrequency signal is detected with a coil (like an antenna) within the scanner system. To improve image quality by enhancing the signal-to-noise ratio (SNR), a local coil applied to the chest (surface coil) over the region of the heart can be used (as opposed to the usual coil surrounding the entire body). A surface coil (approximately 20 cm in diameter) is placed on the chest over the heart region. The advantage of the surface coil is that for regions of the heart closest to the coil, the SNR is superior to that obtained with a conventional body coil that surrounds the whole thorax. However, homogeneity of surface coil generated images is poor, and some regions will be detected with less SNR than a body coil. Many magnetic resonance scanner vendors are currently investigating the use of specialized cardiac coils, which provide the advantages of a surface coil but give homogeneous coverage of the heart.

Vessel Wall Imaging

Most approaches to angiography with magnetic resonance imaging have concentrated on imaging the blood within the vessel lumen. In the vicinity of a stenotic region, the magnetic resonance signal tends to drop out, probably related to turbulence (creating a signal void), and the detailed appearance of the stenosis is lost.[13] In the coronary arteries, the blood velocities are lower than in most other major vessels, and the region of signal loss is expected to be considerably lower. Thus, definition of the stenotic portions of the coronary arteries is better than the stenotic portions of larger arteries. Conversely, the small size and the motion of the coronary arteries makes them more difficult to image. One of magnetic resonance's advantages over standard coronary cine methods is that it has the potential to image the vessel wall in addition to luminal blood. Additionally, magnetic resonance can theoretically register signals from the some of the components of atherosclerotic plaque including lipid and fibrous tissue. Calcification gives no signal. Magnetic resonance has the potential to image thrombus. However, to realistically perform such measurements, image resolution will have to improve substantially from the present day value, of about 1 mm^3.

Clinical Expert or Technical Expert User

It is essential to consider the expertise of the person operating the scanner and analyzing the images so as to design the appropriate procedure to optimize data acquisition and analysis. For example, one should consider whether the operator has technical expertise such as a technologist or physicist, or clinical expertise such as a cardiologist. In the event that a technical expert performs the scan, the procedure should be designed to give the reviewing cardiovascular specialist all of the needed information without requiring that the patient return for further examinations. Thus, a technologist performed study, should give global coverage of the coronary arteries without requiring expert clinical knowledge at the time of examination. However, if a cardiologist is to perform the examination, then individual images can be obtained with a limited number of user-defined orientations until the cardiologist is satisfied that the salient features of the coronary arteries have been imaged. In this mode, successive images are usually planned from previous ones. In the event that a scan did not show a required coronary feature, it would be repeated.

Contrast Enhancement

In peripheral magnetic resonance angiography, the acquisition sequences are designed to image moving blood with much brighter signal intensity than surrounding tissue. However, such a high level of blood-tissue contrast is not generally achieved in coronary magnetic resonance angiography. Thus, some form of contrast enhancement is typically applied to readily allow visualization of the coronary arteries. Several strategies exist to enhance coronary artery contrast.

T1 or T2 Preparation

Separate from tissue density, there are two magnetic resonance properties of the tissue that determine its signal intensity. These are T1 and T2 relaxation times. These relaxation times are related to various equilibrium states of the tissue in a magnetic field. Thus, a preparation phase can be performed prior to imaging to alter these equilibrium states. Such preparation phases can either attempt to suppress myocardium or blood pool signals and thus highlight the coronary blood signal. T1 and T2 preparation phases are feasible due to the different T1 and T2 values between myocardial tissue and blood in the coronary arteries.[14,15]

Contrast Agent

A blood pool contrast agent could be introduced into the blood stream prior to magnetic resonance imaging. Contrast agents typically shorten the T1 and T2 relaxation times, producing a bright signal even when the cardiac slice is imaged in a rapid manner. Thus, if the contrast agent remains in the blood pool, the resultant signal can be preferentially enhanced.

Fat Signal Suppression

Typically, the coronary arteries lie in groves on the cardiac surface that, in adults, tend to contain deposits of adipose tissue. Thus, fat yields signals that interfere with the coronary images. Suppression of the fat signal will improve the contrast of coronary arteries images. Fat signal suppression can usually be accomplished with a preparation radiofrequency pulse sequence applied immediately prior to imaging.[3,16]

Myocardial Suppression

Myocardial signal can also interfere with adequate visualization of the coronary arteries. Myocardial signal can be preferentially suppressed, improving image quality. Subjecting the heart to low-level radiofrequency radiation results in preferential suppression of myocardial signal while the blood signal remains unaffected. Contrast produced in this way is referred to as magnetization transfer contrast (MTC)[10,17] because there is an exchange of magnetization levels between the various states of the tissues (molecules bound versus unbound).

Myocardial Blood Pool Suppression

In addition to thin tomographs, the slice selection procedure of magnetic resonance imaging can be adapted to other spatial geometries. Specifically, large blood pool regions such as the left ventricle can be targeted and the blood signal suppressed prior to imaging. This approach has been used for a projection imaging scheme where two thick-slice images were acquired encompassing a coronary artery: one image was obtained with ventricular blood not suppressed and one obtained with ventricular blood suppressed. Because blood in the coronary arteries always traverses the left ventricle, the coronary artery blood is similarly imaged with and without signal suppression. Digital subtraction of the two acquisitions depicts the coronary artery with high contrast.[18]

Discussion

Presently, magnetic resonance imaging of the coronary arteries is under development, and although the results are very encouraging the technology has not yet developed into a clinically reliable tool. One goal of coronary magnetic resonance angiography is to reduce the need for diagnostic catheter coronary angiography. This would have a twofold benefit: 1) virtual elimination of patient mortality and morbidity, and 2) reduction in costs (per examination) for detection of coronary artery disease. An idealized magnetic resonance coronary angiography procedure should be accomplished in a time interval shorter than 15 minutes. The examination could be performed by a technologist and the results reviewed by a clinical expert in a matter of minutes. The examination would reveal the position and extent of all stenoses. Ultimately, each plaque might be characterized by its composition and size. While such characterization possibilities are still remote, it is clear that technical development already underway is progressing towards this end. A comparison of the properties of the various magnetic resonance coronary artery imaging approaches are given in Table 1.

TABLE 1

Coronary Imaging Techniques: Comparison of Properties

Imaging technique (acquisition time)	Maximum slices/No. of heart beats	Minimum acquisition time (min)	Typical respiratory mode (BH time)	Minimum time to image 100 slices (min)	Signal normalized to SS GE (%)	Cardiac blur per slice (mm)
SS GE (6 msec)	1/256	4.3	gating	430	100	0.10
MS GE (6 msec)	100/256	4.3	gating	4.3	100	0.10
Turbo GE (100 msec)	6/16	0.29	single BH (16 sec)	4.5	6	1.70
Spiral GE (15 msec)	40/16	0.27	single BH (16 sec)	0.8	97	0.25
EPI (50 msec)	10/4	0.07	single BH (4 sec)	0.67	90	0.85

BH indicates breath-hold; SS GE: single slice gradient echo; MS GE: multislice gradient echo; Turbo GE: turbo gradient echo; Spiral GE: spiral gradient echo; EPI: echo planar imaging. Assumptions: 256² resolution, heart rate = 60 beats per minute, imaging time ≤600-msec period after systole. To estimate the cardiac blurring value, the heart is assumed to move by 10 mm over the 600-msec imaging period and that blurring is linearly proportional to the acquisition time. While all properties shown were derived using certain simplifying assumptions, the signal estimates in particular can only be used as an approximation because there are many variables that contribute to signal strength and are beyond the scope of this chapter.

At first it may appear to be a daunting task to process the large amount of image data generated. However, as a rule, computing power doubles every 18 months, and there are computers already available that are capable of the task of rapidly processing such data and generating reasonably high-resolution coronary artery images. Thus, as progress is made in the areas of magnetic resonance image acquisition and data viewing, the computing environments are also progressing in terms of speed and ease of use, simplifying the data management task.

Summary

Magnetic resonance imaging approaches can be applied to visualize the coronary arteries with a resolution currently in the range of 1^3 mm. Technique development continues in the areas of image acquisition, processing, and contrast. Improvements in imaging speed and resolution are expected, making the possibility of replacing some catheter coronary angiography procedures more distinct. Whether coronary magnetic resonance angiography develops with clinical or technologist expert users is presently uncertain, but in either event, patient tolerance will probably dictate that the examination time will be less than 15 minutes. In the broader picture, to be most cost efficient magnetic resonance imaging must live up to its expectation of providing a "one-stop shop" modality (ie, angiography, function, perfusion, and myocardial viability assessed in a single examination session of about 1 hour). The likelihood of this happening within the next 5 years is excellent. When the one-stop shop concept is available, cardiac diagnostics should change dramatically and the magnetic resonance approach could save considerable funds for the evolving, technically optimal, health care system.

References

1. Edelman RE, Manning WJ, Burstein D, et al. Coronary arteries: Breath-hold magnetic resonance angiography. *Radiology* 1991;181:641–643.
2. Manning WJ, Li W, Edelman RR. A preliminary report comparing magetic resonance coronary angiography with conventional angiography. *N Engl J Med* 1993;328:828–832.
3 Meyer CH, Hu B, Nishimura DG, et al. Fast spiral coronary artery imaging. *Magn Reson Med* 1992;28:202–213.
4. Mansfiled P, Morris, PG. *Magnetic Resonance Imaging in Biomedicine*. London: Academic Press; 1982.

5. McKinnon GC. Ultrafast interleaved gradient-echo-planar imaging on a standard scanner. *Magn Reson Med* 1993;30:609–616.
6. Doyle M, Scheidegger MB, de Graaf RG, et al. Coronary artery imaging in multiple one second breath holds. *Magn Reson Imaging* 1993;10: 3–6.
7. Doyle M, Mulligan SA, Matsuda T, et al. Outflow refreshment angiography: A bright blood bright static tissue technique. *Magn Reson Imaging* 1992;10:887–892.
8. Doyle M, Walsh EG, Blackwell GG, et al. Multiple contiguous slice coronary artery imaging without breath holding. Proceedings of American Society for Artificial Internal Organs Cardiovascular Science and Technology Conference. Washington, DC, 1994.
9. Sachs TS, Meyer CH, Hu B, et al. Real-time motion detection in spiral magnetic resonance using navigators. *Magn Reson Imaging* 1994;32: 639–645.
10. Wang Y, Christy PS, Korosec FK, et al. Coronary magnetic resonance with a respiratory feedback monitor: The 2D Imaging Case. *Magn Reson Med* 1995;33:116–121.
11. Keller PJ, Drayer BP, Fram EK, et al. Magnetic resonance angiography with two-dimensional acquisition and three-dimensional display. *Radiology* 1989;173:527–532.
12. Rossnick S, Laub G, Braeckleet R, et al. Three dimensional display of blood vessels in magnetic resonance. Proceedings of the IEEE Computers in Cardiology Conference.
13. Anderson CM, Saloner D, Tsuruda JS, et al. Artifacts in maximum-intensity-projection display of magnetic resonance angiograms. *AJR* 1990;154:623–629.
14. Bottomley PA, Foster TH, Argerisnger RE, et al. A Review of normal tissues hydrogen NMR relaxation times and mechanisms from 1–100 MHz: Dependence on tissue type, magnetic resonance frequency, temperature, species, excision, and age. *Am Assoc Phys Med* 1984;11:425–448.
15. Wright GA, Nishimura DG, Macovski A. Flow-independent magnetic resonance projection angiography. *Magn Reson Med* 1991;17:126–140.
16. Doyle M, Matsuda T, Pohost GM. SLIP: A lipid suppression technique to improve contrast in inflow angiography. *Magn Reson Med* 1991;21: 71–81.
17. Li D, Paschal CB, Haacke EM, et al. Coronary arteries: Three-dimensional magnetic resonance imaging with fat saturation and magnetization transfer contrast. *Radiology* 1993;187:401–406.
18. Wang SJ, Hu BS, Macovski A, et al. Coronary angiography using fast selective inversion recovery. *Magn Reson Med* 1991;18:417–423.

Chapter 18

Nuclear Magnetic Resonance Imaging as Applied to Carotid and Peripheral Atherosclerotic Vascular Disease

Thomas M. Grist, MD and Patrick A. Turski, MD

Introduction

Noninvasive vascular imaging using magnetic resonance imaging (MRI) has made significant strides towards accurate evaluation of the vessel wall and lumen in patients with atherosclerotic vascular disease. Initial reports were directed at imaging the vessel wall using conventional spin-echo techniques, and several investigators realized the potential of MRI to image atherosclerotic plaque.[1] However, these techniques were not widely accepted because the influence of flowing blood on image quality was not well understood, and signal from the lumen was variably seen in the images. This resulted in variable contrast between the vessel wall and the lumen. Techniques directed at imaging the vessel wall, rather than the lumen, have been termed "black blood" magnetic resonance angiography (MRA) techniques.

MRA techniques were not widely accepted until "bright blood" techniques using gradient-echo imaging were developed. The bright blood techniques image flowing blood as positive contrast within the lumen of the vessel, a situation that is more comparable to conventional angiographic techniques. These gradient-echo techniques, when combined with a thin-slice acquisition and com-

TMG supported in part by NIH grant K08-HL02848.

From: Fuster V, (ed.) *Syndromes of Atherosclerosis: Correlations of Clinical Imaging and Pathology.* Armonk, NY: Futura Publishing Company, Inc.: © 1996.

puter algorithms capable of forming a projectional angiogram from the data, have been rapidly embraced by a number of investigators and clinicians interested in studying the carotid and peripheral vascular systems. At many institutions, the bright blood MRA techniques have supplanted a significant fraction of conventional angiograms that would otherwise be performed in patients with atherosclerotic vascular disease.

Currently, MRA techniques are used to image the vessel lumen, whereas MRI studies are often performed in the same patient to evaluate the effects of the disease on the tissue supplied by the vessel. For example, MRI studies of the brain aimed at identifying areas of ischemic disease often accompany MRA studies of the carotid bifurcation. Therefore, when combined with MRI,

MRA has become a powerful tool for the evaluation of atherosclerotic vascular disease and its effects on the end organ.

As the tools for obtaining magnetic resonance images improve through hardware and software enhancements, investigators are beginning to readdress the issue of imaging the atherosclerotic plaque directly, or investigating the influence of blood flow dynamics on the genesis of atherosclerotic disease. For example, investigators have recently reported techniques for high-resolution plaque imaging of the carotid bifurcation.[2,3]

With these historical factors in mind, the objectives of this chapter are threefold. First, to briefly review MRA techniques as applied to carotid and peripheral vessels. Second, we review the most recent clinical studies assessing the diagnostic accuracy of MRA for imaging the vessel lumen and assessing the degree of stenosis in the carotid and peripheral vascular systems. Finally, we review the contributions of MRA and MRI of atherosclerotic plaque to the investigation of plaque morphology.

Magnetic Resonance Angiography Technique

The capability for studying fluid flow with magnetic resonance has long been recognized.[4,5] However, not until recently have the advances in MRI been applied to imaging the blood vessels, therefore leading to the development of MRA.[6-9] MRA is a technique that depends on selective imaging of moving blood in multiple thin, two-dimensional imaging sections. A series of contiguous two-dimensional thin slices may then be assembled to form a three-dimensional imaging volume. Signals from the blood vessels are maximized, while signals from the stationary tissues are suppressed. This allows the use of various computer reconstruction algorithms to reformat images from a volume of tissue into images similar to those provided by conventional angiography. In addition, the individual imaging sections are inspected for the presence of intraluminal abnormalities, or for evaluating the distribution of atherosclerotic plaque.

Magnetic Resonance Imaging

Magnetic resonance images are formed when a patient is placed inside the bore of a strong static magnetic field. When a patient is placed inside the bore, the protons in the body tend to align along the same direction as the applied static magnetic field. The fraction of protons that align with the magnetic field is related to the magnetic field strength. The protons rotate, or "precess" around an axis that is parallel to the applied magnetic field.

If an additional radiofrequency (RF) magnetic field is applied, the additional energy causes the protons to tip away from the major axis of the applied static magnetic field. As the strength of the applied RF field increases, the tip angle, or nutation angle, increases. When the externally applied RF field is turned off, the protons begin to lose energy and relax back towards their equilibrium state, oriented along the same direction as the externally applied static magnetic field. During this process of relaxation, the signals from the protons may be detected with radiofrequency antennas or coils placed around the patient. It is these signals that make up the magnetic resonance images. The process of excitation of the protons with an externally applied RF field is repeated at short intervals in order to form images. For conventional anatomic imaging, RF fields are applied every 0.5 to 2 seconds. For fast imaging techniques like magnetic resonance angiography, the RF fields are applied every 10 to 50 msec.

In order to form cross-sectional images of the body, the spatial position of the distribution of protons in the body must somehow be encoded to form a two-dimensional image. In order to spatially encode the position of these protons, additional external time-varying magnetic fields are applied. These time-varying magnetic fields serve to systematically alter the frequency of precession of the protons depending on their spatial position in the body. Computers are used to reconstruct the position of the protons in tissue, which is dependent on the frequency of precession. The spatial encoding process requires multiple applications of the RF and time-varying magnetic fields in order to encode the spatial position of every proton in the body accurately. The repetitive application of these fields results in the typical 4–12-minute acquisition times for most magnetic resonance images.

Most anatomic images of the body acquired using MRI are formed by using a spin-echo technique, where a RF pulse is applied to tip the protons perpendicular to the applied static magnetic field, which is also called a 90° pulse. For spin-echo imaging, the 90° pulse is rapidly followed by a 180° RF pulse that causes refocusing of signal (also called an "echo") that is then spatially encoded. In order to contribute to the formation of image, a proton must experience successive 90° and 180° pulses. In these typical images of the stationary tissues, signal from flowing blood is not present because the moving protons travel to a new position after the application of the 90° pulse and therefore do not experience both of the RF pulses.

Thus, techniques to form angiographic images of the blood vessels were not routinely implemented until pulse sequences capable of forming an echo after the application of only a single RF pulse were developed. These techniques are called gradient-echo pulse sequences because detectable signals are formed by manipulating the time varying magnetic field gradients to form echoes. Because only a single RF pulse is needed to generate a signal from the protons, gradient-echo pulse sequences may be repeated much more rapidly than spin-echo pulse sequences. This accounts for the shorter time between RF pulses, which for gradient-echo imaging is typically 10–50 msec.

Time-of-Flight Magnetic Resonance Angiography Technique

Because the RF pulses in gradient-echo imaging may be applied in rapid succession, the stationary protons occupying a given slice do not have sufficient time to relax to their equilibrium state parallel to the static magnetic field. As mentioned above, the signal available from a number of protons in tissue is directly related to the fraction of the protons at their equilibrium state. Therefore, if the protons are not allowed to fully relax, they are unable to yield maximal signal after several successive RF pulses applied at short intervals. These protons are described as being "saturated," and are unable to contribute signal to the image. Therefore, the signals in the stationary tissues of gradient-echo images used in MRA acquisitions are typically low (Figure 1A). However, protons in blood that flow into the imaging plane are fully relaxed, because they have not experienced the RF pulses that are applied at the slice location. These protons are fully magnetized in their equilibrium

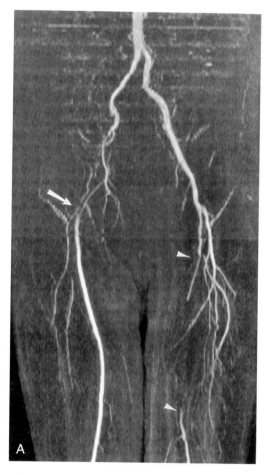

FIGURE 1. *Two-dimensional time-of-flight magnetic resonace angiography (2D TOF MRA) examination of the distal aorta through superficial femoral arteries in a patient with occlusions of the right external iliac and left superficial femoral arteries.* **A:** *Anterior to posterior projection of the 2D TOF MR angiogram demonstrates the occlusion of the external iliac with reconstitution of blood flow on the right at the level of the common femoral artery (arrow). On the left, there is an occlusion of the superficial femoral artery with reconstitution distally (arrowheads) near the adductor canal. This image represents the results of two 8-minute acquisitions of 100 2.9-mm thick axial slices each.*

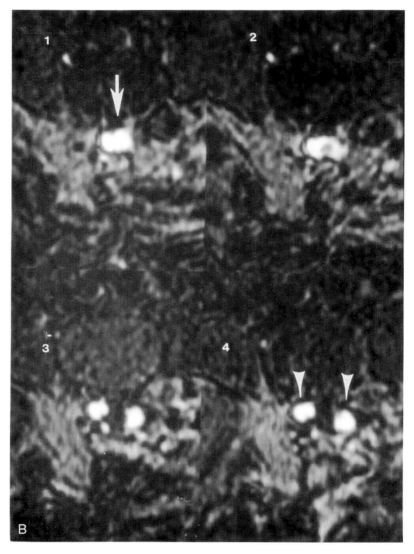

FIGURE 1 (continued). B: *Four of the axial gradient-echo 2D TOF images used to form the image in Figure 1A. The images are obtained at the level of the aortic bifurcation (arrow) and demonstrate the proximal common iliac arteries (arrowheads). Note the suppression of background signal as well as the high signal intensity within the vessel lumen caused by the inflow of unsaturated protons into the imaging slice.*

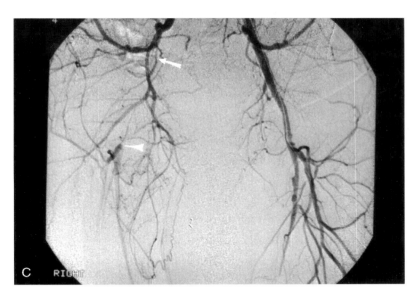

FIGURE 1 (continued). C: *Contrast-enhanced digital subtraction angiogram demonstrating the right external iliac occlusion (arrow) with reconstitution of the common femoral artery (arrowhead). Note the poor opacification of the superficial femoral artery due to the delay in contrast appearance through the extensive collateral network.*

state, and do not experience saturation unless they travel within the acquisition plane for an extended period of time. Therefore, the protons in blood yield maximal signal and appear very white on the individual source images of MRA acquisitions (Figure 1B). This effect has been called "time-of-flight" because the vascular signal is related to the velocity of blood flowing into the imaging plane, or the "time-of-flight" through the imaging slice of individual protons in the blood.

Phase Contrast Technique

Phase contrast MRA techniques provide several versatile methods for imaging the blood vessels using MRI.[10-13] The phase contrast techniques are analogous to Doppler ultrasound methods where the image is generated by observing the phase shifts of signals, rather than the magnitude of the signals. As described above, after the application of an RF pulse, the protons in the body are tipped away from the axis of the static magnetic field into a plane transverse to the static magnetic field. The protons then precess or rotate around the axis of the static magnetic field. The phase of the proton describes the position (from 0°-360°) of the proton as it rotates in the plane transverse to the applied static magnetic field. Moving spins experience different phase shifts in the presence of the applied magnetic fields used in MRA. Therefore, flowing spins may be discriminated from stationary spins by their phase shifts. For phase contrast MRA, the strength and orientation of the applied magnetic field is varied in order to encode different phase shifts for flowing protons relative to stationary protons. The operator then chooses the appropriate magnitude and direction of these velocity selective gradients in order to highlight the anatomy of interest. For example, optimal aortic signal will be obtained with velocity encoding values of 100–200 cm/sec in normal subjects, while velocity encoding values of 30–50 cm/sec yield the best results for imaging the renal arteries. Note that the velocity encoding values on magnetic resonance differ from duplex Doppler ultrasound because the magnetic resonance signals are averaged both in time and space relative to Doppler.

One potentially significant application of phase contrast magnetic resonance techniques to the analysis of atherosclerosis lies in the fact that the method is capable of providing information regarding hemodynamic measurements such as fluid shear. Moore et al[14] used a magnetic resonance velocity measurement method to determine wall shear stress in 15 postmortem human infrarenal abdominal aortas. Sites of low shear stress measured by MRI correlated with areas of intimal thickening identified on pathologic examination. The results demonstrated that sites of high shear stress tended to be spared from the development of atherosclerosis.

Atherosclerotic Plaque Imaging

Magnetic Resonance Imaging of Atherosclerotic Plaque

Time-of-flight and phase contrast MRA techniques are directed towards imaging the blood flow within the vessel lumen, rather than imaging the atherosclerotic plaque directly. However, data from recent studies suggest that luminal diameter is only an indirect predictor of stroke, but rather plaque characteristics play an important role in the pathogenesis of thrombo-embolic stroke.[15,16] Plaque morphology, the presence of hemorrhage, and the existence of plaque ulceration all significantly influence the likelihood of thromboembolic stroke. Therefore, imaging techniques directed at evaluating the atherosclerotic plaque directly may be extremely useful for predicting thromboembolic events.

The groundwork for MRI of atherosclerosis was initially laid by Kaufman et al[17] in an ex-vivo study of iliac artery specimens. Early in vivo work was directed towards atherosclerotic plaque imaging was initially implemented in the aorta, where the size of the vessel and the vessel wall were sufficient to demonstrate the presence of aortic plaque in severe aortic disease.[1] Herfkens[18] performed the first in vivo study of atherosclerosis in a retrospective review of abdominal magnetic resonance images for the presence of aortic plaque, which was confirmed by arteriography or computed tomographic (CT) scanning in 13 patients. In the past, the spatial resolution attainable with MRI has been limited, and therefore no significant application to atherosclerotic plaque imaging was appreciated. However, more recent developments in high-resolution, fast spin-echo imaging techniques have allowed the visualization of atherosclerotic plaque directly.[2,3] These techniques, called "black blood" MRI, allow good contrast between the vessel wall and lumen. More recently, Merickel et al[19] used spin-echo MRI in conjunction with an image processing technique in order to quantify atherosclerosis in the infrarenal abdominal aorta using MRI. The authors demonstrated a twofold increase in wall volume per unit vessel length, corresponding to intimal thickening, before luminal narrowing was detected. The observed intimal thickening preceded occlusion of the lumen, and the authors suggested that the technique may provide an important early indicator of the future development of atherosclerosis.[19] These techniques are currently considered investigational, and it is unknown whether the MRI technique will have sufficiently high resolution to identify disturbances in plaque content that predict the risk of thromboembolic events.

Several investigators have demonstrated the potential to characterize atherosclerotic plaque using MRI. Maynor et al[20] initially showed that fibrous plaques and adipose tissue had unique spectral features at 7.0 T, differing primarily in the ratios of their water and various fat components. Chloroform extractions revealed a typical cholesteric ester spectrum for the fibrous plaque in contrast to the triglyceride spectrum of the adipose tissue.[20] Gold et al,[21] in work evaluating ex vivo fresh specimens of the human aorta at 1.5 T, showed that vessel wall and plaque components could be identified by their magnetic resonance characteristics, and these features correlated with the histologic appearance. Plaque components such as fibrous tissue, calcification, lipids, and areas of hemorrhage were identified using the technique. Vinitski et al[2] used the data obtained from spectral analysis of carotid atherosclerotic plaques to improve conspicuity between plaque and the surrounding adventitial fat and the blood pool in spin-echo imaging.

Carotid Artery MR Imaging

Technique

A number of magnetic resonance techniques have been implemented for the evaluation of extracranial carotid arterial disease. However, the most commonly implemented techniques in the clinical environment include two-dimensional time-of-flight (2D TOF) and single or multiple slab three-dimensional time-of-flight (3D TOF).

Figure 2 demonstrates lateral views of the left and right carotid bifurcations using two different techniques. Figure 2A shows the images obtained using a 2D TOF acquisition method, where multi-

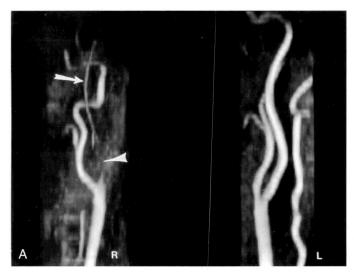

FIGURE 2. *Time-of-flight magnetic resonance angiogrophy (TOF MRA) examinations of a patient with a normal left carotid arterial system and a high-grade stenosis of the right internal carotid artery.* **A:** *Two-dimensional time-of-flight (2D TOF) examination demonstrates a normal-caliber left common, internal, and external carotid arterial system. In addition, the normal vertebral artery is seen. On the right, the examination demonstrates a high-grade stenosis of the right internal carotid artery as evidenced by the signal void of the proximal internal carotid artery (arrowhead). The 2D TOF acquisition is sensitive to slow flow, and therefore demonstrates slow flow in the distal internal carotid artery (arrow). Note that the vertebral artery on the right had been excluded from the processed image by selecting only the carotid artery for reprojection.*

ple 1.5-mm slices were acquired sequentially, acquisition parameters included a repetition time (TR)=45 msec, echo time
(TE)=6.9 msec, imaging field of view (FOV)=24 cm, image
matrix size=256"128, 1 excitation, flip angle=60°. The 2D TOF acquisition covered the area from the common carotid artery approximately 4 cm below the bifurcation through the petrous
portion of the internal carotid artery. There is uniform inflow and
normal caliber vessels including the left common carotid, external
carotid, and internal carotid arteries. Examination of the right
carotid system demonstrates that there is a high-grade stenosis involving the internal carotid artery just beyond the bifurcation. This
high-grade stenosis is associated with "string sign" showing a thin
internal carotid artery lumen with associated slow flow in the distal internal carotid artery.

The advantages of the 2D TOF acquisition are primarily related to its sensitivity to slow blood flow, as shown in Figure 2A.

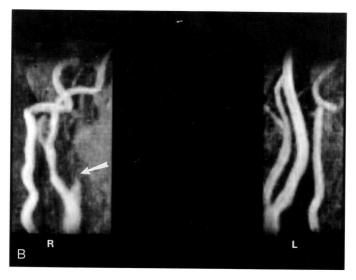

FIGURE 2 (continued). B: *Three dimensional time-of-flight (3D TOF) acquisition in the same patient. Note the widely patent left common, internal, and external carotid artery system. Note however that the 3D TOF
acquisition must be acquired over a shorter vessel segment length in order to insure adequate inflow into the entire imaging volume using the
three-dimensional acquisition technique. On the right, the internal
carotid artery appears completely occluded (arrow). No distal reconstitution of signal within the distal internal carotid artery is seen because of
the relatively slow flow in the distal internal carotid artery.*

Because the acquisition consists of multiple thin (1.5 mm or less) axial sections, blood must only flow at a rate of 3.3 cm/sec for full refreshment, using a repetition time of 45 msec. This fact explains the enhanced sensitivity of the 2D TOF acquisition to the slow arterial flow associated with the "string sign" in Figure 2A. The limitations of the 2D TOF acquisition relate to the fact that only through-plane flow is well visualized. If a blood vessel is traveling within the plane of acquisition, the relatively large flip angle (typically 60°) rapidly suppresses flow signal within the acquisition slice. This phenomena is commonly referred to as "in-plane flow saturation" and is most problematic in areas where it is necessary to visualize branch vessels. A second important limitation of the 2D TOF acquisition is the fact that relatively long echo times are used during image acquisition. The long TE results in increased sensitivity of 2D TOF study to complex flow occurring at or distal to regions of stenoses. Complex flow in these regions creates areas of signal loss on the magnetic resonance images that make exact determination of the luminal diameter difficult (Figure 3). In addition to the long TE, the relatively large volume element size and thickness of the slices in 2D TOF images also increase the sensitivity of the technique to signal loss at the site of complex flow.

The three-dimensional time-of-flight (3D TOF) image acquisition technique has several advantages and limitations relative to 2D TOF methods. Because information from the entire imaging volume is acquired every repetition time in the 3D TOF image acquisition, the imaging volume can be partitioned into thinner slices. In addition, this acquisition technique places fewer demands on the MRI hardware, and therefore the TE can be shortened relative to 2D TOF image acquisition techniques. These two factors result in overall higher spatial resolution and reduced sensitivity to complex flow occurring at the site of stenotic lesions in the vessels.[22-24]

However, the 3D TOF acquisition has several limitations relative to 2D TOF studies. Because information is acquired over the entire imaging volume every TR, flowing blood must flow relatively great distances in order to fully refresh the imaging volume. Therefore, smaller vascular segment lengths are imaged in order to insure complete inflow throughout this segment, as shown in Figure 2B. In addition, the 3D TOF acquisitions use a smaller flip angle to further reduce the likelihood of suppression of slowly flowing blood. Despite these efforts, the 3D TOF images are not well suited for imaging slow flow, as shown in Figure 2B. In the right carotid artery, the

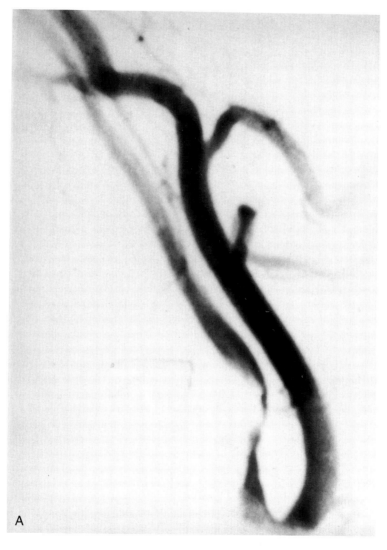

FIGURE 3. *Severe stenosis of right internal carotid artery.* **A:** *Digital subtraction angiogram demonstrates the severe stenosis of the internal carotid artery.*

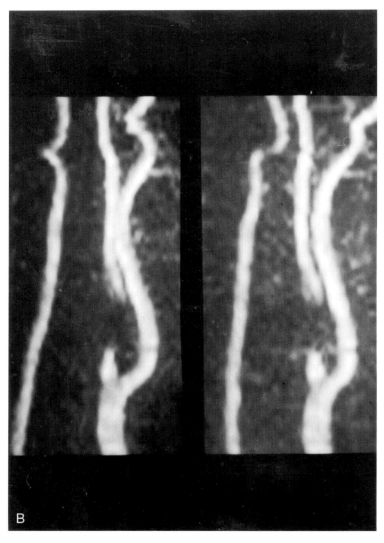

FIGURE 3 (continued). B: *Two-dimensional time-of-flight (2D TOF) acquisition shows complete signal loss at the site of the severe internal carotid artery stenosis. The signal loss at the site of the stenosis is caused by the complex, turbulent flow at the site of the stenosis and just distally. 2D TOF acquisitions are most sensitive to turbulent flow, while three-dimensional techniques are less sensitive, and therefore overestimate stenosis diameter to a lesser degree than two-dimensional acquisitions.*

distal "string sign" is not well visualized due to the suppression of slowly flowing blood that is better seen in the 2D TOF acquisition. The principle advantage, however, of the 3D TOF acquisitions are the fact that small pixels and a short TE are used, and this decreases the overall sensitivity to complex flow occurring near and distal to a stenosis. An example is shown in Figure 4A, which demonstrates a right internal carotid artery stenosis. The individual source images from the 3D TOF acquisition can be reviewed or reformatted in or-

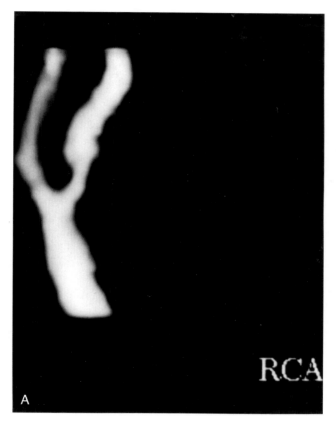

FIGURE 4. *Internal carotid artery stenosis: Measurement of stenosis diameter on three-dimensional time-of-flight (3D TOF) image acquisition.* **A:** *Surface rendered 3D TOF image acquisition demonstrating a stenosis of the proximal internal carotid artery. The maximum intensity projection and surface rendering algorithms contribute to the tendency towards overestimation of the stenosis on magnetic resonance angiography (MRA) studies.*

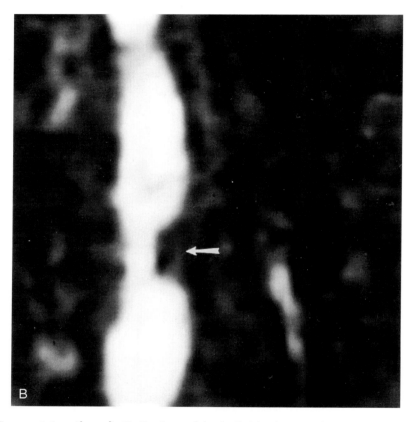

FIGURE 4 (continued). B: *Review of the individual source images or sagittal reformatted images aid in visualizing the vessel lumen at the site of the stenosis in same patient as A. Luminal area and precise luminal diameter measurements available from the three-dimensional data may help to more accurately quantify the degree of stenosis (arrow).*

der to examine the exact luminal diameter of the stenosis (Figure 4B). Because the 3D TOF acquisition is less sensitive to complex flow related signal loss, the vessel lumen is often adequately seen, particularly while reviewing the individual source images.[24]

Because the 2D TOF and 3D TOF MRA techniques each have certain drawbacks, Parker et al[25] recently proposed a hybrid method that uses a multiple overlapping thin slab acquisition (MOTSA) in order to form magnetic resonance angiograms. In this technique, multiple thin 3D TOF acquisitions are obtained and the images are registered so that a large region of vessel can be examined. The advantages of this technique include the fact that the high spatial resolution of the 3D TOF acquisition is maintained, while simultaneously retaining many of the benefits of the slow-flow sensitivity associated with a 2D TOF acquisition.

Additional quantitative blood flow velocity and volumetric

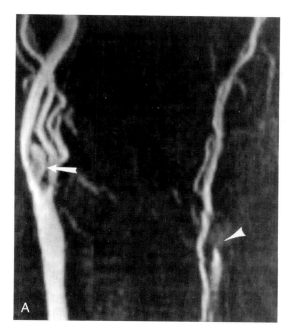

FIGURE 5. *Left carotid artery occlusion.* **A:** *Two-dimensional time-of-flight magnetic resonance angiography (2D TOF MRA) demonstrates a complete occlusion of the left common carotid artery (arrowhead). On the right, there is a large ulceration involving the proximal internal carotid artery (arrow).*

flow rate information can also be obtained using MRA techniques in clinical use.[26–28] These techniques, which rely on two-dimensional and three-dimensional phase contrast magnetic resonance acquisitions, can provide information regarding the velocity and direction of blood flow. An example is shown in Figure 5A, where magnetic resonance images from a patient with a complete occlusion of the left carotid artery and a large ulceration involving the right internal carotid artery are shown. The magnetic resonance images in Figure 5B demonstrate a large infarct in the middle cerebral artery distribution on the left. Figure 5C demonstrates 2 phase contrast (PC) MRA acquisitions obtained in the transaxial plane at the circle of Willis. In this patient with a left carotid occlusion, the images demonstrate extensive collateral flow from the right internal carotid artery as well as the left posterior communicating artery. The phase contrast techniques are particularly valuable for determining the presence of collateral flow pathways because the images may be sensitized to the speed and direction of blood flow.

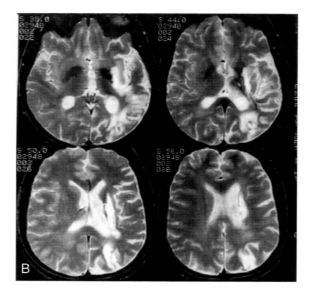

FIGURE 5 (continued). B: *Magnetic resonance images demonstrate a large infarct in the middle cerebral artery territory distribution on the left. Magnetic resonance images of the brain are often performed in conjunction with the MRA examination in order to access the effects of carotid vascular disease on the end-organ.*

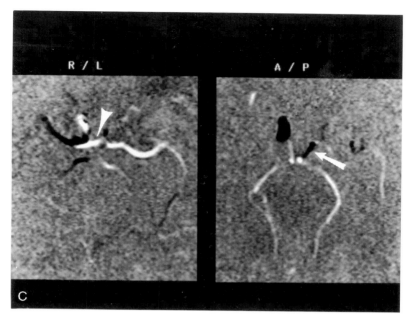

FIGURE 5 (continued). C: *Phase contrast MRA study performed at the circle of Willis to assess collateral flow. Two images from the phase contrast magnetic resonance angiogram are shown. Both images were obtained at the circle of Willis, in the transaxial plane. The image labeled R/L demonstrates a velocity image with flow encoded that moves in the right to the left direction as white pixels, while flow moving from left to right is black. The images demonstrate that left middle cerebral artery flow is provided via the anterior communicating artery from the right carotid system (arrowhead). The images labeled A/P show flow in the posterior cerebral arteries as well as the posterior communicators. In this image, flow moving posterior to anterior is encoded as black, whereas flow moving anterior to posterior is white. Note the reversal of flow (arrow) in the left posterior communicating artery, a major source of collateral flow to the left middle cerebral artery in this patient.*

Diagnostic Accuracy of Carotid Manetic Resonance Angiography

Table 1 summarizes the recent literature regarding the diagnostic accuracy of several carotid MRA trials comparing the accuracy of carotid MRA with conventional angiography. Diagnostic accuracy ranged from 87% to 100%, and for these studies sensitivi-

TABLE 1

Summary of the Results of Several Clinical Trials Studying the Diagnostic Accuracy of Carotid MRA

Reference	Year	MRA Method	No. patients/vessels	Agreement[a] (percent)	Accuracy[b] (percent)
Masaryk[42]	1988	2D TOF	14/14	15	15
Wagle[43]	1989	3D TOF	11/11	NR	100
Edeman[44]	1990	2D or 3D TOF	17/33	39	100
Kido[45]	1991	2D PC	31/60	53	100
Laster[46]	1991	2D TOF	NR/200+	90–100 (stenosis-occlusion)	NR
Litt[47]	1991	2D TOF	50/94	63	100
Masaryk[48]	1991	3D TOF	38/75	98	87
Mattle[49]	1991	2D TOF	20/39	92	100
Wilkerson[50]	1991	3D TOF	13/26	92	100
Furuya[51]	1992	3D TOF	22/26	96	100
Pavone[52]	1992	2D TOF	28/54	72	90
Riles[53]	1992	2D TOF	41/75	52	100
Wesbey[54]	1992	2D TOF	25/37	86	97
Anson[55]	1993	2D and 3D TOF	20/40	95	100
Blatter[56]	1993	3D TOF	51/102	89	99
Freeman[57]	1993	Unspecified	17/36	79	92

[a]Concurrence in depicting lesion size vs overestimation or underestimation.

[b]Identification of normal or abnormal vessel.

NR indicates not reported; 2D TOF: two-dimensional time-of-flight; 3D TOF: three-dimensional time-of-flight; 2D PC: two-dimensional phase contrast; MRA: magnetic resonance angiography.

(Adapted from *Magnetic Resonance Angiography: Vascular and Flow Imaging;* AHCPR Pub #95-0004, October, 1994, Health Technology Assessment No. 3, Table 1. US Department of Health & Human Services, Agency for Health Care Policy and Research, Rockville, MD.)

ties of 89% to 100% and specificities of 64% to 100% were observed for MRA. The wide variability of reported accuracy is in large part caused by differences in technique because the studies were performed with markedly different MRI equipment capabilities.

The North American Symptomatic Carotid Endarterectomy (NASCET) and European Symptomatic Carotid Trial (ESCT) studies have shown the beneficial affect of carotid endarterectomy in patients symptomatic for carotid disease who have a carotid stenosis >69%.[29,30] In addition, ECST showed no benefit of carotid endarterectomy for stenoses <30%.[29] These two studies show convincing evidence that different therapeutic approaches are necessary for treating carotid stenosis, and the decision regarding therapy may be based on the degree of stenosis. In addition, if the patients from the NASCET trial with 70% to 99% stenoses are further stratified into finer groups, there is a correlation between the postsurgical risk of stroke and the degree of stenosis. Therefore, it appears that accurate measures of stenosis severity may play an important role in determining the need for surgery in these patients.

The criteria in the NASCET and ECST trials is essentially based on percent diameter stenosis measurements obtained with conventional arteriography, which is a "battered gold standard" for detecting the luminal area. The deficiencies of conventional angiography have been pointed out in a number of publications,[31,32] and principally lie in the fact that the conventional arteriogram is a projectional image.

MRA, however, has the potential to provide more accurate information regarding the actual luminal diameter of a given stenosis. Because the MRA information is acquired in a three-dimensional volume, true area measurements can be performed. Likewise, the projectional MRA images may be reformatted into thin sections through the areas of stenosis in order to provide a better determination of the true luminal diameter (Figure 4). Anderson[24] recently showed that reviewing the source images from the magnetic resonance angiograms is crucial to reducing the scatter associated with grading stenoses. Using a 3D TOF acquisition, the investigators measured the percentage of diameters internal carotid artery stenosis on source images as well as the maximum intensity pixel (MIP) angiograms. Measurements were made from sagittal (n=150) and transverse (n=140) 3D TOF magnetic resonance angiograms. The diameter measurements with MRA were compared with those from conventional angiography. The investigators found that the accuracy for correctly identifying a stenosis on MRA was significantly higher for interpretation of the source images ($P<0.05$). The loss of intravascular signal frequently encountered on standard MRA MIP intensity pixel projection displays was not seen on the source images accept in stenoses exceeding 85%.

Other approaches will likely reduce the sensitivity of MRA to signal loss at the sites of complex flow near and just distal to the stenoses. For example, we recently reported an magnetic resonance acquisition technique that uses a velocity selective preparation pulse in conjunction with a fast, very short TE gradient-echo readout.[33] This pulse sequence has been shown to be insensitive to signal loss at a stenosis, caused in large part to the short echo time of the image formation technique, as well as the fact that the velocity selective preparation pulse effectively "decouples" spin dephasing during readout from spin dephasing that occurs during the vessel image contrast formation. Saloner et al[34] described a method to reduce the effects of complex flow at the carotid bifurcation using a diastolic gated acquisition, a technique that also significantly reduces artifacts due to turbulent flow. In addition, as gradient coil hardware improves, investigators have shown reduced sensitivity of MRA acquisition sequences to the complex flow at sites of stenosis by implementing MRA acquisitions with very short echo times.[35]

These two developments are important to the eventual application of MRA to the surgical planning of patients presenting for carotid endarterectomy. For example, earlier work by Mittl et al[36] found that even in cases in which magnetic resonance angiography and ultrasound both indicated a stenosis exceeding 70%, a nonsurgical stenosis could still be found at conventional angiography. This study highlights the fact that previous MRA techniques were somewhat limited in determining the percent diameter stenosis accurately. Additional techniques that provide true luminal diameter will be important to the eventual acceptance of MRA used in conjunction with ultrasound as a noninvasive preoperative evaluation of patients being considered for endarterectomy. Importantly, although MRA may not delineate the exact stenosis diameter, the technique may provide the same patient outcome after the imaging procedure as conventional angiography, especially when combined with ultrasound evaluation of the bifurcation. Several outcomes studies of this type have been proposed and are now being performed.

Peripheral Vascular Disease

Atherosclerotic vascular disease involving the peripheral arterial vascular system is a common and important cause of patient morbidity. Patients suspected of having peripheral vascular disease often are initially identified by noninvasive duplex Doppler sonography examinations, followed by imaging using conventional iodinated contrast angiography to identify the length and location of stenotic or occlusive disease. Conventional iodinated contrast angiography has several limitations, foremost is the invasiveness of the procedure, as well as the need for relatively high doses of iodinated contrast injected into the arterial system with the commensurate complications of nephrotoxicity and contrast-induced allergy.

Therefore, a noninvasive technique capable of evaluating the anatomic distribution and length of arterial occlusive disease may have significant value in the evaluation of patients with suspected peripheral vascular disease. Magnetic resonance techniques for evaluating peripherial vascular disease are evolving rapidly, and will likely supplant a large number of conventional diagnostic angiographic procedures in the near future. To date, all of these techniques are directed towards imaging the vessel lumen, rather than the atherosclerotic plaque involving the vessel wall. Many of the same principles used for time-of-flight and phase contrast MRA acquisitions in the carotid vascular system are used with similar success in the peripheral vascular system. Important, however, is the fact that determination of the exact degree of stenosis is not as essential in the peripheral vascular system as compared with carotid vascular system. In general, the most important determinant of the type of therapeutic intervention performed is the length and location of stenosis and/or occlusion, because in short segments, stenoses and occlusions are both amenable to percutaneous angioplasty procedures.

Techniques for Magnetic Resonance Angiography in the Peripheral Vasculature

Several important obstacles to imaging the peripheral vasculature are present. First, the extremities are long, making imaging times fairly lengthy. In addition, the length of the arteries has precluded the development of more efficient acquisitions in the coronal plane. Secondly, typical velocities in the popliteal artery are 50 cm/sec in systole, but only 5 cm/sec average throughout the cardiac cycle. In normal subjects, the reversal of flow during diastole in the triphasic waveform also serves to cause artifacts and reduce the net forward flow. Flow beyond hemodynamically significant lesions may average <1 cm/sec. Third, collateral formation often results in flow moving in directions opposite to the conventional direction, therefore complicating the use of presaturation slabs.

Two-dimensional time-of-flight sequences are the most commonly used acquisition technique for evaluation of the peripheral vascular system (Figure 1). Typically 300–400 thin (2–3 mm) transaxial slices are acquired, extending from the foot through the aortic bifurcation. A spatial presaturation band is placed inferior to the imaging slice in order to suppress venous flow signal, therefore allowing unobstructed views of the arterial system. Acquisition parameters for 2D TOF in the extremities include a TR=30 msec; TE=6.9; flip angle=60°; matrix size=256"128. These parameters result in images that are acquired every 5 seconds, therefore, acquisition of the entire data set requires approximately 60–90 minutes. In practice,

MRA using the 2D TOF techniques is often limited to a specific diseased segment identified with noninvasive studies. This can help to reduce the overall examination time. Images above the knee are usually acquired using the body coil for signal detection, whereas images below the knee are acquired using a dedicated extremity coil. Improvements in coil design and pulse sequence optimization are expected to significantly reduce the overall image acquisition time in the future, and it is not unreasonable to expect peripheral MRA examinations to be performed in <1 hour in the near future.

Advantages of the 2D TOF technique are related to it's sensitivity to slow flow and relative ease of implementation. In addition, the technique provides a full three-dimensional data set, therefore allowing the clinician to view the arterial anatomy at any angle, without the need for an additional acquisitions. Limitations of the 2D TOF technique include; 1) the spatial resolution is limited by the slice thickness, which is relatively large; 2) the use of the large (60°) flip angle is necessary for image signal-to-noise ration considerations, but results in suppression of signal within vessels that run parallel to the image acquisition slice; 3) the use of a spatial pre-saturation band tends to suppress retrograde and collateral that is often seen in patients with significant peripheral occlusive disease; 4) flow within the lumen of the vessel at sites of stenoses is not visualized using the technique, making exact delineation of the stenosis difficult; and 5) ghost artifacts due to vessel pulsatility tend to compromise image quality in normal vascular segments.

The limitations of 2D TOF in the extremities have been addressed by several investigators who have proposed alternate data acquisition schemes. Recently, Prince and co-workers[37-39] proposed a contrast-enhanced 3D TOF MRA technique that relies on the intravenous administration of gadolinium-DTPA contrast during the rapid acquisition of a 3D TOF study. This technique relies on the fact that gadolinium-DTPA is nearly physiologically inert, and therefore not frequently associated with typical complications of nephrotoxicity and contrast allergy. The intravenous infusion begins shortly before the MRA image acquisition, and continues until approximately 15 seconds prior to the end of the MRA imaging procedure. This results in principle "arterial phase" of the contrast agent during the image acquisition, and is insensitive to flow effects described earlier, since the examination essentially depicts any vessel occupied by contrast enhanced blood. Although the gadolinium used for this technique introduces an additional cost, the overall cost of this technique may be substantially lower due to the fact that the image acquisition method is very quick, and therefore, the technical costs associated with scanner usage are reduced.

Two-dimensional phase contrast (2D PC) techniques have also been shown to be useful for the evaluation of peripheral vascular disease.[40] Swan[40] recently described a cardiac gated phase contrast technique that is useful for evaluating lower extremity arterial disease, particularly in the pelvis, which is often plagued by artifacts due to vessel tortuosity and saturation of signal in vessels oriented parallel to the image acquisition slice. The phase contrast technique is also helpful for demonstrating collateral vessels in occlusive disease, as well as for evaluating the patency of bypass grafts that are often oriented in planes parallel to the image acquisition plane.[41]

The 2D PC acquisitions are customarily acquired in the coronal plane. A modified cine phase contrast acquisition is used. The cine 2D PC examination is performed using a thick slab acquisition, with in-plane spatial resolution of 256"192. A slab thickness of 70–99 mm is chosen in order to encompass the peripheral vasculature. A different value of velocity encoding (VENC) is chosen for each patient. The VENC is either determined qualitatively based on the age of the patient, cardiac output, and degree of inflow on 2D TOF examinations, or quantitatively determined using a "VENC prescan." The purpose of the VENC prescan is to determine the exact blood flow velocity throughout the cardiac cycle in order to more accurately determine what the appropriate VENC is for that particular patient. The modified cine 2D PC examination is also called a VENC-optimized phase contrast examination, because the VENC is varied throughout the cardiac cycle depending on the VENC prescan. Typical VENCs used range from 30–70 cm/sec. Other parameters include a TR=34 msec; TE=11 msec; flip angle 15°–25°; 2 NEX; 256"192 matrix; and 32-cm field of view.

Diagnostic Accuracy of Peripheral Magnetic Resonance Angiography

Table 2 lists the results of several early studies evaluating the accuracy of 2D TOF MRA techniques for evaluating the peripheral vascular system. Mulligan and coworkers[58] initially described the performance of a 2D TOF MRA protocol for diagnosing stenotic disease compared with conventional angiography. The authors found that the MRA evaluation of the clinical significance of stenoses agreed with the XRA in only 71% of the lesions. However, this initial report involved only 12 patients and used a 2D TOF technique that was significantly compromised by hardware and software limitations of the MRI equipment at the time. For example,

TABLE 2

Summary of Selected Reports of MRA vs. CA Applied to Study of Peripheral Vascular System

Reference	Year	MRA Method	No. patients	Study vessel(s)	Agreement[a] (%)	Accuracy[b] (%)
Mulligan[58]	1991	2D TOF	12	Iliac, femoral popliteal art.	71	67
Gehl[59]	1991	3D TOF	16	Hemodialysis fistulae	13	100
Owen[60]	1992	2D TOF	73	Infrarenal aorta to feet	82[c]	100
Hertz[61]	1993	2D TOF	19	Distal aorta, iliac femoral, popliteal, crural arteries	83	100
Spritzer[62]	1993	2D gradient-recalled echo	54	Inferior vena cava distal to popliteal veins	NR	96
Yucel[63]	1993	2D TOF	25	Distal aorta through popliteal trifurcation	84	100

[a]Concurrence in depicting lesion size vs overestimation

[b]Identification of normal or abnormal vessel

[c]MRA demonstrated additional patent vessel segments not seen by CA in 9 patients

NR indicates not reported; MRA: magnetic resonance angiography; CA: 2D TOF: two-dimensional time-of-flight; 3D TOF: three-dimensional time-of-flight.

(Adapted from *Magnetic Resonance Angiography: Vascular and Flow Imaging;* AHCPR Pub #95-0004, October, 1994, Health Technology Assessment No. 3, Table 5. US Department of Health & Human Services, Agency for Health Care Policy and Research, Rockville, MD.)

the TE was long (16 msec), resulting in significant signal loss at the sight of stenoses due to complex flow-induce dephasing. Yucel et al[63] demonstrated that a technically more advanced 2D TOF MRA approach had a sensitivity of 89% and a specificity of 95% for identifying stenoses exceeding 70% in diameter. The investigators noted that the 2D TOF technique tended to overestimate the stenosis degree relative to conventional angiography in 10 of 67 segments, but the stenosis was underestimated in only 3 of 67 segments. Hertz et al[61] demonstrated improved accuracy of the 2D TOF technique in a series of 19 patients who were studied using conventional angiography as the gold standard. The authors showed good correlation between the MRA and conventional arteriograms for defining stenosis diameter ($r=0.84$ $P<0.001$).

Because 2D TOF MRA procedures are uniquely sensitive to very slow flow, MRA may offer an advantage over conventional arteriography for evaluating the distal runoff in the leg and foot, areas that are often difficult to evaluate because of problems encountered in delivering contrast to these distal vessels. A recent report demonstrated the value of MRA in detecting radiographically occult runoff vessels in patients with threatened limb loss.[41] In this study of the runoff vessels in 23 patients, MRA detected 22% more runoff vessels and significantly altered interventional plans in 4 patients. This technique is currently being evaluated in a multicenter clinical trial.

Summary

In summary, magnetic resonance techniques to evaluate the carotid and peripheral vascular system are reaching a stage of adolescence: significant development of the methodology has occurred, yet substantial additional progress will likely be made. The MRA techniques described above are rapidly becoming accepted as clinically practical, cost effective methods to evaluate the carotid and peripheral vascular systems. Although potentially important methods to observe atherosclerotic plaque directly have been introduced, magnetic resonance plaque imaging techniques have not been widely disseminated.

References

1. Wesbey GE, Higgins CB, Hale JD, et al. Magnetic resonance applications in atherosclerotic vascular disease. *Cardiovasc Intervent Radiol* 1986;8:342–350.
2. Vinitski S, Consigny PM, Shapiro MJ, et al. Magnetic resonance chemical shift imaging and spectroscopy of atherosclerotic plaque. *Invest Radiol* 1991;26:703–714.
3. Yuan C, Tsuruda JS, Beach KN, et al. Techniques for high-resolution MR imaging of atherosclerotic plaque. *J Magn Reson Imaging* 1994;4: 43–49.
4. Hahn H. Spin echoes. *Phys Rev* 1950;80:580–594.
5. Carr H, Purcell E. Effects of diffusion on free precession in nuclear magnetic resonance experiments. *Phys Rev* 1954;94:630–638.
6. Axel L. Blood flow effects in magnetic resonance imaging. *AJR* 1984; 143:1157–1166.
7. Gulberg G, Wehrli F, Shimakawa A, et al. MR vascular imaging with a fast gradient refocusing pulse sequence and reformatted images from transaxial sections. *Radiology* 1987;165:241–246.
8. Dumoulin C, Hart H. Magnetic resonance angiography. *Radiology* 1986;161:717–720.

9. Laub G, Kaiser W. MR angiography with gradient motion refocusing. *JCAT* 1988;12:377–382.
10. Dumoulin C, Yucel E, Vock P. Two and three dimensional phase contrast MR angiography of the abdomen. *JCAT* 1990;14:779–784.
11. Bryant D, Payne J, Firmin D, et al. Measurement of flow with NMR imaging using a gradient pulse and phase difference technique. *JCAT* 1984;8:588–593.
12. Firmin D, Nayler G, Kilner P. The application of phase shifts in NMR for flow measurement. *MRM* 1990;14:230–241.
13. Spritzer C, Pelc N, Lee J, et al. Rapid MR imaging of blood flow with a phase-sensitive, limited-flip-angle, gradient recalled pulse sequence: Preliminary experience. *Radiology* 1990;176:255–262.
14. Moore JE Jr, Xu C, Glagov S, et al. Fluid wall shear stress measurements in a model of the human abdominal aorta: Oscillatory behavior and relationship to atherosclerosis. *Atherosclerosis* 1994;110:225–240.
15. O'Leary D, Polak J. High-resolution carotid sonography:past, present, and future. *AJR* 1989;153:699–704.
16. Ricotta L. Plaque characterization by B-mode scan. *Surg Clin North Am* 1990;70:191–199.
17. Kaufman L, Crooks L, Sheldon P, et al. Evaluation of NMR imaging for detection and quantification of obstructions in vessels. *Invest Radiol* 1982;17:554–560.
18. Herfkens R, Kiggins C, Hricak H, et al. Nuclear magnetic resonance imaging of atherosclerotic disease. *Radiology* 1983;148:161–166.
19. Merickel MB, Berr S, Spetz K, et al. Noninvasive quantitative evaluation of atherosclerosis using MRI and image analysis. *Arterioscler Thromb* 1993;13:1180–1186.
20. Maynor CH, Charles HC, Herfkens RJ, et al. Chemical shift imaging of atherosclerosis at 7.0 Tesla. *Invest Radiol* 1989;24:52–60.
21. Gold GE, Pauly JM, Glover GH, et al. Characterization of atherosclerosis with a 1.5-T imaging system. *J Magn Reson Imaging* 1993;3:399–407.
22. Haacke EM, Masaryk TJ, Wielopolski PA, et al. Optimizing blood vessel contrast in fast three-dimensional MRI. *Magn Reson Med* 1990;14:202–221.
23. Schmalbrock P, Yuan C, Chakeres DW, et al. Volume MR angiography: Methods to achieve very short echo times. *Radiology* 1990;175:861–865.
24. Anderson CM, Lee RE, Levin DL, et al. Measurement of internal carotid artery stenosis from source MR angiograms. *Radiology* 1994;193:219–226.
25. Parker L, Yuan C, Blatter D. MR angiography by multiple thin slab 3D acquisiton. *Magn Reson Med* 1991;17:434.
26. Huston JD, Ehman RL. Comparison of time-of-flight and phase-contrast MR neuroangiographic techniques. *Radiographics* 1993;13:5–19.
27. Tasciyan TA, Banerjee R, Cho YI, et al. Two-dimensional pulsatile hemodynamic analysis in the magnetic resonance angiography interpretation of a stenosed carotid arterial bifurcation. *Med Phys* 1993;20:1059–1070.
28. Vanninen R, Koivisto K, Tulla H, et al. Hemodynamic effects of carotid endarterectomy by magnetic resonance flow quantification. *Stroke* 1995;26:84–89.
29. Group ECSTC. MRC European Carotid Surgery Trial: Interim results

for symptomatic patients with severe (70–99%) or with mild (0–29%) carotid stenosis. *Lancet* 1991;337:1235–1243.

30. Collaborators NASCET: Beneficial effect of carotid endarterectomy in symptomatic patients with high-grade carotid stenosis. *N Engl J Med* 1991;325:445–453.

31. Zir L, Miller S, Dinsmore R, et al. Intra-observer variability in coronary angiography. *Circulation* 1977;53:627.

32. Deter K, Wright E, Murphy M, et al. Observer agreement in evaluating coronary angiograms. *Circulation* 1975;52:979.

33. Korosec F, Grist T, Polzin J, et al. MR angiography using velocity-selective preparation pulses and segmented gradient-echo acquisition. *MRM* 1993;30:1–10.

34. Saloner D, Selby K, Anderson CM. MRA studies of arterial stenosis: Improvements by diastolic acquisition. *Magn Reson Med* 1994;31:196–203.

35. Haacke EM, Lin W. Technologic advances in magnetic resonance angiography. *Curr Opin Radiol* 1991;3:240–247.

36. Mittl RL Jr, Broderick M, Carpenter JP, et al. Blinded-reader comparison of magnetic resonance angiography and duplex ultrasonography for carotid artery bifurcation stenosis *Stroke* 1994;25:4–10.

37. Prince M, Yucel E, Kaufman J, et al. Dynamic gadolinium-enhanced three-dimensional abdominal MR arteriography. *JMRI* 1993;3:877–881.

38. Prince MR, Narasimham DL, Stanley JC, et al. Gadolinium-enhanced magnetic resonance angiography of abdominal aortic aneurysms. *J Vasc Surg* 1995;21:656–669.

39. Prince MR. Gadolinium-enhanced MR aortography. *Radiology* 1994; 191:155–164.

40. Swan J, Grist T, Weber D, et al. MR angiography of the pelvis with variable velocity encoding and a phased-array coil. *Radiology* 1994; 190:363–369.

41. Owen RS, Carpenter JP, Baum RA, et al. Magnetic resonance imaging of angiographically occult runoff vessels in peripheral arterial occlusive disease. *N Engl J Med* 992;326:1577–1581.

42. Masaryk T, Ross J, Modic M: Carotid bifuraction: MR Imaging. *Radiology* 1988;166:461–466.

43. Wagle W, Dumoulin C, Souza S. 3DFT MR angiography of carotid and basilar arteries. *AJNR* 1989;10:911–919.

44. Edelman R, Mattle H, Wallner B. Extrancranial carotid arteries: Evaluation with "black blood" MR angiography. *Radiology* 1990;177:45–50.

45. Kido D, Panzer F, Szumowski J: Clinical evaluation of stenosis of the carotid bifurcation with magnetic resonance angiographic techniques. *Arch Neurol* 1991;48:484–489.

46. Laster R, Acker J, Halford H. Carotid bifurcation evaluation with vascular MR imaging. *J Magn Reson Imaging* 1991;1:205. Abstract.

47. Litt A, Eidelman E, Pinto R. Diagnosis of carotid artery stenosis: Comparison of 2DFT time-of-flight MR angiography with contrast angiography in 50 patients. *AJNR* 1991;12:149–154.

48. Masaryk A, Ross J, DiCello M. 3DFT MR angiography of the carotid bifurcation: Potential and limitations as a screening examination. *Radiology* 1991;179:797–804.

49. Mattle H, Kent C, Edelmann R. Evaluation of the extracranial carotid

arteries: Correlation of magnetic resonance angiography, duplex ultra-sonography, and conventional angiography. *J Vasc Surg* 1991;13:838–845.

50. Wilkerson D, Keller I, Mezrich R: The comparative evaluation of three-dimensional magnetic resonance for carotid artery disease. *J Vasc Surg* 1991;14:803–811.
51. Furuya Y, Isoda H, Hasegawa S: Magnetic resonance angiography of extracranial carotid and vertebral arteries, including their origins: Comparison with digital subtraction angiography. *Neuroradiology* 1992;35:42–45.
52. Pavone P, Marsili L, Catalano C. Carotid arteries: Evaluation with low-field strength MR angiography. *Radiology* 1992;184:401–404.
53. Riles T, Eidelman E, Litt A. Comparison of magnetic resonance angiography, conventional angiography, and duplex scanning. *Stroke* 1992;23:341–346.
54. Wesbey G, Bergan J, Moreland S. Cerebrovascular magnetic resonance angiography: A critical verification. *J Vasc Surg* 1992;16:619–632.
55. Anson J, Heiserman J, Drayer B. Surgical decisions on the basis of magnetic angiography of the carotid arteries. *Neurosurgery* 1993;32:335–343.
56. Blatter D, Bahr A, Parker D. Cervical carotid MR. Angiography with multiple overlapping thin-slab acquisition: Comaprison with conventional angiography. *AJR* 1993;161:1269–1277.
57. Freeman J, Free T, Rayne H. Assessing extracranial carotid stenosis: Magnetic resonance angiography, duplex scanning, and digital angiography. *South Dakota J Med* 1993;46:53–56.
58. Mulligan S, Matsuda T, Lanzer P. Peripheral arterial occlusive disease: Prospective comparison of MR angiography and color duplex US with conventional angiography. *Radiology* 1991;178:695–700.
59. Gehl H, Bohandorf K, Gladziva V. Imaging of hemodialysis fistulas: Limitations of MR angiography. *JCAT* 1991;15:271–275.
60. Owen R, Cau R, Carpenter J. Symptomatic peripheral vascular disease: Selection of imaging parameters and clinical evaluation with MR angiography. *Radiology* 1993;187:627–635.
61. Hertz S, Baum R, Ower R. Comparison of magnetic resonance angiography and contrast angiography in peripheral artery stenosis. *Am J Surg* 1993;166:112–116.
62. Spritzer C, Norconk JJ, Sostman H. Detection of deep venous thrombosis by magnetic resonance imaging. *Chest* 1993;104:54–60.
63. Yucel E, Kaufman J, Geller S. Atherosclerotic occlusive disease of the lower extremity: Prospective evaluation with two dimensional time-of-flight MR angiography. *Radiology* 1993;187:637–641.

Chapter 19

The Use of Magnetic Resonance Imaging to Study Lesion Development and Progression in Rabbits In Vivo

Russell Ross, Phd, Chun Yuan, Phd,
Elaine W. Raines, MS, Eiji Kaneko, MD,
and Michael P. Skinner, MD

Introduction

The composition of advanced atherosclerosis appears to be critical to subsequent clinical sequelae. Thus, noninvasive imaging of lesions of atherosclerosis in humans has been a goal of the clinician. However, because of limits of resolution of existing instrumentation, this goal has been elusive. In particular, evaluation of the progression of individual lesions of atherosclerosis is difficult and has generally been monitored by angiography, which is invasive and provides little data on the artery wall or the lesion itself. Because there can be compensatory dilation of any artery, despite thickening of the wall caused by atherosclerosis, angiographic detection of lesion progression may not be possible until the lesion has reached a size such that the artery can no longer compensate. Of particular concern is the fact that lipid-rich fibrous plaques, which are at higher risk for complications such as fissuring, hemorrhage, or thrombosis, cannot be differentiated from more stable fibrous plaques that are richer in connective tissue.

This work was supported in part by National Heart, Lung, and Blood Institute grant HL18645 and an unrestricted grant for cardiovascular research from Bristol-Myers Squibb Company.

From: Fuster V, (ed.) *Syndromes of Atherosclerosis: Correlations of Clinical Imaging and Pathology.* Armonk, NY: Futura Publishing Company, Inc.: © 1996.

Because of its noninvasive nature and ability to image the lumen and the wall, magnetic resonance imaging (MRI) is a particularly promising approach to follow lesions in vivo. Initial MRI of atherosclerotic vessels demonstrated a gross anatomic correlation between the morphology of the plaques in the MRI and histologic examination.[1-3] Since these early studies, image analysis protocols have been developed that distinguish vascular hemodynamics and specific structure of arteries.[4] These analyses take advantage of the fact that MRI shows superior soft tissue contrast and is sensitive to both stationary and moving subjects. Most studies were performed ex vivo to obtain high-resolution imaging.

MRI of Atherosclerotic Rabbits

In current studies, high-resolution MRI was achieved using a phased array volume coil and a standard MRI scanner to examine lesion progression in rabbits in vivo. MRI was used to examine advanced lesions of atherosclerosis serially and noninvasively in the abdominal aorta of six New Zealand white rabbits fed a moderately atherogenic diet (0.2% cholesterol, 5% peanut oil) for 14 to 16 months after repeat pullback balloon injury of the abdominal aorta 1 and 13 weeks after initiation of the diet.[5-7]

MRI of Normal, Stenotic, and Aneurysmal Vessels

The rabbits were serially imaged 9 to 16 months after injury and initiation of the diet. Four of the animals demonstrated clear stenosis of their lumens, and two had aneurysmal dilatation. Animals were visualized by time-of-flight (TOF) angiography (Figure 1). Ventral images of the abdominal aorta and iliac bifurcation demonstrated narrowing of the lumen in the animals with advanced lesions, in contrast with marked dilatation in the two animals with lesions having aneurysmal change. Axial views of the lesion areas from these animals demonstrated an increased thickening of the artery wall, compared with a rabbit on a normal chow diet (Figure 1).

MRI Detection of Lesion Progression and Plaque Fissure

It was possible to follow lesion progression via MRI in the stenotic animals. In one animal, lesions imaged 25 weeks apart demonstrated an increase in the thickening of the artery wall. Using

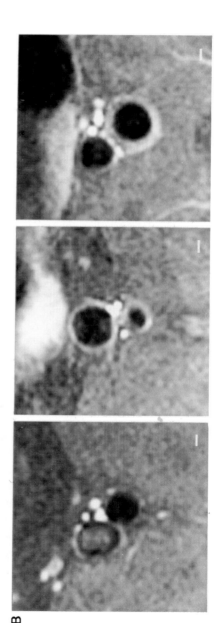

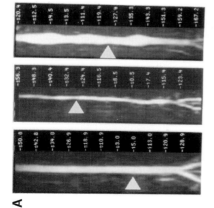

FIGURE 1. *MRI of normal, stenotic, and aneurysmal vessels. The abdominal aortas from two rabbits containing advanced lesions of atherosclerosis were imaged 14 months after injury and initiation of the atherosclerotic diet and compared with the abdominal aorta of a control animal of equivalent size fed a normal diet. In each panel, the same normal aorta is shown on the left, a diseased and stenotic aorta is displayed in the middle, and a diseased and aneurysmal aorta is shown on the right. **A.** Magnetic resonance TOF angiography of a ventral view (2D TOF, flip angle = 40°, TR = 46 msec/TE = 4.6 msec/FOV = 12 cm/matrix = 256×128). The bar (right) is 1 cm. Arrowheads indicate the sites from which the axial views were obtained in B. **B.** Axial views of PDW images acquired with fat suppression. Two-dimensional fast spin echo (TE = 6000 msec/TE = 24 msec/FOV = 9 cm/matrix = 256×256/echo train length = 8). Sites from which these images were taken are denoted by arrows in the TOF images. Scale (on images) is 1 mm.*

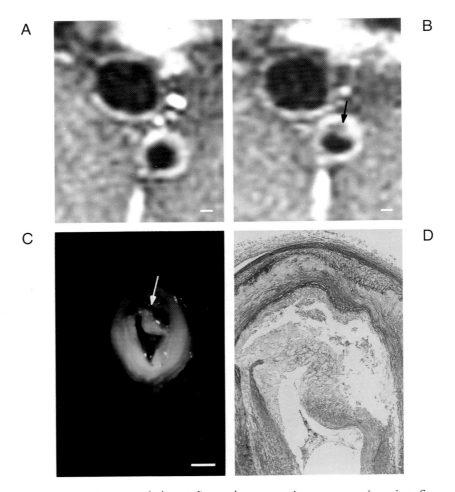

FIGURE 2. *Detection of plaque fissure by magnetic resonance imaging. Serial PDW images were acquired as described in Figure 1 and are an identical distance from the bifurcation in the same animal at two timepoints approximately 7 weeks apart. A branch at the 7 o'clock position provides an internal landmark. Axial sections are derived from a region where there is clear progression of stenosis as seen by magnetic resonance TOF angiography.* **A.** *PDW image at 12.5 months after diet initiation.* **B.** *PDW image obtained 7 weeks after the image in A. A dark region (arrow) developed spontaneously in the ventral wall of the artery that shows a hemorrhagic defect in a necrotic core, as seen in gross specimen C.* **C.** *Dissection microscopy of vessel segment imaged in B. A hemorrhagic defect in the necrotic core of a fibrous plaque (arrow) is apparent in the ventral wall of the artery and corresponds to the opaque region seen when imaged in vivo.*

the relative location of a lesion to the iliac bifurcation (reliably located by two-dimensionl TOF) and local features, such as branches and lymphatics as anatomic landmarks, it was possible to evaluate serial images at the same site. Figure 2 demonstrates by MRI an increase in thickness of the artery wall 25 weeks after the first image. The second image correlated with features of the lesion seen by dissection microscope of a segment of the artery taken at the same level 1 day later. Sites of lipid accumulation, focal necrosis, and intimal thickening observed in the histologic section correlated with changes in the MRI. Regions containing necrosis tended to appear dark, and those rich in collagen and extracellular matrix appeared light gray.

In this animal, a plaque fissure could be detected using serial proton density-weighted (PDW) images. As shown in Figure 2, a thickened artery could be seen 12.5 months after initiation of the diet (Figure 2A). A dark region (indicated by the arrow, Figure 2B) appeared 7 weeks after the initial image, which developed spontaneously in the ventral wall of the artery. Examination of the gross specimen (Figure 2C) showed a hemorrhagic defect in a necrotic core obtained by dissection microscopy of the vessel segment imaged in Figure 2B. A clear break in the collagen-rich fibrous cap was seen with histologic examination of this same site (Figure 2D).

Discussion

By developing the phased array volume coil, it has become possible to improve the resolution of the MRI method to approximately 0.4 mm while preserving a good signal level. This resolution allows definition of some of the fine structure of advanced lesions of atherosclerosis in vivo. It has also become possible to follow the progression of these lesions in vivo in the rabbit abdominal aorta and iliac arteries. Recently, images of equal quality have been obtained in nonhuman primates (unpublished data). It should be possible to adapt these approaches to human disease, particularly for more peripheral arteries, such as the carotid artery and superficial femoral artery. MRI also provides the opportunity for longitudinal studies to

*(B). This animal died while being scanned due to an overdose of anesthesia and could not be perfusion fixed. Consequently, the lumen contour was not preserved. **D.** Histology of the vessel segment imaged in B and observed under the dissecting microscope in C. The slide is from the area of defect seen by dissection microscopy in C. The immersion fixed vessel was paraffin embedded and sectioned and stained with Masson's trichrome (collagen blue, cells pink). The magnification ×100.*

examine lesion formation and progression in experimental animals and, ultimately, in humans. Furthermore, MRI might be used to evaluate the effects of therapy, such as the use of antioxidants or hepatic hydroxymethyl glutaryl coenzyme A (HMG-CoA) reductase inhibitors to induce lesion regression or prevent lesion formation.

Previous studies using MRI required ex vivo examination to achieve resolutions comparable to that obtained with the phased array volume coil at sites in vivo with relatively little motion (eg, abdominal aorta and iliac arteries). Examination of arteries where there is greater motion still presents further technical problems (eg, breathing affecting the thoracic aorta, or the heartbeat affecting the coronary arteries). Active or passive cardiac gating and faster data acquisition schemes might solve motion problems.

In summary, images acquired in vivo correlate with the fine structure of advanced lesions subsequently examined histologically, including the fibrous cap, necrotic core, and fissuring. Thus, MRI provides the potential to identify lesions noninvasively with characteristics such as more lipid-rich lesions associated with plaque fissuring and dissection. Such identification would have significant impact on possible prevention of clinical sequelae associated with these lesions.

References

1. Mohiaddin RH, Sampson C, Firmin DN, et al. Magnetic resonance morphological, chemical shift and flow imaging in peripheral vascular disease. *Eur J Vasc Surg* 1991;5:383–396.
2. Merickel MB, Berr S, Spetz K, et al. Noninvasive quantitative evaluation of atherosclerosis using MRI and image analysis. *Arterioscler Thromb* 1993;13:1180–1186.
3. Gold GE, Pauly JM, Glover GH, et al. Characterization of atherosclerosis with a 1.5T imaging system. *J Magn Reson Imaging* 1993;3:399–407.
4. Berr SS, Hurt NS, Ayers CR, et al. Assessment of the reliability of the determination of carotid artery lumen sizes by quantitative image processing of magnetic resonance angiograms and images. *Magn Reson Imaging* 1995;13:827–835.
5. Skinner MP, Yuan C, Mitsumori L, et al. Serial magnetic resonance imaging of experimental atherosclerosis detects lesion fine structure, progression and complications in vivo. *Nature Med* 1995;1:69–73.
6. Hayes CE, Hattes N, Roemer PB. Volume imaging with MR phased arrays. *Magn Reson Med* 1991;18:309–319.
7. Yuan C, Mitsumori LM, Skinner MP, et al. Magnetic resonance techniques for monitoring the progression of advanced lesions atherosclerosis in rabbit aorta. *Magn Reson Imaging* In press.

Chapter 20

Radioisotopic Imaging of Atheroma

Helmut Sinzinger, MD, Margarida Rodrigues, MD, and Harald Kritz, MD

Introduction

Atherosclerosis and its cardiovascular complications are a major cause of morbidity and mortality. A key problem of the disease is its silent progression over decades towards its acute manifestation, which frequently results in sudden death. Current therapy is directed towards control of risk factors, namely elevated cholesterol, cigarette smoking, and hypertension, that were epidemiologically identified to be causally related to the typical pathoanatomic changes of the disease.

Three mechanisms involved in human atherogenesis are lipid infiltration,[1] cellular invasion and proliferation,[2] and (parietal) thrombus formation.[3] Considerable diversity in the clinical expression of atherosclerosis shows that several mechanisms are acting in the atherogenic process and its clinical manifestation.

Despite the high rate of occurrence of the disease and although the pathomechanisms of atherosclerosis are well known, its early diagnosis is still difficult. The conventional imaging techniques that have developed over the last decade, such as computerized tomography, magnetic resonance imaging, echo Doppler, and angiography allow the identification of morphological changes that occur when the atherosclerotic plaque has already evolved and encroaches on the lumen[4] and the definition of the extent of more advanced atherosclerotic lesions.[5] Angioscopy is a new approach for studying patients with atherosclerosis, however, these techniques

Dr. Margarida Rodrigues is on leave from the Oncology Hospital of Lisbon, Portugal.

From: Fuster V, (ed.) *Syndromes of Atherosclerosis: Correlations of Clinical Imaging and Pathology.* Armonk, NY: Futura Publishing Company, Inc.: © 1996.

are ineffective for detecting atheromatous plaques in their early development.[4,5] Thus, there is a need for a noninvasive method that can identify, assess the extent, and monitor early atherosclerotic lesions at a rather early stage of the disease when the lesions are metabolically most active and when therapeutic interventions could be more beneficial.[4] Intensive research efforts have been directed towards the evaluation of metabolic changes in the arterial wall and the functional staging of atherosclerotic lesions using radionuclides.

This chapter reviews the radioisotopic techniques that have been used for gaining insights into the pathogenetic mechanisms of atherosclerosis and for the early functional imaging of atheroma.

Platelets

Platelet deposits occur at sites where the protective endothelium has been lost from the arterial surface.[6] Different mechanisms such as endothelial injury, the incorporation of a thrombus (either originated by plasmatic coagulation or by platelets alone or mostly by a combined action), and the biochemical effects of intraplatelet substances that are released in response to injury[5] are accepted as key events in the development of both the early and advanced lesions of atherosclerosis and in thromboembolic complications of the disease.

Platelet accumulation can be detected by radiolabeling of platelets if the number of platelets and the duration of reactivity at the imaging site (residence time) are sufficient.[5] Examinations after radiolabeling of platelets also allow the study of platelet behavior, namely the evaluation of the kinetics, measurement of platelet survival, in vivo distribution, and sites of sequestration of platelets.[7] For platelet labeling, several radionuclides and tracers (Table 1) have been studied during the last decades. More recently, the possibility of labeling platelets with ^{123}I-metaiodobenzylguanidine (MIBG), stable (nonradioactive) rubidium, monoclonal antibodies and [68]Ga (^{68}Ga-oxine, -tropolone and -MPO) were also tried. However, because of the advantageous physical characteristics of [111]In (Table 2) that allow external imaging as well as parallel kinetic monitoring, and the advantages of oxine (namely its comparatively simple handling and general availability) compared with other chelates for radiolabeling platelets with ^{111}In,[7] ^{111}In-oxine is still the radiopharmaceutical of choice for platelet labeling. The radiolabeling of platelets with ^{111}In-oxine is a rather simple technique that can be performed in 45–60 minutes.

TABLE 1

Radionuclides and Complexes Most Frequently Used for Platelet Labeling

Radionuclides	Complexes
^{51}Cr	
^{111}In	Oxine
	Oxine-sulphate
	Tropolone
	Mercaptopyridine-N-oxide (MPO, MERC)
	Acetylacetone
	Chlorotetraphenylporphyrin
^{99m}Tc	Oxine
	Hexamethylpropylaminooxime (HMPAO)
	Phytate

The accumulation of radiolabeled platelets at atherosclerotic lesions has been demonstrated in various parts of the vascular tree (Table 3). Platelet uptake is generally used to quantify the severity of the atherosclerotic ulceration or the tendency towards thrombosis. Platelets incorporate into lesions and accumulate only in active thrombus. The prevalence of positive images varies extremely from young stroke patients (>70%) to intermittent claudication patients (<15%). No correlation to the clinical extent of the disease (as assessed by angiography) was found.[5]

Surprisingly, active human atherosclerotic lesions identified by imaging are relatively stable and show minimal changes in activity over periods of at least several weeks unless subject to pharmacological intervention. Platelet labeling has thus also been successfully used for monitoring the efficacy of platelet-inhibitory drugs

TABLE 2

Characteristics of ^{111}In

Half-life—	2.83 days
Major energies of gamma photons—	173 KeV (89%)
	247 KeV (94%)
Gamma camera imaging	
High cost	
LE— > 80% (depending on the complex)	
No specificity of labeling	
Elution rate—0.27% per hour	

TABLE 3

Imaging of Atherosclerosis Using Radiolabeled Platelets

Carotid arteries
Abdominal aorta
Femoral arteries
Aneurysms
Thrombogenicity
Therapeutic monitoring

(Table 4) in atherosclerotic disease and, in particular, in peripheral vascular disease[8–11] and carotid artery disease.[12] Although platelet labeling has long been established, it is not yet widely used. Labeling problems, interpretation, and a variety of other methodological factors[7] are limiting its general application.

Low-Density Lipoproteins

Chronically elevated blood low-density lipoprotein (LDL) levels are among the factors identified that lead to the development of premature atherosclerosis. Exposure of proliferating endothelial cells to ^{125}I-LDL in amounts associated with the premature development of atherosclerosis has been shown to induce a delayed and an exponential increase in endothelial monolayer permeability to macromolecules.[13] Once elevated permeability developed, it persisted, and it was not readily reversible by successive exposure to lower LDL levels. The precise pathomechanism by which elevated LDL concentrations exert their effect remains to be clarified.

TABLE 4

Effect of Drugs Evaluated by Platelet Labeling

Aspirin
Dipyridamole
Codergocrine (Hydergine[R])
Dihydroergotoxin
Sulfinpyrazone
Prostaglandins
Nitric oxide donors
Calcium channel blockers
Angiotensin-converting enzyme inhibitors
Clofibrate

LDL labeling was introduced about a decade ago by Lees et al.[14] Since then, radiolabeling of autologous LDL became a useful technique for in vivo monitoring of both vascular LDL and liver LDL metabolism.[5] Various radionuclides (^{131}I, ^{125}I, ^{123}I, ^{99m}Tc, ^{111}In, and ^{67}Ga) have been used for labeling of LDL. Short-lived isotopes such as ^{123}I or ^{99m}Tc provide images with better quality than longer-lived isotopes, whereas these are preferable to obtain kinetics data.

Normally, no uptake of radiolabeled LDL can be seen in the vascular system.[15] However, under a variety of experimental conditions, an increased entry of LDL into the arterial wall in vitro[16] and in vivo[15] has been demonstrated. Autologous ^{123}I-labeled LDL was shown[15] to allow localization of areas with an increased LDL entry as well as to allow monitoring of kinetics in patients suffering from clinically manifest atherosclerosis. The imaging itself seemed to be independent of the lipoprotein profile, reflecting an increased local LDL lesion influx only.[15] A relevant LDL retention was found only in lipid and foam cell rich lesions, while advanced lesions such as fibrous plaques showed much less or sometimes almost no uptake at all.[5]

The accumulation of lipids within the arterial plaque and not at the surface (where fissures and ruptures occur) does not allow direct imaging of the plaque rupture with radiolabeled lipids or lipoproteins. Because platelets accumulate at the surface of arterial lesions, platelet imaging could be useful. However, the long residence of platelets at the arterial lesions and also the necessity of performing imaging at the precise time of occurrence of the fissure makes it rather unlikely that platelet imaging may contribute to the diagnostic identification and monitoring of plaque rupture.

Recently, imaging and kinetic analysis with radiolabeled LDL allowed the characterization of the surface lining as well as the estimation of the foam cell content of the lesions in an experimental model of atherogenesis in cholesterol-fed rabbits (Figure 1A to 1C) as well as in humans (HS, unpublished data). Imaging with radiolabeled LDL may thus be a simple approach for identifying certain vascular areas characterized by an enhanced lipid entry and for assessing the disease activity. Preliminary results of studies performed in patients under dietary as well as drug treatment indicate that radiolabeled LDL may also be promising for giving information about the efficacy of a treatment regimen in patients suffering from atherosclerosis and hyperlipidemia.

LDL-apheresis is widely accepted as an efficacious and safe therapy for patients suffering from severe familial hypercholesterolemia. It reduces atherogenic LDL from about 40% up to 75%,

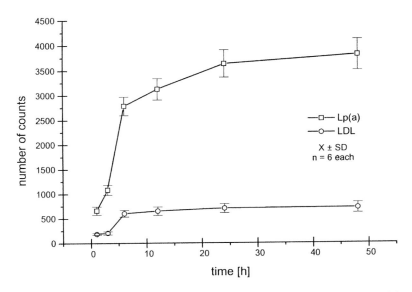

FIGURE 1A. *Accumulation of* [125]*I-LDL and* [125]*I-Lp(a) in intact areas of the rabbit arterial wall.*

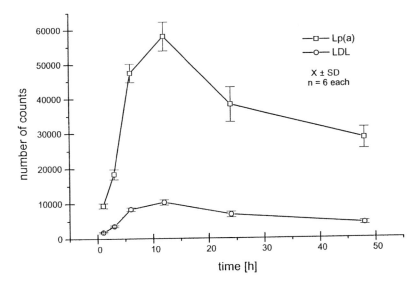

FIGURE 1B. *Accumulation of* [125]*I-LDL and* [125]*I-Lp(a) in deendothelialized areas of the rabbit arterial wall.*

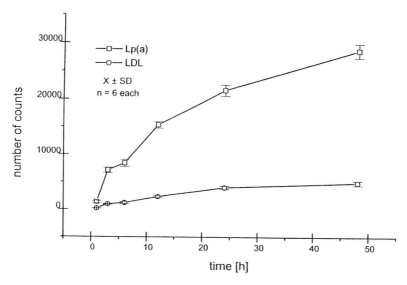

FIGURE 1C. *Accumulation of ^{125}I-LDL and ^{125}I-Lp(a) in reendothelialized areas of the rabbit arterial wall.*

induces regression of many clinical symptoms (eg, xanthoma or angina pectoris) as early as after a few weeks of therapy, and improves both in vitro and in vivo platelet function. LDL-apheresis can be monitored effectively by this approach.

Lipoprotein(a)

There is strong evidence that high plasma levels of lipoprotein(a) (Lp(a)), a genetic variant of plasma LDL, are an important risk factor for premature development of atherosclerosis.[17] Most of the atherogenicity of Lp(a) seems to depend on processes occurring in the arterial intima. However, the pathophysiological mechanism(s) whereby an increased concentration of Lp(a) contributes to disease remains to be elucidated. The atherogenicity of Lp(a) may reside mainly in its affinity for fibrin in lesions, which leads to accumulation of lipid in fibrous plaques. Increased fibrin deposition and high levels of Lp(a) may be thus synergistic factors in atherogenesis.[18]

A higher entrapment of ^{125}I-Lp(a) was found[19] in foam cell-rich areas at the shoulder of the lesion rather than in a more central region. It is likely that (chemically) modified Lp(a) particles enter preferentially into the macrophages resident in the intima and media, and promote their transformation into foam cells.

Lp(a) seems to be transferred into the arterial wall by a mechanism similar to that of LDL. However, Lp(a) was found to accumulate in the arterial wall to a much higher extent than LDL in cholesterol-fed rabbits (Figure 1A to 1C) (HS, unpublished data).

In humans, extensive information concerning radiolabeled Lp(a) is not yet available. Preliminary studies (HS, unpublished data) in hypercholesterolemic patients show a high uptake of ^{125}I-Lp(a) by the liver, which seems to indicate that the use of radiolabeled Lp(a) will not lead to a sufficient uptake from the vessels to allow detection and quantification of the activity of atherosclerotic lesions. Further research is required to evaluate the specific indications and the value of radiolabeled Lp(a) and (mildly) oxidized Lp(a) for studying experimental and human atherosclerosis.

Modified Low-Density Lipoproteins

One of the processes involved in atherogenesis that has been studied extensively in vitro and in vivo is the oxidative modification of LDL. It was first proposed that modification of LDL was a prerequisite for macrophage uptake.[20] It is now well known that modified LDL, and especially oxidized LDL, is taken up via a scavenger receptor of monocyte-derived macrophages. The scavenger receptor, in contrast to the classic LDL receptor, shows no regulation and does not recognize native LDL.[21] By the subsequent accumulation of cholesteryl ester the macrophages transform into foam cells. The findings that massive accumulation of foam cells is observed in early atherosclerotic lesions supports the hypothesis that unlimited uptake of the oxidatively modified LDL by macrophages is involved in the development of atherosclerosis in vivo.

Several forms of biologically modified LDL recognized by scavenger receptors do exist, eg, oxidized-, acetylated-, glycosylated- and malonylated-conjugated-LDL. Oxidation can be induced by incubating it under appropriate culture conditions (Table 5).[21] Many different products are generated during the oxidative modification of LDL and presumably each of these may have diverse biological effects. Releasing products of oxidized LDL, among others, are chemotactic for monocytes and T lymphocytes, inhibit the motility of macrophages, and are highly cytotoxic to various cells, including endothelial cells,[22] which potentiate the pathological accumulation of cholesterol in the arterial plaque.

Measures to protect LDL and to inhibit oxidative modification of LDL in order to retard the initiation and/or progression of atherosclerotic lesions are an exciting area for future research.

TABLE 5

Induction of LDL-oxidation

Incubation with cells
(action of cellular oxygenase, generation
of active oxygen in the cell)

Endothelial cells
Smooth muscle cells
Macrophages
Fibroblasts
Platelets

Incubation with catalysts of lipid peroxidation
transition metals (eg, copper, iron)

Monocytes

The role of monocytes in cholesterol-induced atherosclerosis of animals as a result of tissue reaction after injury to the endothelium is well established. There is now evidence that one of the earliest events implicated in the pathogenetic process of atherosclerosis is the adherence of circulating monocytes to the intact endothelial lining of the artery, followed by migration of adherent monocytes through endothelial junctions into the subendothelial space where they demonstrate phagocytic capabilities and begin to accumulate lipid, finally being transformed into lipid-laden macrophage foam cells. The factors predisposing to monocyte adhesion in vivo as well as the monocyte kinetics and their in vivo distribution remain, however, poorly understood.

In vitro studies confirmed monocyte migration into atherosclerotic arteries. For in vivo studies, the use of radiolabeled monocytes is still at a very early stage and has been limited by their radiosensitivity (doses higher than 20 μCi ^{111}In/10^8 monocytes decrease cell viability starting as early as 6 hours after labeling) and several severe technical problems, namely the contamination of monocytes isolated from blood with adherent platelets and other white blood cells, and thus the methodology necessary to harvest a sufficient number of monocytes (about 1.10^9) in high purity for the scintigraphic imaging using monocytes. Because of the quite small number of cells that can be obtained, in vivo quantification may be rather difficult. Limited data are available, however, show that imaging of lesions (monkey, human) is possible and that they colocalize frequently with LDL-positive areas.

In the future, the study of autologous monocytes may contribute to the monitoring of cellular movement into the arterial wall. Loading monocytes with modified LDL using a double tracer (^{123}I and ^{111}In) technique for radiolabeling is currently under investigation.

Fibrinogen

Fibrinogen is involved in atherothrombotic events and in the development of cardiovascular disease. It has a half-life of about 3 to 4 days, being catabolized to fibrin(ogen) degradation products. Fibrin and its related fragments seem to contribute to atherogenesis via multiple mechanisms and to be involved in the initiation of atherosclerotic lesions, namely by causing endothelial cell disorganization, being associated with stimulation of smooth muscle cell proliferation, binding to plasma lipoproteins, and attracting macrophages, which leads to lipid accumulation.

Cases of arterial thrombi detected in vivo with [125]I-, [131]I-, or ^{123}I-labeled fibrinogen were reported. However, early expectations about the study of atherosclerosis with radiolabeled fibrinogen were not fulfilled by later clinical use. In patients with either cerebral or peripheral vascular disease, no usefulness could be found. Detection of coronary thrombi is limited to anecdotal single reports.

Fibronectin

Fibronectin is abundant in human atherosclerotic intimal lesions, especially in developing fibrous plaques, as well as in experimentally induced atherosclerotic lesions.[23] [131]I-, [111]In-, and ^{125}I-labeled fibronectin were shown to accumulate in experimental arterial lesions. However, as no positive human imaging data are available and any accumulation will always be unspecific, it is rather unlikely that this glycoprotein will have a great diagnostic future.

Porphyrins

The mechanism of uptake of various porphyrins by atherosclerotic lesions has not yet been clarified. A selective unspecific accumulation of a hematoporphyrin derivative in rabbit and nonhuman primate atheromatous lesions was originally reported.[24] Biodistribution showed an enhanced uptake by the liver, spleen, kidney, and bone marrow.

A varying lesional composition might result in a different porphyrin uptake pattern. It seems very likely that these unspecific labels will not be successful for imaging atherosclerotic lesions.

Human Immunoglobulin G

Foam cells, monocytes, and macrophages trapped in the subendothelial space express abundant Fc receptors that selectively bind IgG, most probably by Fc-receptor interaction.[25] Polyclonal IgG and specifically its Fc subunit are preferentially bound to the atherosclerotic plaque, most particularly in young lesions in which the foam cell is most abundant.[26] The use of radiolabeled human immunoglobulin G (HIG) and Fc fragments has been explored in an attempt to image experimental and human atheroma.

In an experimental model of atherogenesis in cholesterol-fed rabbits, ^{111}In-polyclonal HIG accumulation was higher in de- and reendothelialized areas (Table 6), foam cells, at the edge of lesions and hyperlipidemia (Table 7). In 43 patients with clinically manifested atherosclerotic lesions in the carotid arteries, ^{111}In-polyclonal HIG identified 86% of the lesions shown by ultrasonography. However, it did not correlate to the extent and the clinical stage of the disease as shown by ultrasonography. In a preliminary study in patients with cerebrovascular disease, ^{99m}Tc-HIG scintigraphy identified 75% (3 out of 4 arteries) of atheromatous lesions.[27] These data indicate that imaging with radiolabeled HIG, although unspecific, is promising for providing valuable information concerning metabolic aspects of atherosclerosis. However, autoantibodies produced against biologically modified lipoproteins may compete with IgG for Fc-receptor binding,[26] which may hamper the interpreta-

---

TABLE 6

HIG Accumulation in the Rabbit Arterial Wall

	HIG
Endothelialized areas	0.009±0.0003 (n=11)
Deendothelialized areas	0.032±0.0130 (n=10)
Reendothelialized areas	0.029±0.0050 (n=7)

*uptake in % of injected dose/g tissue
X±SD, n=6 each, **P<0.001

TABLE 7

HIG Uptake* and Sudan III-Staining in the Rabbit Arterial Wall

	Positive	Negative
Aortic arch	0.029±0.006	0.008±0.0001**
Thoracic aorta	0.012±0.005	0.005±0.0003**
Abdominal aorta	0.024±0.003	0.007±0.0003**

*uptake in % of injected dose/g tissue
X±SD, n=6 each, **P<0.001

tion of results obtained with radiolabeled HIG. Whether radiola-beled-IgG, radiolabeled Fc fragments, or radiolabeled polymers of Fc may be of benefit in the future for the early diagnosis and de-termination of the clinical stage and extent of atherosclerosis in hu-mans still needs further study.

Peptides

Accumulation of SP-4 (a synthetic ApoB peptide fragment)[28] labeled with ^{123}I,[29] [125]I,[30] and [99m]Tc[31] was found in rabbit athero-sclerotic plaque. SP-4 seems to be able to detect metabolically ac-tive atherosclerotic plaque and to be potentially useful for imaging atherosclerosis in vivo. Administration of other peptides in humans has not yet been studied. The mechanism of uptake of peptides by atherosclerotic lesions and their binding site has not yet been iden-tified.

Monoclonal Antibodies

Monoclonal antibody technology offers the opportunity to ob-tain targeting agents with high specificity and affinity. Investigation of the use of lipoprotein-specific antibodies, antibodies against the LDL receptor and their respective fragments and peptides contin-ues. The ^{99m}Tc labeling to lys-cys-thr-cys-cys-ala aminoacids and linking them to molecular (minimal) recognition units may be also of great value, namely for thrombus imaging.

Radiolabeled monoclonal antibodies may be a promising non-invasive and specific approach for imaging atherosclerotic lesions in the future. Monoclonal antibodies may also have potential use as targeting vehicles for antiatherosclerotic drugs.

Positron Emission Tomography

^{68}Ga-labeling of platelets (MPO platelets, oxine platelets, tropolone-platelets), ^{68}Ga-labeling of LDL (native LDL, oxidized LDL, glycosylated LDL, malonylated LDL),

^{68}Ga-labeling of Lp(a) (oxidized Lp(a)), and ^{68}Ga-labeling of oxine monocytes has been investigated for thrombus or atherosclerosis imaging. The ^{68}Ge/^{68}Ga generator is a relatively cheap source of positron emission tomography (PET) radiopharmaceuticals and a promising alternative to the cyclotron for clinical applications. Thus, expectations exist about PET becoming a routine clinical tool, capable of providing functional imaging of vascular lesions with high resolution.

However, the resolution of the PET system and the high radiation dose delivered to the spleen are limiting factors for ^{68}Ga-PET imaging. Also, the half-life of ^{68}Ga (68 minutes) is too short for monitoring the accumulation of ^{68}Ga radiopharmaceuticals in lesions, and also limits the time for the preparation of the Ga complex.

Application of PET studies to humans and further research for improving ^{68}Ga radiopharmaceuticals are necessary for evaluating the specific applications and the potential advantages of this new procedure for the study of vascular lesions.

Conclusions

The clinical introduction of specific drugs designed to reduce the incidence and complications of vascular disease has increased the demand for and interest in a clinical imaging approach that would allow rapid diagnosis of human atherosclerosis, determination of the activity of the disease in a subclinical stage, and therapy monitoring.

In recent years, a large number of different scintigraphic techniques, using specific or unspecific radiolabeling agents, have been implemented for studying the main mechanisms of atherogenesis and for the functional imaging of vascular lesions, with varying degrees of success. Other than ^{111}In-oxine platelets imaging, which has been long established, no general recommendations and procedures exist. Methodological problems and insufficient knowledge concerning the in vivo behavior of almost all the agents studied are limiting their widespread clinical use.

With these methodologies it is now possible to gain insight and achieve better understanding of the spontaneous course of the pathogenetic mechanisms of atherosclerosis for a certain vascular segment. Furthermore, these procedures seem to be a simple and rather promising approach for diagnosing patients suffering from atherosclerosis, namely for detecting the disease at an early pre-clinical state, as well as for assessing the disease activity and for monitoring the efficacy of therapeutic interventions. Overall, nuclear medicine methodologies appear to have a fascinating future in the study of the vascular system. However, further studies to evaluate the specific indications and value of these noninvasive techniques for evaluating atherosclerosis in vivo are needed.

References

1. Anitschkov NN. Experimental arteriosclerosis in animals. In: Cowdry EC, ed. *Arteriosclerosis: Survey of the Problem*. New York: MacMillan; 1933:271–322.
2. Virchow R. Phlogose und Thrombose im Gefaßsystem. In: *Gesammelte Abhandlungen zur wissenschaftlichen Medizin*. Berlin: Hirsch; 1856.
3. Rokitansky Cv: *Über einige der wichtigsten Krankheiten der Arterien*. Vienna: KuK Hofund Staatsdruckerei; 1852.
4. Prat L, Torres G, Carrió I, et al: Polyclonal ^{111}In-IgG, ^{125}I-LDL and ^{125}I-endothelin-1 accumulation in experimental arterial wall injury. *Eur J Nucl Med* 1993;20:1141–1145.
5. Sinzinger H, Virgolini I. Nuclear medicine and atherosclerosis. *Eur J Nucl Med* 1990;17:160–178.
6. Harker LA, Ross R, Glosmet JA. The role of endothelial cell injury and platelet response in atherogenesis. *Thromb Hemost* 1978;39:312–321.
7. Rodrigues M, Sinzinger H. Platelet labeling—methodology and clinical applications. *Thromb Res* 1994;76:399–432.
8. Mustard JF, Moore S, Packham MA, et al. Platelets, thrombosis and atherosclerosis. In: Sinzinger H, Auerswald W, Jellinek H, Feigl W, eds. *Progress in Biochemical Pharmacology*. Basel: S. Karger; 1977:312–325.
9. Sinzinger H, Fitscha P: Epoprostenol and platelet deposition in atherosclerosis. Lancet 1984; i: 905–906.
10. Sinzinger H, Fitscha P, O'Grady J et al: Synergistic effect of prostaglandin E1 and isosorbide dinitrate in peripheral vascular disease. Lancet 1990; i: 627–628.
11. Sinzinger H, Kaliman J, Fitscha P, et al. Diminished platelet residence time on active human atherosclerotic lesions in-vivo-evidence for an optimal dose of aspirin? *Prostaglandins Leukot Essent Fatty Acids* 1988;34:89–93.
12. Weiss K, Gludovacz D, Sinzinger H. Additive action of calcium blockers and ASA on platelets. In: Schrör K, ed. *Prostaglandins and Other Eicosanoids in the Cardiovascular System*. Basel: S. Karger; 1985: 511–514.
13. Guretzki HJ, Gerbitz KD, Olgemöller B, et al. Atherogenic levels of low density lipoprotein alter the permeability and composition of the endothelial barrier. *Atherosclerosis* 1994;107:15–24.

14. Lees S. External imaging of human atherosclerosis. *J Nucl Med* 1983;24:154–161.
15. Sinzinger H, Bergmann H, Kaliman J, et al. Imaging of human atherosclerotic lesions using ^{123}I-low-density lipoprotein. *Eur J Nucl Med* 1986;12:291–292.
16. Alavi M, Moore S. Measurement of ^{125}I-I-LDL entry into ballooned rabbit aorta using average plasma value. *Arteriosclerosis* 1985;5:413.
17. Scanu AM. Genetic basis and pathophysiological implications of high plasma Lp(a) levels. *J Intern Med* 1992;231:679–683.
18. Smith EB. Fibrinogen and atherosclerosis. *Wien Klin Wochenschr* 1993;105:417–424.
19. Kreuzer J, Lloyd M B, Bok D, et al. Lipoprotein(a) displays increased accumulation compared with low-density lipoprotein in the murine arterial wall. *Chem Phys Lipids* 1994;67/68:175–190.
20. Goldstein JL, Ho YK, Basu SK, et al. Binding site on macrophages that mediates uptake and degradation of acetylated low density lipoprotein, producing massive cholesterol deposition. *Proc Natl Acad Sci USA* 1979;76:333–337.
21. Steinberg D, Parthasarathy S, Carew TE, et al. Beyond cholesterol. Modifications of low-density lipoprotein that increase its atherogenicity. *N Engl J Med* 1989;320:915–924.
22. Witztum JL. Role of oxidised low density lipoprotein in atherogenesis. *Br Heart J* 1993;69:12–18.
23. Stenman S, van Smitten K, Vaheri A. Fibronectin and atherosclerosis. *Acta Med Scand* 1980;642:165–170.
24. Spears JR, Shopshire D, Paulin S. Fluorescence of experimental atheromatous plaques with hematoporphyrin derivative. *J Clin Invest* 1983;71:395–399.
25. Fowler S, Shio H, Haley NJ. Characterization of lipid-laden aortic cells from cholesterol-fed rabbits. IV. Investigation of macrophage-like properties of aortic cell populations. *Lab Invest* 1979;41:372–378.
26. Demacker PNM, Dormans TPJ, Koenders EB, et al. Evaluation of indium-polyclonal immunoglobulin G to quantitate atherosclerosis in Watanabe heritable hyperlipidemic rabbits with scintigraphy: Effect of age and treatment with antioxidants or ethinylestradiol. *J Nucl Med* 1993;34:1316–1321.
27. Prat L, Roca M, Rubio J, et al. ^{111}In-platelets and [99]mTc-human polyclonal immunoglobulin (HIG) scintigraphy in patients with cerebrovascular disease. *Rev Esp Med Nucl* 1993;11:163.
28. Shih IL, Lees RS, Chang MY, et al. Focal accumulation of an apolipoprotein B-based synthetic oligopeptide in the healing rabbit arterial wall. *Proc Natl Acad Sci USA* 1990;87:1436–1440.
29. Hardoff R, Braegelmann F, Zanzonico P, et al. Imaging atherosclerosis with I-123 SP4. *J Nucl Med* 1992;33:845.
30. Hardoff R, Zanzonico P, Braegelmann F, et al. Autoradiographic identification of atherosclerosis with I-[125] SP4. *Circulation* 1992;86:78.
31. Vallabhajosula S, Goldsmith SJ, Buttram S, et al. Noninvasive imaging of atherosclerotic lesions in rabbits with Tc-99m labeled peptides. *Circulation* 1992;86:709.

Chapter 21

Radiopharmaceutical Imaging of Atherosclerosis

Robert S. Lees, MD and Ann M. Lees, MD

Introduction

Imaging atherosclerotic plaques by radiopharmaceutical techniques has the potential to allow characterization of such lesions by their metabolic activity. This approach contrasts with traditional methods of detecting atherosclerotic lesions either by their space-occupying characteristics or by the disturbance of laminar blood flow that is produced by luminal encroachment (Figure 1). For example, catheter-based arterial angiography outlines luminal narrowing (Figure 1, A), and the ability of the method to detect plaques depends almost entirely on the presence of luminal encroachment. B-mode ultrasound, and with lower resolution, magnetic resonance imaging (MRI), detect plaques by their bulk (Figure 1, B). When luminal encroachment approaches three quarters of the cross-sectional area of the vessel, blood flow becomes unstable, and at higher degrees of stenosis, frankly turbulent (Figure 1, C). Such flow disturbances can be detected by Doppler ultrasound and magnetic resonance angiography (MRA). However, all of these techniques locate only advanced atherosclerosis. Detection of early plaques, which produce little or no luminal encroachment (Figure 1, D), and evaluation of plaque stability must depend on other plaque properties such as metabolic activity. This activity includes, but may not be limited to, extracellular low-density lipoprotein (LDL) trapping, smooth muscle cell migration and proliferation, and inflammatory responses such as monocyte recruit-

This work was supported by grants from the National Heart, Lung and Blood Institute, Diatech Incorporated, and the Boston Heart Foundation.

From: Fuster V, (ed.) *Syndromes of Atherosclerosis: Correlations of Clinical Imaging and Pathology.* Armonk, NY: Futura Publishing Company, Inc.: © 1996.

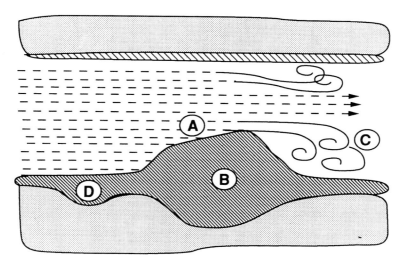

FIGURE 1. *Schematic cross section of an atheromatous artery showing properties that allow in vivo detection by traditional methods. **A.** Luminal narrowing, detectable by contrast angiography and magnetic resonance angiography (MRA). **B.** Lesion mass, detectable by B-mode ultrasound and magnetic resonance imaging (MRI). **C.** Disturbed blood flow, demonstrable by Doppler ultrasound and MRA. **D.** An early lesion, which does not have sufficient mass to be seen by ultrasound or magnetic resonance and that does not encroach on the lumen sufficiently to disturb blood flow. Such lesions are invisible to the diagnostic modalities listed in A-C.*

ment, foam cell development, and invasion by lymphocytes and granulocytes.

Symptoms do not appear until relatively late in the course of atherosclerosis. The clinical silence occurs because the early changes of atherosclerosis involve enzymatic fragmentation of the internal elastic lamina that leads to dilation of the vessel. This process preserves the lumen even as the arterial wall is thickened and deformed by the disease.[1] The ability to track metabolic activity in plaques would allow detection of atherosclerotic lesions at a stage of development too early to be seen by traditional methods. This is an optimal time to treat, before extensive permanent damage to the artery wall has occurred. Radiopharmaceutical imaging also makes it possible to follow the course of plaques, and thus could play a major role in evaluating the efficacy of treatment by diet and/or drugs.

Pathological studies such as PDAY (Pathological Determinates of Atherosclerosis in Youth)[2] offer clear evidence that occult inflammatory attack on the arterial wall occurs in young people. PDAY showed that the aortic wall of subjects who died in accidents in the first three decades of life often exhibits cellular infiltration, foam cell formation, smooth muscle cell proliferation, and may even have calcification, necrosis, and plaque hemorrhage.[2,3] These processes, as noted above, are usually accompanied by enzymatic destruction of the internal elastic lamina, producing vessel dilation and allowing the growing atherosclerotic lesion, under perfusion pressure in vivo, to expand outward, leaving a round and grossly intact lumen, which may be larger than the original lumen until late in the course of the disease.[1]

Evaluation of metabolic activity would also be very useful for differentiating between unstable and stable plaques. Plaque instability can be difficult, if not impossible, to detect by traditional means, which reveal nothing about plaque composition. Yet unstable plaques lead to sudden and catastrophic events, including myocardial infarction and stroke.[4] Large collections of foam cells in the shoulders of plaques are thought to be a major contributing factor to plaque instability because they lack the tensile strength of fibrous tissue. The metabolic activity of foam cells is high, making them excellent targets for imaging techniques, which are sensitive to such activity.

Many methods have been used to detect early atherosclerosis.[5,6] These include ultrasound, ultrafast x-ray computed tomography, magnetic resonance imaging (MRI), and of course arterial angiography. To date, all of these techniques have suffered from insensitivity, insufficient resolution, or inability to detect vessels other than superficial ones, eg, the carotid arteries in the neck or the femoral arteries in the groin. Recently, intravascular ultrasound has produced excellent high-resolution images of early nonstenotic or mildly stenotic atherosclerotic lesions in the coronary arteries; unfortunately this technique is highly invasive and not feasible for detection and follow-up of disease in asymptomatic patients.

About 15 years ago, we and our colleagues began a quest to identify early atherosclerosis by its intense metabolic activity, which begins well before the lumen is even mildly compromised. We asked ourselves what was different about the arterial wall in early atherosclerosis, what change in composition or function we might exploit to image the early changes of the disease, preferably by noninvasive means.

We knew from the work of many investigators[7–10] that plasma LDL accumulated in well-established lesions. A study by Minick and colleagues[11] suggested that LDL might accumulate in the earliest lesions as well. Their model was the balloon-catheter deendothelialized rabbit aorta, a model first described by Baumgartner in the rat.[12] When the aortic endothelium is removed with a balloon catheter, endothelial cells slowly grow out from branch arteries to re-cover the vessel. After healing has progressed for a few weeks, but before it is complete, the aorta has both reendothelialized islands with regenerating endothelium at the edges, and still deendothelialized areas. Minick and his group had set out to test the hypothesis of Ross and Glomset[13] that the intimal thickening and lipid accumulation associated with arteriosclerosis occur primarily in still deendothelialized areas. To their surprise, they found that both lipid accumulation and intimal thickening were primarily associated with the edges of regenerating endothelial islands.[11] What was most interesting was the focal nature of the lipid accumulation, which they located by Oil O staining. Oil Red O stains nonpolar lipids such as cholesterol esters. Even in normal chow-fed rabbits, they could detect cholesterol ester accumulation in areas of active endothelial regeneration at the edges of the healing islands, but there was little or no Oil Red O staining either in still deendothelialized or completely healed areas.

We hypothesized that the focally accumulated cholesterol ester seen in the healing rabbit aorta was delivered to the lesions by plasma LDL, and furthermore, that the accumulation was determined by events occuring within the arterial lesion itself, rather than by high plasma cholesterol concentrations. If this were so, LDL might represent a marker for arterial lesions, and if suitably radiolabeled, might be used to locate such lesions by external imaging.

To test our hypothesis, we began by interrogating the same rabbit model used by Minick et al.[11] While the lipids of LDL are not unique, the protein moiety, apolipoprotein B (apo B), is present only in lipoproteins of low and very low density,[14] and lipoprotein(a).[15] Therefore, as a probe, we labeled LDL in the protein moiety with iodine-125 (^{125}I). We hoped to determine by en face radioautography whether LDL would accumulate in the same locations where Minick et al had found cholesterol ester, that is, at the edges of regenerating endothelial islands. We balloon-catheter-deendothelialized only the abdominal aorta, leaving the thoracic aorta uninjured.[16] A series of rabbits were injected with ^{125}I-LDL and technetium-99m (^{99m}Tc)-albumin at times ranging from 24 hours to 12 weeks after balloon deendothelialization. The radiolabeled proteins were allowed to circulate for 24 hours before the animals were killed. By counting the abdominal and thoracic aortas before radioautography, we found that the accumulation of LDL, but not albumin, was directly related to the extent of healing. Like albumin, ^{125}I-labeled high-density lipoproteins also did not accumulate significantly.

Because some studies using the balloon-catheter-deendothelialized and healing aorta model of atherosclerosis are performed within a few days after deendothelialization, it is important to emphasize that we found that LDL accumulation was relatively low in the first 2 weeks after abdominal-aortic deendothelialization. In animals between 4 and 8 weeks after ballooning, LDL accumulation was at its peak. As healing continued and the islands coalesced, LDL accumulation fell; it reached levels seen in normal arteries at 12 weeks, when healing was complete.

Radioautographic results corresponded to the quantitative data. Radioautographs showed little or no focal accumulation of LDL in the first 2 weeks after deendothelialization. Thereafter, focal accumulation at the edges of regenerating endothelial islands was marked (Figure 2), and occurred in the same location that Minick et al had found accumulation of cholesterol ester. The accumulation of ^{125}I-LDL in the healing aorta at 4–5 weeks after deendothelialization was great enough to be seen when the intact rabbit was imaged with a standard planar gamma camera.[17]. LDL accumulation in the still-deendothelialized areas was diffuse, rather than focal. By 8 to 9 weeks after deendothelialization, healing islands began to coalesce. Once healing was complete, both focal and diffuse LDL accumulation disappeared. It was particularly striking that for each reendothelializing island, the site of focal LDL accumulation moved outward as the healing edge moved outward, and the site where LDL would have accumulated a week or two earlier was now refractory to LDL accumulation.

The above studies were done at varying times after deendothelialization, but animals were always killed 24 hours after injection of radiolabeled LDL. Subsequently we carried out studies in which the time after deendothelialization was kept constant, and the time of sacrifice after radiolabel injection was varied from 2.5 to 40 hours.[18] In these studies, focal LDL accumulation at the edges of the islands reached a peak at 4 hours after injection, and remained constant thereafter for up to 40 hours, even as the blood pool radioactivity declined, indicating that focally accumulated LDL was tightly bound. In contrast, ^{125}I-LDL which accumulated diffusely in deendothelialized areas of the artery was in equilibrium with, and decreased in parallel with the fall-off of radiolabel in the blood.

The rabbit experiments were followed by studies of human subjects with carotid atherosclerosis.[19] One hundred milliliters of blood were collected from each patient; LDL was prepared under

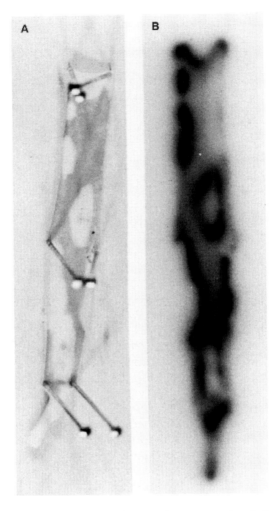

FIGURE 2. *Photograph and en face radioautograph of the abdominal aorta of chow-fed New Zealand white rabbit 5 weeks after balloon catheter deendothelization. The aorta was harvested 24 hours after a single injection of 1 mg of* ^{125}*I-LDL. Thirty minutes before sacrifice, Evans Blue dye was injected to stain still deendothelialzed areas.* **A.** *In the photograph of the opened aorta these areas are dark. The light areas show the extent of regenerated endothelium, which originates from unballooned aortic branch arteries. A small portion of the unballooned thoracic aorta, which also did not stain with Evans Blue, is barely visible at the top of the photgraph. The aortic bifurcation is at the bottom.*

sterile conditions, radiolabeled, filtered through a 0.22-μm filter, and reinjected intravenously. Patients were imaged with a gamma camera at several times after injection. At 48 hours, when the blood concentration of radiolabeled LDL had decreased somewhat, accumulation of ^{125}I-LDL could be seen in atherosclerotic lesions in the carotid arteries of three patients. Results for a fourth patient, who had been identified by angiography to have peripheral, but not carotid disease were negative.

These studies demonstrated the potential for imaging atherosclerosis with radolabeled LDL. Unfortunately, ^{125}I-LDL is a poor radiopharmaceutical for imaging purposes. The isotope has a long half-life (60 days), which results in a significant radiation dose to the patient. In addition, LDL itself has a long biological half-life in plasma, which makes the blood in the vessel radioactive for a prolonged period. Thus, the high radioactivity in the luminal blood pool of the arteries under examination may obscure some lesions. We addressed the first question, that of a suitable isotope, by turning to [99m]Tc. This isotope is the most widely used imaging agent in nuclear medicine, because of its short half-life (6 hours), its favorable, relatively clean, single gamma emission at 140 keV, and its low cost and convenience. It is provided by a technetium generator, a radiation-shielded column containing silica-bound molybdate, which spontaneously decays to ^{99m}Tc-pertechnetate. The latter, unlike molybdate, does not bind to the silica column and is readily eluted with sterile saline solution. Technetium in this form can be reduced and coupled to a variety of molecules. The use of ^{99m}Tc-labeled radiopharmaceuticals allows the use of a planar gamma camera or a tomographic instrument; patients absorb a very small amount of radiation, both in comparison with other isotopes and to ordinary transmission x-ray angiography.

Before carrying out studies with ^{99m}Tc-LDL, we had to develop a method for labeling LDL with the isotope. Labeling with ^{99m}Tc is usually done under acidic conditions, but such conditions cause irreversible aggregation of LDL, so a method for labeling LDL under alkaline conditions was needed. Making use of the survey of technetium-labeling conditions of Jones et al[20] we were able to label

---

FIGURE 2. (continued) *B*. *An en face radioautograph of the same aorta, on the **right**, was obtained after 3 weeks of exposure at −70˚C. It shows intense focal accumulation of radiolabel in areas which correspond to the edges of regenerating endothelial islands outlined in the photograph, and less, more diffuse accumulation in unhealed areas. Methods used are described in Reference 16.*

LDL with ^{99m}Tc under conditions that did not denature the lipopro-tein[21] The ^{99m}Tc-LDL was then tested in the deendothelialized rab-bit model. After the deendothelialized aorta had healed for 4 to 5 weeks, ^{99m}Tc-LDL was injected and allowed to circulate for several hours. The rabbit was then placed under a gamma camera and an image of the aortic lesions was obtained. When the aorta was har-vested, it was apparent that the gamma camera images corre-sponded with lesions in the aorta.[17]

The next step was to test ^{99m}Tc-LDL in human subjects with atherosclerosis. These studies were carried out in the same way as the ^{125}I-LDL human imaging studies, with preparation and radio-labeling of the patient's own LDL. Over a period of several years, we imaged 17 patients.[22] Clear-cut plaque images were obtained in pe-ripheral vessels, including the carotid, iliac, and femoral arteries of four of the patients. In four other patients there was suggestive ev-idence of focal accumulation of radiolabel in the coronaries; how-ever, the level of blood pool background radioactivity was too high to be certain of coronary accumulation. All the patients had prior angiograms that demonstrated atherosclerosis. However, the gamma camera images were read by three experienced nuclear medicine physicians without knowledge of the angiographic data. Only images that were called positive by all three nuclear medicine specialists were reported as positive.

The most information was obtained from six patients who had carotid endarterectomies immediately after the ^{99m}Tc-LDL imaging studies. The carotid specimens obtained from these patients showed two to four times more radioactivity in the most athero-sclerotic areas of the specimens in comparison with the least in-volved areas, even in specimens where the total radioactivity was too low to permit imaging. This finding was consistent with the fo-cal accumulation of ^{125}I-LDL seen in our earlier radioautographs of deendothelialized rabbit aortas.[16]

The most interesting finding in the carotid specimens was that their histologic composition appeared to correlate with the ability to obtain an external image. The five specimens that did not pro-duce a gamma camera image were mature, fibrocalcific plaques. The one carotid specimen that was associated with an image had many foam cells and a recent plaque hemorrhage (Figure 3). This was the first confirmatory evidence that radiolabeled LDL could lo-cate metabolically active, unstable atherosclerotic plaques.

Clearly, technetium was an excellent isotope for gamma cam-era imaging. However, even before the ^{99m}Tc-LDL human studies were completed, it was apparent that the prolonged high blood pool background that resulted from the long biological half-life of

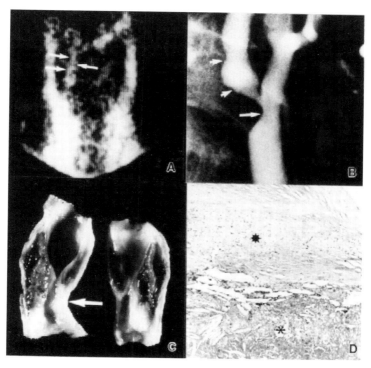

FIGURE 3. *Scintigraphic, angiographic, and pathological data from a patient with carotid atherosclerosis. **A**. Gamma camera image obtained 9 hours after intravenous injection of 13 mCi of ^{99m}Tc-LDL. Framed bilaterally by the patient's external jugular veins, the right carotid bifurcation shows extensive sequestration of ^{99m}Tc-LDL (arrows), while the left carotid has little or no uptake. **B**. Angiogram of the patient's right carotid bifurcation, which demonstrates extensive atherosclerosis and a tight stenosis at the origin of the internal carotid artery. The left carotid (not shown) had only minimal disease. **C**. Photograph of the right carotid endarterectomy specimen, showing tight stenosis (arrow) and recent plaque hemorrhage. **D**. Photomicrograph of the endarterectomy specimen, showing foam cells (star), cholesterol crystals, large thin-walled neovascular sinuses, and necrotic debris (asterisk). Reprinted with permission from Reference 22.*

LDL in the plasma made gamma camera visualization of plaques difficult except in a few patients. We also realized that the use of LDL as an imaging agent was not practical. It had to be prepared from each patient's blood, which took several days, and it had no shelf-life; that is, it had to be freshly made for each study.

Knowing that peptide hormones are rapidly cleared from the blood, we decided to test the possibility that some surface-accessible, apo B-derived, peptide sequences short enough to be synthesized easily would not only clear rapidly from the circulation, but would also share with intact LDL the property of focal accumulation in arterial lesions. Around 1985, we began to design 18–21 amino acid synthetic peptides to be tested for focal accumulation in deendothelialized rabbit arterial lesions. To our knowledge, this was the beginning of the concept that short synthetic peptides based on biologically-occurring amino acid sequences might be useful radiopharmaceutical imaging agents. We also synthesized a control peptide that we believed would not show focal accumulation, based on the LDL receptor-binding domain of apo E, for which the complete primary structure was already known. There were two reasons why we believed that the LDL receptor-binding domain was not involved in the focal accumulation of LDL in arterial lesions. First, patients with homozygous familial hypercholesterolemia, which is characterized by a complete lack of LDL receptors, develop symptomatic atherosclerosis as early as 4 to 6 years of age. Second, we had previously tested methyl LDL, which is not recognized by the LDL receptor,[23] in the deendothelialized rabbit model and found that it accumulated focally at least as well as native LDL.[24]

At the time that we began the synthetic peptide work, the complete sequence of apo B was not yet known. Thus, our first test peptide, SP-1, based on a partial sequence that was not later confirmed, did not show any focal accumulation. Control peptides, SP-2 and SP-3, based on the LDL receptor-binding domain of apo E, also did not accumulate focally. In 1986, when the complete primary sequence of apo B was published,[25–27] we designed a test peptide, SP-4, based on the known sequence. Because the LDL receptor-binding domain of apo B was near the C-terminus of the protein, we modeled the new test peptide on the first surface accessible domain at the opposite, N-terminal, end of the molecule, as described by Forgez et al.[28] SP-4 included amino acids 1000 through 1016 of apo B, with a tyrosine added to allow radiolabeling of the peptide with[125]I. (All the peptides had an added tyrosine to facilitate labeling).[29]

New imaging studies of arterial lesions in the deendothelialized rabbit aorta were performed with ^{125}I-labeled SP-2 and SP-4 [29]. As usual, deendothelialized arteries were allowed to heal for 4–5 weeks in order to ensure maximal LDL accumulation. After injection, the labeled peptide was allowed to circulate for 24 hours. By that time, <0.5% of the injected dose remained in plasma. Nevertheless, radioautographs from rabbits injected with SP-4 showed intense focal accumulation of radiolabel at the healing edges of re-generating endothelial islands. In contrast, radioautographs from rabbits injected with SP-2 showed only diffuse accumulation in the deendothelialized areas. We later synthesized a peptide based on the LDL receptor-binding domain of apo E (SP-11) that also did not accumulate focally in deendothelialized rabbit arterial lesions.[30,31] The results suggested that these short apolipoprotein-based pep-tides had secondary structures in plasma similar to the same amino acid sequences in the whole lipoprotein, a possibility that would support the use of such peptides to probe the functions of different domains of apo B.

SP-4 was also tested in Watanabe Heritable Hyperlipidemic (WHHL) rabbits. These animals, with a defect in the LDL receptor, develop spontaneous atherosclerosis. Radioautography showed that ^{125}I-SP-4 accumulated focally in WHHL atherosclerotic lesions (Figure 4).

After the initial studies with SP-4, we became interested in what elements of the peptide structure conferred on it the ability to accumulate focally in arterial lesions. We explored the structure-function relationships by replacing individual amino acids with other amino acids of similar size, charge and polarity,[30] and found that such conservative substitutions did not abolish the ability of peptides modeled on SP-4 to accumulate focally in healing rabbit arterial lesions. Thus, a particular pattern of charge and hydropho-bicity, rather than a particular amino acid sequence, appear to me-diate focal accumulation.

We next turned to the question of how to label SP-4 with ^{99m}Tc, and how to do so without changing the peptide's specificity for ar-terial lesions. Neither of these problems had yet been solved. The solution was provided by Dr. Richard T. Dean of Diatech, Inc., who with his colleague, Dr. John Lister-James, synthesized several tech-netium-chelating agents for labeling peptides.[32] The goal was to at-tach a chelating sequence that would bind ^{99m}Tc tightly to the peptide without altering its pertinent biological properties. Two different chelating complexes were chosen for testing in hypercho-lesterolemic rabbits. The SP-4 peptides with the added chelating se-quences were called P199 and P215. Drs. Stanley Goldsmith and Shankar Vallabhajosula at Mt. Sinai Hospital in New York showed, with both in vivo and ex vivo imaging, that P199 concentrated in the aortic arch of hypercholesterolemic rabbits, where atheroscle-rotic involvment was greatest. P215 gave similar results.[32] There was almost no accumulation of radiolabeled peptide in the aortic arch of normal rabbits. The studies provided evidence that the ad-dition of these chelating ligands did not significantly alter the bio-

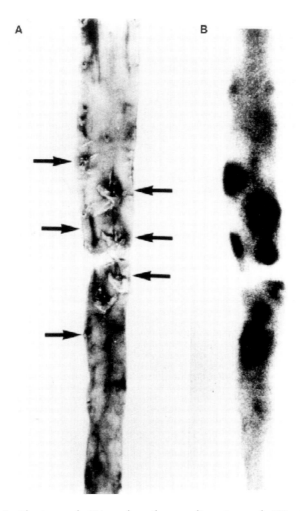

FIGURE 4. *Photograph (**A**) and en face radioautograph (**B**) of the opened aorta of a chow-fed Watanabe Heritable Hyperlipidemic rabbit. The aorta was harvested 24 hours after a single injection of 1 mg of ^{125}I-labeled SP-4, a short synthetic peptide derived from the native sequence of apolipoprotein B. Several discrete atherosclerotic lesions are visible in the photograph (arrows). In the radioautograph, intense focal accumulation of radiolabel corresponds with atherosclerotic lesions visible in the photograph.*

logical properties of SP-4 that were essential for successful imaging of atherosclerosis.

After the animal studies, human studies in patients with carotid atherosclerosis were begun and are still in progress. The studies have been carried out at MetroWest Medical Center in Natick and Framingham, Massachusetts, in collaboration with Dr. Arnold Miller; in New York at Columbia University College of Physicians and Surgeons in collaboration with Dr. J.P. Mohr; at New York Hospital in collaboration with Dr. Jeffery Borer; and at Mount Sinai in collaboration with Dr. Vallabhajosula and his colleagues.

Patients with carotid disease were again chosen for the following reasons: 1) the carotid bifurcation is a fairly large structure that is relatively superficial and easy to image with the gamma camera; 2) unstable carotid lesions often make themselves known through transient cerebral ischemic attacks or transient monocular blindness, thus allowing surgical intervention before irreversible brain damage occurs; 3) carotid endarterectomy, the preferred treatment, provides a pathology specimen that includes most of the plaque; it can be examined grossly and microscopically and correlated with the imaging data; 4) carotid atherosclerosis is very common, and its surgical treatment is successful and frequently used, so that clinical trial data are relatively easily and rapidly obtained.

The Phase I/II trial is to include at least 30 patients, of whom 17 have been studied as of the end of December 1994. The data management plan is as follows. The images will be read by three experts in nuclear medicine, who will be blinded to the clinical and pathological data. The interpretation of each image must be by consensus. Likewise, the endarterectomy specimens will be analyzed by pathologists with no knowledge of the imaging results. After both components of the data are analyzed separately, the imaging and pathology results for each patient will be associated with that patient's clinical history. An overall calculation of the sensitivity and specificity of the images for predicting the histologic composition, stability, and relationship of the lesions to the clinical symptoms will be determined.

Some preliminary observations can be made from images obtained to date. Planar images, similar to those that we obtained with ^{125}I-LDL and ^{99m}Tc-LDL may be informative, but single photon emission computed tomography (SPECT) images appear to predict the activity and extent of the lesions most clearly (Figure 5). We are hopeful that the completed study will provide much useful new information on how best to characterize the metabolic activity of atherosclerotic plaques in vivo.

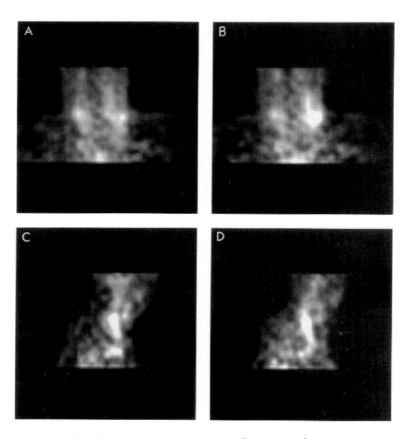

FIGURE 5. *Single photon emission computed tomography (SPECT) images begun 30 minutes after intravenous injection of 20 mCi of ^{99m}Tc-labeled P215, the SP-4 peptide modified by addition of a technetium-binding ligand.[32] The patient was a 79-year-old man with rapidly progressive bilateral carotid stenosis.* **A** *and* **B** *represent two consecutive coronal slices through the plane of the patient's carotid arteries, with the patient facing the camera. The right carotid bifurcation, on the left side of the images, shows moderate accumulation of ^{99m}Tc-P215, while the left carotid shows marked accumulation of radiolabel.* **C** *shows a sagittal view of the right carotid, with the patient's right shoulder towards the camera, and* **D** *shows the left carotid from the same view point. These images confirm the presence of extensive active atheroma bilaterally.*

In summary, we have developed a radiopharmaceutical technique for assessment of atherosclerotic plaques by gamma camera imaging, using plaque metabolic activity as the target. The technique uses intravenous injection of a radiolabeled probe, and thus, is minimally invasive. In early experiments, radiolabeled LDL was used to test feasibility. Once it became apparent that the approach had validity, a more practical radiolabeled probe was developed. The method now uses small synthetic apo B-based peptide radiolabeled with ^{99m}Tc. The advantages of the ^{99m}Tc-labeled peptide include fast clearance from plasma coupled with rapid sequestration of radiolabel in atherosclerotic plaques, selectivity for foam cell filled plaques, low antigenicity, low dose of radioactivity to the patient, and low cost. Because the probe is synthetic, there is no question of biological contamination with any pathogens. Clinical trials of the peptide in patients with carotid disease, while incomplete, appear promising. If the final analysis confirms the early results, we plan to extend the study to unstable coronary disease, as well as to atherosclerotic lesions elsewhere in the body.

References

1. Glagov S, Weisenberg E, Zarins CK, et al. Compensatory enlargement of human atherosclerotic coronary arteries. *N Engl J Med* 1987;316:1371–1375.
2. PDAY Research Group. Natural history of aortic and coronary atherosclerotic lesions in youth. *Arterioscler Thromb* 1993;13:1291–1298.
3. Wissler RW, the PDAY collaborating investigators: New insights into the pathogenesis of atherosclerosis as revealed by PDAY. *Atherosclerosis* 1994:108(suppl):S3-S20.
4. Fuster V, Stein B, Ambrose JA, et al. Atherosclerotic plaque rupture and thrombosis. *Circulation* 1990:82(suppl II):II-47–II-59.
5. Lees RS, Myers GS. Noninvasive diagnosis of arterial disease. In: Stollerman GH, ed. *Advances in Internal Medicine*. Volume 27. Chicago: Year Book Medical Publishers; 1982:475–509.
6. Lees RS. Non-invasive detection of vascular function and dysfunction. *Curr Opin Lipidology* 1993;4:325–329.
7. Kao VC, Wissler RW. A study of the immunohistochemical localization of serum lipoproteins and other plasma proteins in human atherosclerotic lesions. *Exp Mol Pathol* 1965;4:465–479.
8. MacMillan RC, Adams CWM, Ibrahim MZM. Histochemical identification of plasma proteins in the human aortic intima. *J Pathol Bacteriol* 1965;89:225.
9. Woolf N, Pilkington TRE. The immunohistochemical demonstration of lipoproteins in vessel walls. *J Pathol Bacteriol* 1965;90:459–463.
10. Smith EB, Slater RS. The chemical and immunological assay of low density lipoproteins extracted from human aortic intima. *Atherosclerosis* 1970;11:417.
11. Minick CR, Stemerman MB, Insull W, Jr. Role of endothelium and hy-

percholesterolemia in intimal thickening and lipid accumulation. *Am J Pathol* 1979;95:131–158.

12. Baumgartner HR. Eine neue Methode zur Erzeugung von Thromben durch gezielte überdehnung der Gefasswand. *Z Gesamte Exp Med* 1963;137:227–249.

13. Ross R, Glomset JA. The pathogenesis of atherosclerosis. *N Engl J Med* 1976;295:369–377, 420–425.

14. Hatch FT, Lees RS. Practical methods for plasma lipoprotein analysis. *Adv Lipid Res* 1968;6:1–68.

15. Utermann G. The mysteries of lipoprotein [a]. *Science* 1989;246:904–910.

16. Roberts AB, Lees AM, Lees RS, et al. Selective accumulation of low density lipoproteins in damaged arterial wall. *J Lipid Res* 1983;24:1160–1167.

17. Lees RS, Lees AM, Fischman AJ, et al. External imaging of active atherosclerosis with ^{99m}Tc-LDL. In Glagov S, et al., eds. *Pathobiology of the Human Atherosclerotic Plaque*. New York: Springer-Verlag; 1990:841–851.

18. Chang MY, Lees AM, Lees RS. Time course of ^{125}I-labeled LDL accumulation in the healing, balloon deendothelialized rabbit aorta. *Arterioscler Thromb* 1992;12:1088–1098.

19. Lees RS, Lees AM, Strauss HW. External imaging of human atherosclerosis. *J Nucl Med* 1983;24:154–156.

20. Jones AG, Orvig C, Trop HS, et al. A survey of reducing agents for the synthesis of tetraphenylarsonium oxytechnetiumbis (ethanedithiolate) from [^{99}Tc] pertechnetate in aqueous solution. *J Nucl Med* 1980;21:279–281.

21. Lees RS, Garabedian HD, Lees AM, et al. Technetium-99m low density lipoproteins: Preparation and biodistribution. *J Nucl Med* 1985;26:1056–1062.

22. Lees AM, Lees RS, Schoen FJ, et al. Imaging human atherosclerosis with ^{99m}Tc-labeled low density lipoproteins. *Arteriosclerosis* 1989;9:461–470.

23. Weisgraber KH, Innerarity TL, Mahley RW. Role of the lysine residues of plasma lipoproteins in high affinity binding to cell surface receptors on human fibroblasts. *J Biol Chem* 1978;253:9053–9062.

24. Fischman AJ, Lees AM, Lees RS, et al. Accumulation of native and methylated low density lipoproteins by healing rabbit arterial wall. *Arteriosclerosis* 1987;7:361–366.

25. Knott TJ, Pease RJ, Powell LM, et al. Complete protein sequence and identification of structural domains of human apolipoprotein B. *Nature* 1986;323:734–738.

26. Yang C-Y, Chen S-H, Gianturco SH, et al. Sequence, structure, receptor-binding domains and internal repeats of human apolipoprotein B-100. *Nature* 1986;323:738–742.

27. Law SW, Grant SM, Higuchi A, et al. Human liver apolipoprotein B-100 cDNA: Complete nucleic acid and derived amino acid sequence. *Proc Natl Acad Sci USA* 1986;83:8142–8146.

28. Forgez P, Gregory H, Young JA, et al. Identification of surface-exposed segments of apolipoprotein B-100 in the LDL particle. *Biochem Biophys Res Comm* 1986;140:250–257.

29. Shih I-L, Lees RS, Chang MY, et al. Focal accumulation of an

apolipoprotein B-based synthetic oligopeptide in the healing rabbit arterial wall. *Proc Natl Acad Sci USA* 1990; 87:1436–1440.

30. Taylor JW, Shih I-L, Lees AM, et al. Surface-induced conformational swithching in amphiphilic peptide segments of apolipoproteins B and E and model peptides. *Int J Peptide Protein Res* 1993;41:536–547.

31. Lees RS, Shih I-L, Taylor JW, et al. Apolipoprotein (apo) B peptide analogs accumulate in arterial lesions. *Clin Res* 1990;38:483a. Abstract.

32. Dean RT, Lister-James J, Lees RS, et al. Peptides in biomedical sciences: Principles and practice. In: Martin-Comin J, et al., eds. *Radiolabeled Blood Elements: Recent Advances in Techniques and Applications.* New York: Plenum Press; 1994:195–199.

Chapter 22

Radionuclide Labeled Monoclonal Antibody Imaging of Atherosclerosis and Vascular Injury

D. Douglas Miller, MD, CM

Introduction

The technique of monoclonal antibody (MoAb) production, which was developed in 1975, has had a significant impact on the diagnosis and clinical management of patients with neoplastic processes,[1,2] and has been extended to the noninvasive detection and therapy of cardiovascular disease.[3,4] The initial application of cardiovascular MoAb scintigraphy was directed towards the detection of venous[5-8] and coronary[9] thrombosis using indium-111 (^{111}In) or technetium-99m (^{99m}Tc) labeled antifibrin antibodies.

More recently, MoAb have been developed to react with platelet surface membrane antigens, usually glycoproteins, which are expressed on the surface of activated platelets after degranulation.[10,11] There are extensive data supporting the diagnostic value of radiolabeled MoAb directed against platelet membrane antigens such as the fibrinogen receptor IIB/IIIA glycoprotein complex found in intravascular thrombi.[12-16] A novel class of MoAb within a cluster of differentiation with high in vitro and in vivo specificity for translocated α-granule membrane proteins of activated platelets has also been developed.[16,17] Two such MoAb, S-12 and KC4 (anti-PADGEM), recognize and bind to different epitopes of the α-granule membrane glycoprotein GMP-140 (Mr = 140,000) that expresses more than 10,000 membrane sites per platelet after degranulation, have been radiolabeled for imaging of thrombosis[18,19] and vascular intervention injury sites[20,21] in animals and humans.

From: Fuster V, (ed.) *Syndromes of Atherosclerosis: Correlations of Clinical Imaging and Pathology*. Armonk, NY: Futura Publishing Company, Inc.: © 1996.

Two approaches, ie, the use of radiolabeled molecular or cellular elements involved in the thrombotic process and the use of monoclonal antibodies to protein antigens located in the thrombus, have been successfully applied. Monoclonal antiplatelet antibody imaging has significant advantages over in vitro autologous platelet labeling techniques for thrombus scintigraphy, including the availability of kit preparations, direct intravenous injection of MoAb fragments (with low immunogenicity), and rapid blood clearance (particularly with antibody fragments). The resulting improvement in image quality permits earlier recognition of intravascular damage and smaller thrombi without the need for blood pool subtraction techniques and blood cell-platelet separation before imaging. The blood pool clearance of MoAb radiopharmaceuticals is principally determined by the half-life of antibody-coated platelets, and not by the antibody or antibody fragment per se. The high specificity of the MoAb-platelet antigen reaction, the capacity to modify the MoAb to enhance blood clearance biokinetics and optimize scintigraphic visualization of the target site,[4] and the availability of ^{99m}Tc labeling kits for use with standard nuclear medicine systems are significant advantages over previous imaging studies with ^{111}In oxine autologous platelets.[22-25]

Pathophysiology of Thrombosis

Thrombus formation after vessel wall injury due to vascular trauma or spontaneous atherosclerotic plaque rupture causes immediate platelet adhesion and aggregation with formation of a platelet plug.[10] Thromboplastin is generated, which converts prothrombin to thrombin, after which soluble fibrinogen is converted to insoluble fibrin and a localized thrombus forms. The interaction of platelet plasma membranes with various substances within or accumulating at the injured vessel site is complex. Platelets are involved at each step of this process, adhering at sites of vascular injury, aggregating on the adherent layer to form a platelet thrombus, and simultaneously secreting vasoactive amines, adenosine diphosphate, platelet-derived growth factor, β-thromboglobulin, and platelet factor-4. Additional recruitment of platelets follows and may transform a hemostatic plug to an occlusive thrombus.

Local agonists such as thrombin stimulate the binding of fibrinogen to platelets and stimulate transfer of membrane-bound calcium into the cytoplasm. The former event results in continued platelet aggregation, whereas the latter triggers the secretion of granular substances and results in the recruitment of additional platelets. Components in this complex hemostatic (or thrombotic) pathway, particularly platelets, fibrinogen, and fibrin, have been used for imaging studies of both venous and arterial thrombotic events.

Preparation of Monoclonal Antibodies for Imaging

Use of the entire immunoglobulin molecule may be disadvantageous to the radiolabeling, biodistribution, and immunoreactivity of the MoAb. This has led to the use of immunoglobulin fragments, particularly the F(ab')$_2$ portion of the immunoglobulin found at the most distal portion of the immunoglobulin G (IgG) "Y" molecular configuration. Pepsin enzymatic digestion separates the nonspecific Fc fragment from the proximal part of the IgG molecule. The two F(ab') fragments are linked by disulfide bonds at the "hinge" region of the immunoglobulin "Y". This F(ab')$_2$ fragment retains its immunoreactivity. Further papain enzymatic cleavage can be used to separate each arm of the immunoglobulin "Y" from the nonspecific Fc portion of the molecule. Although Fc receptors exist in many organs, fragments of the immunoglobulin molecule [either F(ab')$_2$ or Fab] are more specific and thus more frequently used for diagnostic purposes.

Antibodies may be generated against a wide variety of biological macromolecules. The hypervariable (HV) region of the immunoglobulin molecule that determines immunoradioactivity is located in the Fab portion of the molecule. The Fab portion of the molecule contains the constant region of the light chain, a constant region of the heavy chain (C_h1), and the variable (V) region of the molecule. The remainder of the immunoglobulin molecule, the nonspecific Fc fragment, binds to the Fc receptors on macrophages.

The quality of radionuclide monoclonal images depends on the specificity of the antibody receptor interaction. Target-to-background ratios depend on the extent of binding to the target, and the ability to clear or eliminate nonspecific background radioactivity from the intravascular pool. Delivery of a second antibody trapped in liposomes, or the use of chimeric antibodies, has successfully reduced background radioactivity and improved image resolution. In general, a minimum target-to-background ratio of 2:1 must be achieved to permit detection and to be compatible with specificity for the target antigen. In addition, the use of recombinant DNA technology to generate human MoAbs may improve antibody affinity and reduce potential immunogenicity of currently available murine MoAbs.

Thrombus Imaging Antibodies

Antibodies have been raised against two sites (ie, epitopes) on activated platelets found in thrombi, the IIB/IIIA glycoprotein (the fibrinogen receptor) and the α-granule membrane glycoprotein, GMP-140. Glycoprotein IIB/IIIA is present on both resting (circulating) and thrombin-activated platelets (although IIB/IIIA receptor site characteristics change with activation). As such, MoAb that recognize this receptor may bind to both resting and activated platelets. In contrast, GMP-140 is expressed primarily (10,000 sites per platelet by activated platelets, making MoAb against this glycoprotein relatively specific for thrombus-associated (ie, noncirculating) platelets. This MoAb approach exhibits excellent sensitivity during the acute phase of platelet activation and thrombus formation within hours of spontaneous or iatrogenic vascular injury when platelet aggregation and α-granule degranulation are maximal.

In vitro secretion of platelet α-granule contents (ie, platelet-derived growth factor [PDGF], platelet factor-4, etc.) occurs at lower thrombin concentrations than that of platelet dense-granules, the site of serotonin storage.[11,16] Dual-isotope binding studies have demonstrated that with increasing thrombin concentrations, the GMP-140 specific MoAb S-12 (Fab') binds a slightly lower thrombin concentration than that causing serotonin secretion. Although lower level binding of S-12 occurs in postcapillary vascular endothelial cells expressing a similar selectin protein that is found on the Weibel-Palade bodies containing Von Willebrand's factor,[17] S-12 binding at vascular thrombosis sites is specifically attributable to α-granule degranulation (Figure 1). As such, S-12 binding is an indirect marker of PDGF release, giving it relevance in the setting of postangioplasty hyperproliferative responses and restenosis (Figure 2). This concept was studied in experimental[26] and clinical[27] protocols in our laboratory (Figures 3 through 5). These binding properties have also been explored using platelets obtained from the coronary effluent of patients undergoing angioplasty[28] and after acute unstable angina episodes[29] in which increased anti-PADGEM MoAb binding was demonstrated using a nonimaging fluorescence-activated flow cytometric (FACA) assay.

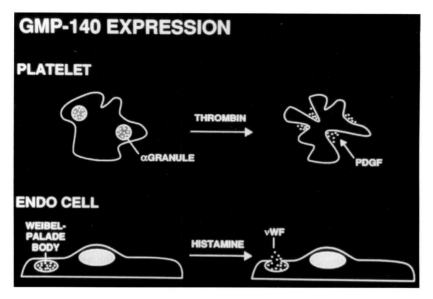

FIGURE 1. *Platelet membrane glycoprotein GMP-140 expression occurs after aggregation and platelet α-granule degranulation that exposes this antigen to the platelet surface through the membrane-connected cannalicular system. The same GMP-140 antigen is expressed by postcapillary endothelial cells after degranulation of the Weibel-Palade bodies releasing von Willebrand's factor. Up to 40,000 GMP-140 antigenic sites are expressed on the surface of a platelet after the degranulation reaction. These sites are recognized by the monoclonal antibodies (ie, S-12 and KC4), which can be labeled with technetium-99m to permit nuclear imaging of vascular injury sites.*

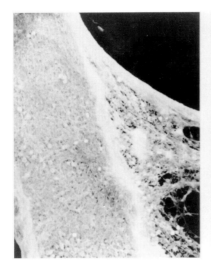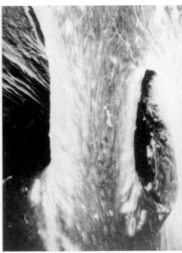

FIGURE 2. *Scanning electron microscopic images of stent struts removed within hours of angioplasty and stent placement (**left panel**), and 6 weeks after stent placement (**right panel**). Acute stent placement is associated with intense platelet and fibrin deposition with platelet degranulation. At 6 weeks, the stent strut is reendothelialized with a paucity of red and white cells adherent to the surface.*

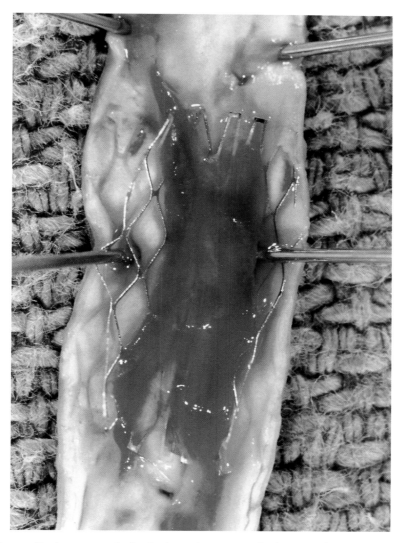

FIGURE 3. *A gross pathological section (magnified 10×) of a recent stent placement site in an atherogenic rabbit aorta. Thrombus material is present adhering to the stent struts that have imprinted the soft atherogenic vascular tissue. In this experimental model, the vessels were widely patent, without angiographic evidence of thrombus in their lumens.*

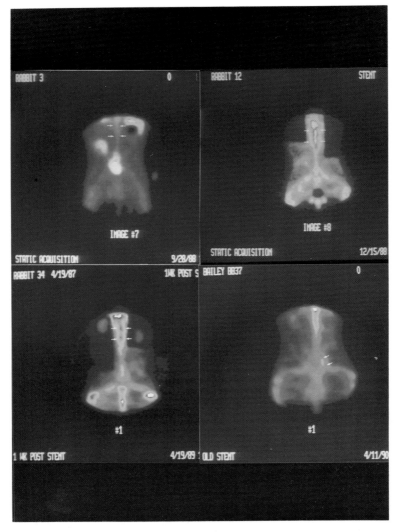

FIGURE 4. *Serial images acquired from different animals at time points prior to (**upper left**), immediately after (**upper right**), 1 week after (**lower left**), and 6 weeks after (**lower right**) intravascular stent placement (see arrows for site of stent implantation). Baseline uptake of technetium-99m (**99mTc) S-12 is minimal prior to stent placement. With stent deployment in the infrarenal aorta, there is intense uptake that persists at a lower level up to 1 week after vascular injury. By 6 weeks after stent placement, minimal residual uptake is identified in the left iliac artery.*

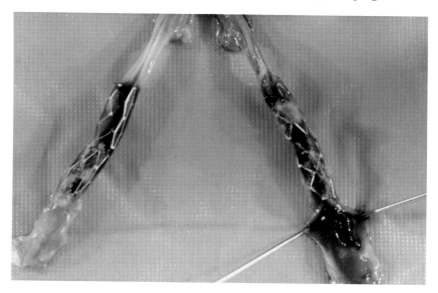

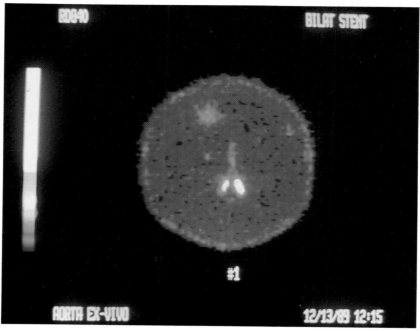

FIGURE 5. *Coating of the stents with polymers that can be impregnated with drugs such as heparin alters local thrombosis and technetium-99m (^{99m}Tc) S-12 monoclonal antibody uptake. **Panel A** demonstrates the gross difference in iliac artery thrombus deposition between coated and uncoated stents in the same animal. Ex vivo images of the same arteries (**panel B**) demonstrated a 2:1 difference in ^{99m}Tc S-12 activity between the uncoated and coated stent sites.*

Imaging of Other Atheromatous Plaque Constituents

Lipid Elements

The atherosclerotic plaque is a metabolically active lesion, characterized by repetitive cycles of endothelial cell injury and repair. The local release of cellular mitogens and growth factors after platelet activation is considered to be the principal mechanism of plaque growth, eventually resulting in a partially occlusive stenosis subject to plaque rupture and complete thrombotic occlusion. The endothelium that proliferates during the repair phase after minor injury has increased permeability to low-density lipoproteins (LDL) and the cholesterol transported by these proteins, resulting in the progressive deposition of atheromatous material in and around cellular elements in the plaque. Sites of reendothelization show marked increases in permeability to LDL,[30] which can be detected in vivo by radionuclide imaging.[31]

Human imaging studies in the iliac and femoral arteries at 1 and 24 hours after injection of 1.5 mCi of [111]In IgG, have demonstrated low blood pool activity (at 24 hours) and IgG localization in sites of atheromatous involvement.[32] This highlights the nonspecific insudation of proteins that may occur in atheroma.

To circumvent this problem of nonspecificity, monoclonal antibodies have been developed against epitopes on the surface of mononuclear leukocytes (macrophages) that accumulate in sites of atherosclerosis.[33] The monoclonal antibody 32.2 has demonstrated an uptake ratio of 4:1 in atherosclerotic regions as compared with normal aortic areas. This was greater than the uptake observed after the injection of nonspecific ^{111}In-labeled intact human IgG, which localizes via the FAC interaction with the FcR in the same lesions. Ex vivo macroautoradiograph studies were reproduced in 50% of rabbits injected with ^{111}In-labeled 32.2 F(ab')$_2$ using in vivo gamma camera scintigraphy. An [111]In MoAb of the IgM class (Z2D3) and an IgG F(ab')$_2$ MoAb with specificity for ground substance in the aorta of atherogenic rabbits have been localized with gamma imaging and macroautoradiography to the healing edge of atheromatous lesions.[34] Ultimately, more specific MoAb imaging of atherosclerotic plaques may be possible with these or other comparable imaging agents.

Nonplatelet Thrombotic Elements

Monoclonal imaging with antibodies to fibrin has been applied for the detection of venous thrombosis[5–7] and coronary thrombi.[9]

Radioisotope MoAb labeling is possible without affecting antigen binding or off-binding kinetics. These antifibrin antibodies recognize specific epitopes on the fibrin molecule and do not bind to fibrinogen. Blood clearance of [99mTc]-labeled antibody is more rapid than that of comparable [111In]-labeled monoclonals, although images become positive at approximately the same time after injection using both isotopes. [99mTc] antifibrin is more easily applied to standard gamma camera imaging, and the possibility of "kit" preparations is appealing.

Monoclonal antibodies (59D8, T2G1S) have been developed that are directed against the beta chain of fibrin in canine models and in patient studies. Antifibrin antibody imaging has been reported in acute canine coronary thrombi studies using [111In]-labeled monoclonal 64C5. Open-chest models have demonstrated left anterior descending coronary artery antifibrin MoAb uptake after intracoronary injection in animals with a clot created by injection of thrombin after arterial intimal injury. Activity ratios in normal versus thrombosed left anterior descending coronary arteries averaged 14:1 at 30 minutes after clot formation. Administration of tissue plasminogen activator (TPA) (0.75 μg/kg per minute) to produce coronary thrombolysis resulted in decreased coronary antifibrin binding.[9] [99mTc] labeled T2G1 Fab' fragments have been used to image chronic arterial thrombi in vascular grafts, aortic aneurysms, and the left ventricle,[35] but is less accurate than [111In] platelet scintigraphy in this setting, possibly due to the paucity of active fibrin.

Conclusions

Despite the increasing availability of imaging techniques to localize and quantify the anatomic burden of atherosclerosis, there remains a need for correlative biological measurements in order to discriminate the potential of a given plaque for clinically important events such as acute thrombosis or postintervention restenosis. Once a coronary event has occurred, the capacity to noninvasively monitor the course of patients with accelerated atherogenesis would facilitate therapeutic monitoring. It is possible, but as yet unproven, that radiolabeled MoAb and other proteins with high specificity for lipid, platelet, and fibrin surface receptor sites will be a useful means to index the biological proliferative or thrombogenic potential of anatomically well-defined atheromatous lesion.

In order to alter the receptor specificity and affinity of MoAb, to improve the range of species reactive with the MoAb, or to modify MoAb biokinetics, genetic engineering techniques such as gene transfection with recombinant DNA can be applied to design new molecules. These chimeric and humanized antibodies, and other modified antibody fragments (ie, single-chain antigen-binding proteins, V_H-domain proteins, etc.) can optimize certain antibody functions or endow new properties to the MoAb.[2] This technique has been successfully used to reduce immunogenicity and improve tissue localization, without altering antigenic specificity. The genetically modified MoAb, and smaller synthetic (oligo) peptides that are rapidly cleared from the background blood pool are now being evaluated in experimental models of thrombosis[4] and atherosclerosis.[36] Platelet IIB/IIIA-directed ^{99m}Tc-labeled peptides have been used to image activated platelets in animal thrombi.[37]

The limitations of MoAb imaging of aortic and coronary vascular injury sites due to adjacent ventricular blood pool and tissue background activity cannot be underestimated. [99m]Tc S-12 MoAb imaging of aortic angioplasty injury sites in rabbits can be significantly degraded by adjacent activity in the kidneys and bladder, the principal sites of MoAb excretion.[21] While peripheral human angioplasty sites can be imaged with [99m]Tc S-12 with good (>2:1) target-to-background activity ratios,[22] anecdotal experiences of S-12 coronary angioplasty imaging have required background subtraction, tomographic (single photon emission computer tomography [SPECT] or positron emission tomography [PET]) imaging, and myocardial left ventricular hypertrophy to distinguish vascular MoAb uptake from slower to clear blood pool activity.

In this context, the combination of highly resolved angiographic or tomographic studies of plaque morphology, and lower resolution scans of highly specific markers of plaque biology is clinically attractive. Fusion images combining computed tomography or magnetic resonance anatomy with SPECT images of radiolabeled MoAb distribution have been successfully implemented for the spatial localization of metastic neoplastic processes.[38] Despite the ongoing challenges associated with resolving small plaques and image degradation associated with cardiac motion, it is probable that fusion imaging will be successfully implemented to assess coronary atherosclerosis, particularly in patients where a clinically definable coronary event (ie, angioplasty, unstable angina, myocardial infarction, etc.) can be used to identify the occurrence of plaque disruption as a guide to the timing of these imaging studies.

References

1. Deland FH. A perspective of monoclonal antibodies: Past, present and future. *Sem Nucl Med* 1989;29:158–165.

2. Serafini AN. From monoclonal antibodies to peptides and molecular recognition units: An overview. *J Nucl Med* 1993;34:533–536.

3. Koblick PD, DeNardo GL, Berger HJ. Current status of immunoscintigraphy in the detection of thrombosis and thromboembolism. *Sem Nucl Med* 1989;29:221–237.

4. Knight LC. Scintigraphic methods for detecting vascular thrombus. *J Nucl Med* 1993;34:554–561.

5. Nedelman MA, Schaible TF, Epps LA, et al. Specificity of ^{99m}Tc labeled antifibrin uptake in an acute venous thrombosis model. *J Nucl Med* 1989;30:787.

6. Bourgeois P, Feremans W, VanGysel JP, et al. ^{111}In-labeled antifibrin antibodies (AFAb) in the diagnosis of vein thrombosis; First results. *J Nucl Med* 1988;29:807.

7. Peltier P, Plamchoa B, Tefaucal P, et al. Imaging venous thrombi using antifibrin monoclonal antibody. *J Nucl Med* 1986;29:806.

8. Rosebrough SF, McAfee JG, Grossman ZD, et al. Thrombus imaging: A comparison of radiolabeled GC4 and T2G1s fibrin-specific monoclonal antibodies. *J Nucl Med* 1990;31:1048–1054.

9. Kanke M, Yasuda T, Matsueda G, et al. Detection of residual coronary thrombi after reperfusion using ^{111}In labeled monoclonal antifibrin antibody. *J Nucl Med* 1986;27:910.

10. Shattil SJ, Bennett JS. Platelets and their membranes in hemostasis: Physiology and pathophysiology. *Ann Intern Med* 1980;94:108.

11. Stenberg PE, McEver RP, Shuman MA, et al. A platelet α-granule membrane protein (GMP-140) is expressed on the plasma membrane after activation. *J Cell Biol* 1985;101:880.

12. Stuttle AWJ, O'Donnell CJ, Virji N, et al. Imaging thrombus with radiolabelled Fab' fragments of a monoclonal antibody to platelets. *J Nucl Med* 1988;29:940.

13. Coller BS, Oster ZH, Meinken GE, et al. Autologous dog platelets (P) reacted with an 111-Indium-labeled monoclonal antibody to GPIIb/IIIa can be used to image thrombi. *Circulation* 1984:II:195.

14. Stuttle AW, Klosok J, Peters AM, Lavender JP. Sequential imaging of post-operative thrombus using the ^{111}In-labeled platelet-specific monoclonal antibody P256. *Br J Radiol* 1989;62:963–969.

15. Som P, Oster ZH, Zamora P, et al. Radioimmunoimaging of experimental thrombi in dogs using technetium-99m labeled monoclonal antibody fragments reactive with human platelets. *J Nucl Med* 1986;27:1315–1320.

16. McEver RP, Martin MN. Monoclonal antibody to a membrane glycoprotein binds only to activated platelets. *J Biol Chem* 1984;259:9799.

17. McEver RP, Beckstead JH, Moor KL, et al. GMP-140, a platelet-granule membrane protein, is also synthesized by vascular endothelial cells is localized in Weibel-Palade bodies. *J Clin Invest* 1989;84:92.

18. Palabrica TM, Furie BC, Konstam MA, et al. Thrombus imaging in a primate model with antibodies specific for an external membrane protein of activated platelets. *Proc Natl Acad Sci USA* 1989;86:1036–1040.

19. Chouraqui P, Davidson M, Thomas C, et al. Effect of thrombus age on uptake of ^{99m}Tc labeled anti-activated platelet monoclonal antibody. *J Nucl Med* 1991;32:1013. Abstract.

20. Miller DD, Boulet AJ, Tio FO, et al. In vivo technetium-99m S-12 antibody imaging of platelet a-granules in rabbit endothelial neointimal proliferation after angioplasty. *Circulation* 1991;83:224–236.

21. Miller DD, Rivera FJ, Garcia OJ, et al. Technetium-99m labeled mono-

clonal anti-platelet antibody [S-12] imaging of vascular injury in human percutaneous transluminal angioplasty. *Circulation* 1992;85:1354–1363.

22. Ezekowitz MD, Snyder EL, Pope C, et al. The use of indium-111 platelet scintigraphy in man: Comparisons with in vitro tests and in vivo platelet function—a five year experience. In: Thakur ML. ed. *Radiolabeled Cellular Blood Elements.* New York: Plenum; 1985.

23. Fuster V, Dewanjee MK, Kaye MP, et al. Noninvasive radioisotope technique for detection of platelet-depositions in coronary artery bypass in dogs and its reduction with platelet inhibitors. *Circulation* 1979:50:1508.

24. Lam JYT, Chesebro JH, Steele PM, et al. Deep arterial injury experimental angioplasty: Relation to a positive Indium-111 labeled platelet scintigram, quantitative platelet deposition and mural thrombosis. *J Am Coll Cardiol* 1986;8:1380.

25. Stratton JR, Ritchie JL. The effects of antithrombotic drugs in patients with left ventricular thrombi: Assessment with indium-111 platelet imaging and two-dimensional echocardiography. *Circulation* 1984;69:561.

26. Miller DD, Guy DM, Tio FO, et al. Monoclonal S-12 anti-platelet antibody imaging predicts angiographic patency and intimal repair following intravascular "stent" placement. *Circulation* 1990;82(suppl III):III-320.

27. Bailey SR, Guy DM, Garcia OJ, et al. Polymer coating of Palmaz-Schatz stent attenuates vascular spasm after stent placement. *Circulation* 1990;82(suppl III):III-541.

28. Palabrica TM, Smith JJ, Aronovitz MJ, et al. Flow cytometric analysis of platelet PADGEM expression during percutaneous transluminal coronary angioplasty. *Circulation* 1990;82:(suppl III):III-655.

29. Palabrica TM, Smith JJ, Aronovitz MJ, et al. Platélet PADGEM expression in the coronary and systemic circulations in stable and unstable coronary artery disease. *Circulation* 1990;82(suppl):2602.

30. Roberts AB, Lees AM, Lees RS, et al. Selective accumulation of low density lipoproteins in damaged arterial wall. *J Lipid Res* 1983;24:1160.

31. Lees AM, Lees RS, Schoen FJ, et al. Imaging human atherosclerosis with ^{99m}Tc-labeled low density lipoproteins. *Arteriosclerosis* 1988;8:461.

32. Fischman AJ, Rubin RH, Delvecchio A, et al. Imaging of atheromatous lesions in the iliac and femoral vessels: Preliminary experience in ^{111}In IgG in human subjects. *J Nucl Med* 1989;30:817.

33. Khaw BA, O'Donnell S, Fischman A, et al. Localization of experimental atherosclerotic lesions with monoclonal antibody. *J Nucl Med* 1989;30:859.

34. Khaw BA, Calenoff E, Chen F, et al. Localization of experimental atherosclerotic lesions with monoclonal antibody Z2D3. *J Nucl Med* 1993;32:1005.

35. Stratton JR, Cerqueira MD, Dewhurst TA, et al. Imaging arterial thrombosis: Comparison of technetium-99m-labeled monoclonal antifibrin antibodies and indium-111 platelets. *J Nucl Med* 1994;35:1731–1737.

36. Hardoff R, Braegelmann F, Zanzonico P, et al. External imaging of atherosclerosis in rabbits using I-123 labeled synthetic peptide fragments. *J Clin Pharm* 1993;33:1039–1047.

37. Knight LC, Radcliff R, Kollmann M, et al. Thrombus imaging with ^{99m}Tc synthetic peptides reactive with activated platelets. *J Nucl Med* 1990;31:757. Abstract.

38. Loats H. CT and SPECT image registration and fusion for spatial localization of metastic processes using radiolabeled monoclonals. *J Nucl Med* 1993;34:562–566.

Chapter 23

The Calcium Story and Electron Beam Computed Tomography

Bruce H. Brundage, MD

Introduction

Imaging the coronary arteries has been a major focus of clinicians interested in cardiovascular disease for a long time. The search for better and, in particular, noninvasive methods has lead to the development of ultrafast x-ray transmission computed tomography, more recently also called electron beam computed tomography (EBCT). Briefly, the technology requires that a powerful electron beam be generated, magnetically focused, angled, and steered to sweep a series of four tungsten targets. The energy of the electron stream striking the tungsten target creates x-ray that is then collimated to pass through the region of interest (the heart) and is measured by an array of detectors opposite the tungsten target. The electron beam can sweep the tungsten target in as short an interval as 50 msec. Images are reconstructed by usual computed tomography algorithms. The rapid image acquisition time eliminates motion artifact related to cardiac contraction (Figure 1).

For the purposes of detecting coronary calcium, EBCT images are obtained in 100 msec and only one tungsten target is used. Scan slice thickness is 3 mm, and 30 to 40 adjacent axial scans are obtained by table incrementation. The scans are usually acquired during one breath-hold and are triggered by the electrocardiographic signal at 80% of the RR interval, which is near the end of diastasis and before atrial contraction to minimize the effect of cardiac motion. The coronary arteries are easily identified by EBCT because of the contrast effect of periarterial fat (Figure 2). Coronary calcium is also easily identified because of its high den-

From: Fuster V, (ed.) *Syndromes of Atherosclerosis: Correlations of Clinical Imaging and Pathology.* Armonk, NY: Futura Publishing Company, Inc.: © 1996.

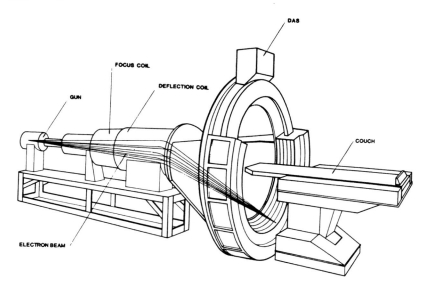

FIGURE 1. *A diagram of the electron beam computed tomography scanner depicts the path of the electron beam. DAS indicates data acquisition system. Provided courtesy of Imatron, Inc., South San Francisco, CA.*

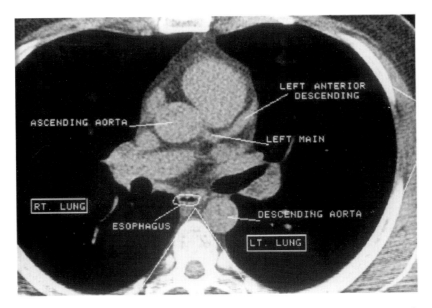

FIGURE 2. *An electron beam computed tomography (EBCT) scan at the level of the left main coronary artery demonstrates a normal left main and anterior descending coronary artery without calcium.*

sity (Figure 3). Most coronary calcium is located in the proximal third of the major vessels.

For many years the standard method for the noninvasive detection of coronary artery disease has been exercise stress testing. The basis for this test is the fact that narrowing of coronary arteries by more than 50% of their luminal diameter will result in myocardial ischemia at high levels of cardiac work. Methods to improve the sensitivity of exercise stress testing have focused on developing better ways to detect ischemia, such as myocardial perfusion scintigraphy with thallium-201 radioisotope. However, clinicians have recognized for many years that someone can have a normal stress test and still subsequently suffer a coronary event such as an acute myocardial infarction or even sudden death within a short interval.[1] This clinical fact perplexed physicians for a long time, until the role of thrombosis in the pathogenesis of acute coronary events, especially acute myocardial infarction, was rediscovered.[2] Furthermore, the understanding of the pathogenesis of coronary thrombosis has been expanded to recognize the role of plaque rupture or fissure in initiating acute coronary syndromes.[3] More recently, clinicians have come to recognize that the so-called

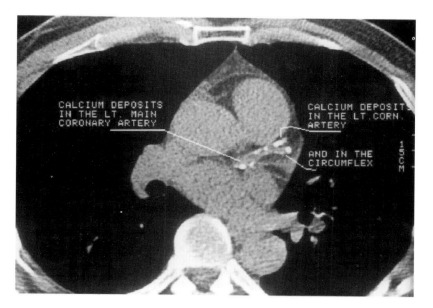

FIGURE 3. *An electron beam computed tomography (EBCT) scan at the level of the left coronary bifurcation demonstrates calcium in the left main, anterior descending, and circumflex coronary arteries. LT indicates left main coronary artery; CORN, coronary.*

culprit lesion associated with acute myocardial infarction is often nonobstructive, ie, produces <50% luminal narrowing.[4] These observations now provide understanding as to why any diagnostic test that relies on the production of myocardial ischemia will fail to detect a nonobstructive lesion that, at a later date, will lead to an acute coronary event. Clearly, a different approach for detecting individuals at risk for future cardiac events is needed.

If the detection of coronary artery calcium is to have clinical value, all of the following questions will have to be answered in the affirmative: 1) is atherosclerosis a progressive process?; 2) can the progression of atherosclerosis be slowed, arrested, or reversed?; 3) can nonobstructive plaques lead to complete thrombotic coronary artery occlusion?; 4) are better methods needed to identify people whose first symptom of coronary artery disease is sudden death or acute myocardial infarction?; 5) does cholesterol level (and other coronary artery disease risk factors) not always correlate with the degree of atherosclerosis?

An estimated 600,000 people die annually in the United States from coronary artery disease. It is also estimated that nearly half of these individuals die suddenly and unexpectedly.[5] Between 25% and 50% of those dying suddenly have not been previously diagnosed as having coronary artery disease, and so have had no chance to benefit from treatment. Therefore, there are between 75,000 and 150,000 people dying each year who could potentially be saved by effective treatment if they could only be identified. In addition, 1,000,000 Americans experience a myocardial infarction each year. It is estimated that at least 300,000 of these individuals had not been diagnosed as having coronary artery disease. If these people could also be identified, effective treatment could be expected to prevent many of these acute infarctions. Therefore, the need for an effective and preferably noninvasive and cost-effective method for detecting coronary atherosclerosis is obvious.

The onset of coronary atherosclerosis occurs relatively early in life. Autopsy studies of American soldiers killed in the Korean and Vietnam Wars have demonstrated that the process is sometimes well-advanced even in the third decade of life.[6,7] More and more plaques are deposited in the intima of the coronary vessels as the years go by. Clinically silent plaque rupture is the rule rather than the exception.[8] Thrombosis is believed to be part of the usual reparative process and is followed by deposition of fibrous tissue and calcium in the plaque. Therefore, calcium is a fortuitous marker of the amount of coronary atherosclerosis. Usually, when coronary atherosclerosis becomes extensive, then clinical events begin to occur (Figure 4). While acute coronary artery events are often associated

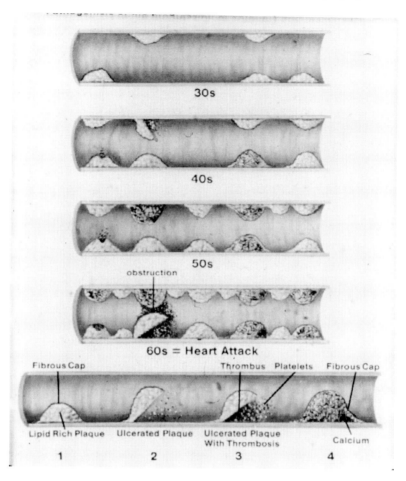

FIGURE 4. *The figure depicts the progression of coronary atherosclerosis with age and the natural history of plaques. Courtesy of Dr. Arthur S. Agatston, University of Miami, Miami Beach, FL.*

with lipid-laden plaques, coronary events usually occur in people with rather extensive coronary atherosclerosis so that some coronary calcium can be expected to be present. It is thought that 80% to 90% of culprit lesions are lipid laden, but they only represent 10% to 20% of all the plaques present.

In addition to the rationale that the detection of coronary artery calcium will be useful in identifying people at risk for acute coronary events, early detection of people with mild coronary atherosclerosis is of potential value also, particularly if the process can be retarded, arrested, or reversed. There are substantial data to indicate that lowering serum cholesterol in patients with known coronary artery disease (secondary prevention) reduces the incidence of nonfatal infarction, fatal infarction, cardiovascular mortality, and all cause mortality.[9] There is much more controversy about primary prevention. In a recent editorial, Hulley states it is time to change direction in our national cholesterol screening and intervention policy and consider ". . . limiting cholesterol screening and intervention to the minority in our population for which the benefits clearly predominate over the harms (those with coronary disease or other reasons for being at a comparable very high risk of coronary heart disease death)."[10] Diagnostic tests that more accurately identify who truly is at risk for coronary events are certainly needed. The detection of coronary calcium by EBCT could be a significant step toward accomplishing this goal.

There are three lines of evidence that support the hypothesis that the detection of coronary artery calcium by EBCT is an effective method for the early detection of coronary atherosclerosis and the identification of individuals at increased risk for experiencing an acute coronary event. These are pathological, angiographic, and outcomes or end-point studies.

Pathological Studies

Blankenhorn[11] first described the strong association between coronary calcium and obstructive coronary artery disease. He performed postmortem radiographs on human hearts and demonstrated that the presence of radiographically detectable coronary calcium correlated with the presence of histologically identified coronary artery obstruction. A study of 1200 autopsies from Charity Hospital, New Orleans, La correlated the percent of the luminal surface of the coronary arteries covered with calcium with the cause of death. From the fourth to the seventh decade of life, patients dying of atherosclerotic causes had a much greater percentage of their coronary arteries covered with calcium than individuals dying from other causes. For example, among people who died in the sixth decade of life from atherosclerotic causes, on average 20% of the surface of their coronary arteries was involved with calcium compared with 6% for people dying of other causes.[12] A more recent pathological study was reported by the Mayo Clinic group. The investigators performed EBCT scanning of postmortem coronary arteries every 3 mm. The arteries were then sectioned every 3 mm, and the cross-sectional area was measured. The relationship between coronary calcium detected by EBCT and cross-sectional area reduction was determined. All but 2.5% of areas free of calcium had <75% cross-sectional area reduction. In fact, the average cross-sectional reduction for the left anterior descending, circumflex, and right coronary arteries was 7.8%, 3.1%, and 14.2%, respectively. In other words, calcium-free areas of the coronary artery are usually free from significant coronary narrowing.[13]

Angiographic Studies

Tanenbaum et al[14] were the first to show a strong association between the presence of EBCT-detected coronary calcium and angiographically significant coronary artery disease. In 1990, Agatston et al[15] confirmed this finding and also demonstrated for the first time that the amount of coronary calcium was useful in predicting who would have significant coronary artery disease (Figure 5). The Mayo Clinic subsequently reported on the comparison of EBCT-detected coronary calcium and coronary angiographic findings in 100 consecutive patients. No patient with angiographically significant coronary artery disease was without detectable coronary

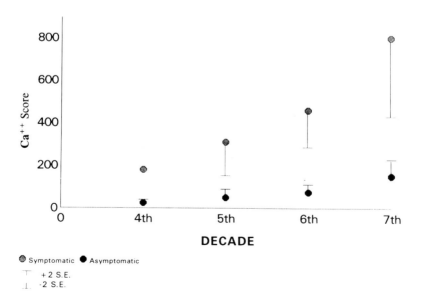

FIGURE 5. *The graph defines the relationship between calcium (Ca++) score and age and presence or absence of clinical coronary artery disease. Adapted with permission from Reference 15.*

calcium by EBCT.[16] Recently, six EBCT centers collected coronary angiographic data on 710 patients who also had EBCT scanning for coronary calcium within 3 months. They found the presence of coronary calcium detected by EBCT was 95% sensitive for predicting the presence of angiographic disease. In patients 50 years of age and older, the sensitivity exceeded 99%. However, specificity for the entire cohort was only 44%.[17] Further analysis of the data demonstrated that determining the number of vessels with calcium improved specificity. Increasing it progressively from 44% for one-vessel calcification to 96% for four-vessel involvement (left anterior descending, circumflex, right and left main coronary arteries).[18] Probability tables were then created correlating the amount and distribution of calcium with the presence of multivessel angiographic disease.[19] These tables indicate that determining the amount of calcium and the number of vessels involved by EBCT may be useful in predicting the presence of multivessel disease. However, this study is limited, as are all angiographic studies, by high prevalence of disease in the angiographic population. Therefore, these probabilities cannot be directly extrapolated to an asymptomatic population, which is the group in whom screening for coronary calcium by EBCT would be most useful.

Outcome Studies

The ultimate information required to determine whether screening for coronary artery calcium will have significant clinical value can only be obtained from prospective studies which employ hard clinical events as endpoints and as the tool of measurement. Several such studies are currently underway. Some results have already been reported from one of these investigations. Over 1400 asymptomatic individuals with several risk factors for coronary artery disease have been followed for over 3 years. All subjects had digital subtraction fluoroscopy on entry into the study to determine whether coronary calcium was present (EBCT was not available at the start of the study, but all surviving subjects had an EBCT scan during the third year of the study). After 1 year, those individuals with fluoroscopically detectable calcium had risk ratios between 3 and 4 for nonfatal infarction, coronary revascularization, and development of angina (Table 1). All were statistically significant.[20] Coronary death was not statistically greater at 1 year, but does approach significance at 2 years.[21] Another follow-up study of 1040 asymptomatic males was performed to determine whether large amounts of calcium posed an increased risk for having significant

TABLE 1

Coronary Heart Disease Events in 1459 Subjects*
with or without Coronary Calcium

Event[†]	Calcium (n=691)	No Calcium (n=768)	Risk Ratio	P Value
I (coronary heart disease death)	3 (0.4%)	3 (0.4%)	1.00	NS
II (nonfatal myocardial infarction)	8 (1.2%)	2 (0.3%)	4.00	0.03
III (coronary revascularization)	10 (1.5%)	3 (0.4%)	3.75	0.03
IV (angina)	27 (3.9%)	10 (1.3%)	3.00	0.001
I, II, III or IV	37 (5.4%)	16 (2.1%)	2.57	0.001

*Follow-up data were not obtained for two subjects (both in the survivor group) of the total study group of 1461 subjects.
†Some subjects had more than one event.
The table compares the incidence of subsequent coronary events in an iinitially asymptomatic cohort of 1459 subjects. Adapted with permission from Reference 20.

obstructive coronary artery disease. Approximately 12% of the study population had large amounts of coronary calcium and approximately 13% of these subjects were found to have significant coronary artery disease within 6 months of being scanned as defined by the development of an acute myocardial infarction, need for coronary revascularization, or evidence of significant obstructive disease (>50% diameter reduction) on a coronary arteriogram.[22] Further follow-up analysis of an expanded cohort is currently in progress.

In summary, the rationale for the need for a noninvasive, cost-effective diagnostic test that can detect the presence of coronary atherosclerosis independent of the production of myocardial ischemia, and yet be capable of predicting when significant obstructive disease is present has been presented. Pathological studies have demonstrated that coronary calcium is virtually always associated with presence of coronary atherosclerosis. Furthermore, the absence of coronary calcium usually excludes the presence of significant coronary obstruction. Both pathological and angiographic studies have shown the greater the amount of coronary calcium the greater the likelihood for significant coronary obstruction. Angiographic studies have also demonstrated that the number of calcified vessels is also important. Four-vessel calcification is highly specific for obstructive multivessel disease. Finally, prospective studies of asymptomatic populations have shown that the presence of coronary calcium is associated with a three- to fourfold increase in the subsequent development of nonfatal myocardial infarction and angina as well as the need for coronary revascularization. Moreover, a pilot study suggests that the greater the amount of calcium the greater this risk. EBCT appears to have great potential as a screening test for detecting subclinical but important coronary artery atherosclerosis.

References

1. Epstein SE, Quyyumi AA, Bonow RD. Sudden cardiac death without warning: Possible mechanisms and implications for screening asymptomatic populations. *N Engl J Med* 1989;312:320–324.
2. DeWood MA, Spores J, Notski R, et al. Prevalence of total coronary occlusion during the early hours of transmural myocardial infarction. *N Engl J Med* 1980;303:897–902.
3. Fuster V, Badimion L, Cohen M, et al. Insights into the pathogenesis of acute ischemic syndromes. *Circulation* 1988;77:1213–1220.
4. Little WC, Constantinescu M, Applegate RJ, et al. Can coronary angiography predict the site of a subsequent myocardial infarction in patients with mild-to-moderate coronary artery disease. *Circulation* 1988;78:1157–1166.
5. Castelli W, Leaf A. Identification and assessment of cardiac risk: An overview. *Cardiol Clin* 1985;3:171–178.
6. Enos WF, Holmes RH, Beyer J. Coronary disease among United States soldiers killed in action in Korea: Preliminary report. *JAMA* 1953;152:1090–1093.
7. McNamara JJ, Molot MA, Stimple JF, et al. Coronary artery disease in combat casualties in Viet Nam. *JAMA* 1971;216:1185–1187.
8. Fuster V, Stein B, Ambrose JA, et al. Atherosclerosis plaque rupture and thrombosis: Evolving concepts. *Circulation* 1990;82:II-47–59.
9. Rossouw JE, Lewis B, Rifkind BM. The value of lowering cholesterol after myocardial infarction. *N Engl J Med* 1990;323:1112–1119.
10. Hulley SB, Walsh JMB, Newman TB. Health policy on blood cholesterol: Time to change direction. *Circulation* 1992;86:1026–1029.
11. Blankenhorn DH, Stern D. Calcification of the coronary arteries. *AJR* 1959;81:772–777.
12. Eggen DA, Strong JP, McGill HC. Coronary calcification: Relationship to clinically significant coronary lesions and race, sex and topographic distribution. *Circulation* 1965;32:948–955.
13. Simons DB, Schwartz RS, Edwards WD, et al. Noninvasive definition of anatomic coronary artery disease by ultrafast computed tomographic scanning: A quantitative pathologic comparison study. *J Am Coll Cardiol* 1992;20:1118–1126.
14. Tanenbaum SR, Koridos GT, Veselik KE, et al. Detection of calcific deposits in coronary arteries by ultrafast computed tomography and correlation with angiography. *Am J Cardiol* 1989;63:870–872.
15. Agatston AS, Janowitz WR, Hildner FJ, et al. Quantification of coronary artery calcium using ultrafast computed tomography. *J Am Coll Cardiol* 1990;15:827–832.
16. Breen JF, Sheedy PF, Schwartz RS, et al. Coronary artery calcification

detected with ultrafast CT as an indication of coronary artery disease. *Radiology* 1992;185:435–439.

17. Georgiou D, Budoff M, Kennedy J, et al. The value of ultrafast CT coronary calcification in predicting significant coronary artery disease compared to angiography: A multicenter study. *Circulation* 1993;88:I-639. Abstract.

18. Budoff M, Georgiou D, Brody AS, et al. The value of receiver operating characteristic (ROC) curve analysis to detect coronary artery disease by coronary calcification on ultrafast CT (UFCT): A multicenter study. *J Am Coll Cardiol* 1994;23:210A. Abstract.

19. Georgiou D, Kennedy JM, Brody AS, et al. Probability of multivessel coronary artery disease in 531 patients based upon ultrafast CT (UFCT) coronary calcification: A multicenter study. *J Am Coll Cardiol* 1994;23:179A. Abstract.

20. Detrano R, Wong ND, Tang W, et al. Prognostic significance of cardiac cine-fluoroscopy for coronary calcific deposits in a high-risk asymptomatic population. *J Am Coll Cardiol* 1994;24:354–358.

21. Detrano R, Tang W, Wong N, et al. Coronary calcium predicts myocardial infarction in asymptomatic subjects after two years of follow-up. *J Am Coll Cardiol* 1995;(special issue):13A.

22. Brundage BH, Rich S, Rassman W, et al. Follow-up of asymptomatic individuals with high coronary calcium scores on UFCT scans. *J Am Coll Cardiol* 1994;23:208A. Abstract.

Panel Discussion III

Imaging Techniques, Tissue Characterization, Angiography, Ultrasound, Angioscopy, Magnetic Resonance Imaging

Dr. Valentin Fuster: Dr. Nissen, you were supposed to talk about intravascular ultrasound and angioscopy, I didn't hear you talking about angioscopy. You don't believe in angioscopy?

Dr. Steven E. Nissen: We don't do a lot of work with angioscopy. The problem with angioscopy is it gives you just one piece of information, namely, what's the color of the material that's in the coronary [artery]. Is it red, and therefore thrombus? Is it white, or is it yellow? And to put a device down the coronary simply to get that information, it's hard to justify. And so we do use it periodically, but not consistently because it doesn't tell us anything about what's the anatomy below the surface. I think angioscopy probably is not going to really make it as a clinical tool, although certainly it's exciting to be able to see the thrombi that we know are there in patients with unstable syndromes.

Dr. Fuster: Dr. Ambrose, you are an expert in the field. What have you learned with angioscopy? Dr. Nissen has not learned much.

Dr. John A. Ambrose: I wouldn't go that far at all. One thing that's interesting about angioscopy is that when you look at a vessel, the amount of yellow plaque that you see. However, because of the thickness of the catheter, it's quite difficult to interrogate the entire stenotic lesion before you do the procedure. Obviously, after the procedure it's something different or if the lesion is not that severe. But the very interesting thing that I have seen is that there's so much yellow plaque in these vessels, and probably some of these are the plaques more susceptible to the acute syndromes. It's just very enlightening to see angioscopically what we can see.

From: Fuster V, (ed.) *Syndromes of Atherosclerosis: Correlations of Clinical Imaging and Pathology.* Armonk, NY: Futura Publishing Company, Inc.: © 1996.

Dr. Fuster: You are talking about yellow plaques, but what about the thrombus aspect?

Dr. Ambrose: Again, my comments were related just to the yellow plaque. Clearly, for thrombus, you can see thrombus much better with angioscopy than with angiography. And perhaps white versus red thrombus may give us some insight into pathophysiology. Nevertheless, angioscopy as a clinically useful tool, it's stretching it a little bit.

Dr. Fuster: Dr. Ambrose, but if you see yellow with angioscopy, and Dr. Nissen sees connective tissue with intravascular ultrasound, you've really got into the vulnerable lesion.

Dr. Ambrose: I think so.

Dr. Fuster: Why have both of you not done the correlation between intravascular ultrasound and angioscopy in the same region? You are giving us the answer to the lesion we are most interested in and the one we want to attack. You do it with angioscopy, Dr. Nissen with intravascular ultrasound.

Dr. Ambrose: I think that a good correlation of angiography versus angioscopy versus ultrasound has not been done.

Dr. Fuster: Well you guys have a project here. Because, actually the main, one of the main issues in this meeting is to identify the vulnerable plaques. So I guess you are really on target if you are able to make the correlation of both. Dr. Rosenfeld?

Dr. Kenneth Rosenfeld: I just make one comment that I didn't make in terms of the liabilities of carotid ultrasound, and that is that there have been numerous investigators who have tried to identify thrombus by intravascular ultrasound. And although it's controversial, I think most people would agree that that is a limitation of this technique, you cannot see thrombus nearly as well as you can see it by angioscopy. Angioscopy is really the only technique that affords that kind of imaging, I think. Do you agree with that?

Dr. Nissen: Yeah, I also agree with that, although interestingly there are two things coming very shortly. We have begun some preliminary studies in animals, and soon in humans with an ultrasound device that's 18/1000" in diameter. So you don't have to worry about getting it into a tight lesion preinterventionally. And then second, we've also been pushing the frequency from 30 MHz to 40 MHz, and we have even done some studies with 50 MHz devices. And at those high frequencies, the subtleties, differences of lipid rich plaques, and thrombi become much more easily identifiable. So we are getting closer to the microscope, if you will, as we push the frequency up higher.

Dr. Robert S. Lees: My colleague, Dr. Miller, a vascular surgeon, has been using angioscopy in situations where nothing else is as good. For instance, after the surgeon has operated on an artery in the leg, and the limb is still cold and blue, the resolution of the angioscope allows you to see at once what is obstructing the vessel. This has been of immense value and life-saving, or limb-saving, since the angioscope is readily available in the operating room, easily visualizes clot, and allows appropriate steps to be taken immediately to save the limb.

Dr. Fuster: It seems to me that the main contribution of intravascular ultrasound thus far has been to tell us that commonly there's extensive disease that we don't see with angiography. Is this correct?

Dr. Nissen: I think that's right. Nevertheless, I think now that we have been able to map the coronary wall, that we have been able to study patients that have been either in the throes of an acute event or having had an acute event within the recent few days, and with the new ultrasound device technology evolving, the potential is to really understand what the plaque morphological features are that are associated with acute events. And I do think that there's a very good chance we will be able to do that. If it's true that the global plaque burden is an important predictor of outcome, and if the morphological aspects of it, if a thin rather than a thick cap, if a sonolucent plaque rather than a fibrotic one, if these are the plaques we have to worry about, I would be hopeful that we could study a patient and predict from their ultrasound what would their likelihood be over the next several years of having an acute event. And that would be really a big step forward, I think.

Dr. Fuster: John, you have seen a large number of patients after myocardial infarction having normal coronary arteries at angiography. Do you think these are patients who really have plaques that would be very apparent by intravascular ultrasound? What's your view?

Dr. Ambrose: I think the example that Dr. Nissen showed was quite remarkable. There was so much plaque at ultrasound in that particular vessel versus angiographically what looked like a completely normal artery. However, I think that with the higher resolution that you have for digital imaging, you commonly do not see vessels that are completely normal unless maybe the patient had used cocaine or there was a Prinzmetal's angina and it was vasospasm. So while I think that was a very interesting example, I would say that with the higher resolution angiography, this is probably a minority of what we see post-myocardial infarction. Nevertheless, intravascular ultrasound, by giving us this three-dimensional look, is a much better way of looking and assessing lesions than angiography.

Dr. Nissen: Dr. Ambrose, it turns out that we've not yet encountered myocardial infarction with normal coronaries. That is to say, in a group of now about 20 such patients that I have studied, every single one of them has had significant plaque burden. But we are up against angiography, what Dr. Seymour Glagov predicted we would be up against. Namely, that even with the highest possible resolution, if the plaque is all remodeled, the adventitia outward, such that the lumen is not narrowed, then no matter how precisely we look at the lumen, it still doesn't show us stenosis at angiography. The other thing that happened recently is we had the opportunity to study a series of patients with normal coronaries who had ergonovine-induced spasm. And 100% of a group of 15 of those patients had a large remodeled plaque right at the site where the ergonovine-induced spasm occured. So I guess I'm wondering whether these symptomatic patients with normal coronaries, if any of them are really normal.

Dr. Ambrose: I think you're probably correct. I guess my point is that seeing now perfectly normal coronary arteries, at least with these higher-resolution systems, is less common than we used to see and things that we could call normal don't look so normal when some of these patients are studied. But clearly ultrasound is giving us a window that angiography is lacking. And clearly the work of Dr. Glagov has been shown to be absolutely correct, and we could not predict that from angiography alone.

Dr. Lees: I would just add one word to the problem of detecting lesions. We don't see half of what goes on. I had the privilege of a visit from a French Philips ultrasound team a few weeks ago. The Philips scientists demonstrated a high-resolution, ultrafast ultrasound machine for imaging peripheral vessels. What they showed, among other things, is, if you will, a Bernoulli effect—a lesion that is not very stenotic in diastole—becomes highly stenotic in systole, when the blood flow velocity goes up three- or fourfold. We don't see that phenomenon in the catheter lab where we've maximally dilated the vessel with nitroglycerin. But when the patient is out and about, this phenomenon probably occurs. Furthermore, if the patient has abnormal coronary vasoreactivity, with exercise and increased blood flow the resulting increase in wall shear will cause the vessel to constrict, and the Bernoulli effect will make it constrict further. So, I don't believe that patients who have an infarct with apparently normal angiograms have normal coronary arteries. I believe that we just don't see the lesions and what happens to them when the patient is walking around.

Dr. Erling Falk: It has been demonstrated that the calculation of percentage in the luminal obstruction by angiography may be inaccurate because of diffuse disease and also because of the compensatory enlargement. But, I think that intravascular ultrasound may not completely overcome the problem of the degree of stenosis because using the lumen reference site proximal of the lesion with intravascular ultrasound you also got the problem with diffuse disease. So, how could we determine the percentage of luminal obstruction using intravascular ultrasound?

Dr. Nissen: I guess the key question is do we really want to? I think there are a couple of things to think about. One is if we have a tomographic image, we have a precise cross-sectional area in the lesion. And given the fact that the capability of the artery for flow is determined by the shape and the size of the lumen, then I would consider the luminal measurements to be the key measurements. Second, if you do have intravascular ultrasound, you can at least determine whether the reference segment you are looking at is normal or abnormal because there are some patients in whom there is focal disease, in which case you know exactly what the size of the normal segment is. And you can use that to gauge the severity of the obstruction. Otherwise, I think we've got to get away from percent stenosis.

Dr. Stephen M. Schwartz: *Question:* These are two-part questions but they are very closely related. The first part is the safety of intravascular ultrasound. A lot of the vessels that would be interesting to look at are nonsymptomatic or minimally symptomatic. I guess I would like some comment on that. The second part, which is maybe the same question, in a way. You said Dr. Nissen, that in the ergonovine-treated patients, 100% had some kind of a lesion. Do you have any idea, between your own data and maybe Dr. Wissler's data, about what the incidence is of nonluminal encroaching lesions in matched patients of this age?

Dr. Nissen: *Answer:* Obviously we don't study asymptomatic patients. So what we get is a funny population. There's not much that we can do about this. With regard to safety, we've performed intravascular ultrasound in a group that we would consider very precious. Namely, transplant recipients, most of whom are normal initially. We have studied now nearly 400 transplant recipients with no morbidity of any kind. So I think that sliding a 1-mm catheter into the coronary [artery] is extremely safe, and I'm very comfortable doing this, even in normals.

Dr. James H. Chesebro: One of the problems we have is detecting thrombus and looking at changes over time which relate to our new antithrombotic drugs, in other words, the importance in quantitating changes in thrombus. I would like to ask the speakers if in the future they anticipate being able to see the thrombus other than by angioscopy.

Dr. Nissen: Briefly, we've had an opportunity in a few patients to do intravascular ultrasound during infusion of agents like urokinase. And it's really remarkable, but you can literally see what happens to the material. Now, we don't always know that it's actually thrombus, unfortunately, but at higher frequencies we will.

Dr. D. Douglas Miller: I think that now that we have radiolabeled all the nucleotides and other hybrid type monoclonals with less immunogeneticity that it will be possible to perform staged serial studies on these patients. In particular, to identify patients perhaps at the highest incidence of early reocclusion following a thrombolytic therapy and possibly patients who are having active release of growth factors and other growth-stimulating substances predisposing to restenosis.

Dr. Ambrose: Going back to angioscopy, I think is excellent and the best technique. Angiography, high-resolution angiography is good; Greg Brown has some very nice images that he has done with the TIMI Study. To identify thrombi, only a minority of very active processes are showing up. Furthermore, the drugs administered are interfering with uptake.

Dr. Helmut Sinzinger: In regard to platelets, at the moment it is not possible. If we work with molecular recognition units, I think a monitoring should be possible in the near future, but at the moment, concerning platelet labeling, I don't see a positive trend.

Discussant A from the Audience: I would like to ask Dr. Brundage a question. I found a very high correlation between ulcerated plaques and calcification in arteries that were not significantly narrowed. I would like to ask, in your study, in your follow-up, whether your patients who went on to develop unstable angina and acute myocardial infarction were restudied and if the site of the occlusion in these acute events was located on plaques that originally were not narrowed and calcified?

Dr. Bruce H. Brundage: The answer is, I don't know.

Dr. Fuster: Thanks. I really like short answers.

Discussant A from the Audience: At the last AHA meeting, there was some data showing that if you had acute lesions you probably didn't see calcification by using various modalitites, angiographic or even, I think it was ultrafast computed tomography. And I was wondering, do you think that the evidence of calcification in the follow-up studies indicates that this is a marker for coronary disease but not of these dangerous lesions?

Dr. Brundage: Certainly, calcification is a marker for coronary disease and that was the point I tried to make in my talk this morning. I think it's, in a sense, a fortuitous marker, and I wouldn't want to make too much more about that. There are young people under the age of 40 that can have angiographically obstructed disease and have clinical events without having coronary calcium. But more than 80% of those people will have only single-vessel disease. So, by the time you develop multivessel disease, by the time you get over the age of 50, not always, but nearly always, calcium is present when there's a significant coronary atherosclerosis.

Dr. Fuster: Did you have your own ultrafast computed tomography done?

Dr. Brundage: Yes, I have.

Dr. Fuster: And what happened? Can you say this publicly?

Dr. Brundage: My coronary arteries—publicly, are clean as a whistle.

Dr. Fuster: And you are very relaxed about it?

Dr. Brundage: I'm very relaxed about it.

Dr. V. Fuster: *Question:* Then I go back to your talk. People at your age, you showed 40% of them who have negative calcification and they have coronary disease, so how can you be so relaxed? So, you can not be relaxed whether the test is positive or negative. I hope this is a fair comment. Is this correct?

Dr. Brundage: *Answer:* Because you restricted us to short answers, I don't agree with you.

Dr. Fuster: All right. That's fair, too.

Discussant B from the Audience: Just one word for the sake of complete truthfullness about calcium. Calcification is one of the very earliest, most constant changes in atherogenesis. Linda Deemer, in your town, has done beautiful work on this at the biochemical level, and Fred Jones, from our town, and his colleague Bob Levy down in Ann Arbor have done extensive experimental and pathological work. Calcium is present in the very early stages of atherosclerosis; the more sensitive the method in which you look for it the more often you're going to see it.

Dr. Brundage: Can I just add a quick point to follow up on that. That is, that people at the NIH have been looking at homozygous familial hypercholesterolemia children under the age of 10, and they show a good correlation between the amount of calcium and the severity of the coronary atherosclerosis.

Dr. Fuster: At autopsy and with surgical experiment we are able to identify and characterize vascular lesions by MRI technology. Do you think in the near future, it will be possible to have an MRI coil inside the coronary arteries and characterize coronary lesions?

Dr. Howard L. Kantor: I think in the chambers of the heart it is something that could be done anytime. That's actually not a big problem. You can make coils as small as any of the devices other people are using right now. In the coronaries, it is also possible and not a problem. The issue in any vascular imaging is the motion of the coil and the resolution of the image. That is, if the coil is moving during the collection of the data, then you are going to blur the available data. If you freeze the data, and Dr. Pohost mentioned some of the technique for freezing data, turns out you reduce the resolution. So there is a lot of work that needs to be done. However, I wouldn't write it off since we're generally developing higher signal-to-noise techniques, and not only the coils but in fact the gradients that generate the resolution are actually getting better.

Discussant C from the Audience: We have actually performed a few of combined studies with intravascular ultrasound and angioscopy to look exactly for what you have mentioned, Dr. Fuster, looking for the vulnerable plaque. Problems we have encountered so far is that, as was mentioned, the resolution of the ultrasound is not high enough. In terms of the use of the angioscope, it's good for determining the color of the plaque as well as for thrombus and the presence or absence of disruption. And now clinically we have been able to predict which lesions could get into trouble at the time of revascularization, at the time of angioplasty. I don't know, Dr. Ambrose, whether you agree that angioscopy can help us determine lesion-specific therapy in terms of changing our approach towards a certain lesion or not?

Dr. Ambrose: I'm not sure it does. Only perhaps in very specific instances.

Dr. Fuster: Final question: Dr. Pohost, when will we have magnetic resonance replacing coronary arteriography for diagnosis? Tell us the date or the year.

Dr. Gerald M. Pohost: The date or the year. I told you that last year, right?

Dr. Fuster: That's why I am asking. You to told me it was last year, right?

Dr. Pohost: (*laughter*) Let's see. It's now 1995. Let's give it until 1998, January.

Dr. Fuster: So, you think it's a long road?

Dr. Pohost: Yes.

Dr. Fuster: Thank you very much.

Chapter 24

Progression and Regression of Coronary Atherosclerosis: A Review of Trials by Quantitative Angioplasty

Jeroen Vos, MD, Peter N. Ruygrok, MD, and Pim J. de Feyter, MD

Introduction

Despite the trend towards an overall reduction in cardiovascular morbidity and mortality, coronary artery disease remains the most common cause of death in western countries.[1] Coronary atherosclerosis is caused by functional and structural changes in the arterial wall, including abnormal vasoconstriction, enhanced interaction of blood cells with the endothelium, accumulation of lipoproteins in the wall, activation of coagulation mechanisms, and migration and proliferation of vascular smooth muscle cells.[2] These changes in the arterial wall eventually lead to obstruction of the lumen of the coronary artery, a process that is modulated by the remodeling capacity of the vessel wall.[3] Coronary angiography has been used to study the atherosclerotic changes of the coronary artery lumen. However, coronary angiography is acknowledged to have limitations, because it evaluates the coronary lumen, rather than the wall. Thus, coronary angiography does not allow the measurement of the total plaque burden, but only accounts for the components of the plaque that intrude into the coronary vessel lumen.[4] Recent clinical trials using angiography have shown that intensive life-style changes or lipid-modifying interventions are able

From: Fuster V, (ed.) *Syndromes of Atherosclerosis: Correlations of Clinical Imaging and Pathology.* Armonk, NY: Futura Publishing Company, Inc.: © 1996.

to slow the progression of coronary atherosclerosis. In this chapter we review the published angiographic trials on the progression/regression of coronary atherosclerosis.

Lipid-Modifying Trials: Classification and Design

We have arbitrarily classified the angiographic trials on progression and regression of coronary atherosclerosis into four groups: a) the early lipid-modifying trials using qualitative (visual panel reading) assessment of the angiograms; 2) lipid-modifying trials using a variety of lipid-lowering drugs, except the statins, using quantitative coronary angiographic assessment; 3) the most recent trials using a statin as monotherapy, and using quantitative coronary angiographic assessment; and 4) the lipid-modifying trials using intensive life-style changes, diet, and exercise and using quantitative coronary angiography.

The design, lipid-modifying intervention, number of patients enrolled in the trial, duration of the intervention, and selection of patients studied are summarized in Table 1. The early lipid-modifying trials (group A) include the NHLBI[5] the CLAS,[6] and the POSCH[7] trials. Notably, the POSCH trial used partial ileal bypass surgery as the lipid-modifying intervention. These patients were followed by serial angiography at 3, 5, 7, and 10 years, which makes this study the largest prospective serial angiographic trial published so far. For the purpose of this chapter only the 3-year follow-up data are presented (Table 1).

The lipid-modifying trials using a variety of drugs (group B) such as colestipol, niacin, resin, cholestyramine, or lovastatin include the FATS,[8] the SCOR,[9] the STARS,[10] the SCRIP,[11] and the HARP[12] trials. The SCRIP trial is arbitrarily assigned to this group, because although the trial used a strategy of multiple risk-factor reduction, in addition, in almost 90% of the patients a lipid-lowering drug intervention was also used. The lipid-modifying trials using a statin as a monotherapeutic intervention (group C) include the MARS,[13] CCAIT,[14] MAAS,[15] and REGRESS[16] trials. Finally the lifestyle change trials (group D) include the Lifestyle,[17] STARS-2,[10] and Heidelberg[18] trial.

The definitions of progression and regression of coronary atherosclerosis which have been used in the various angiographic trials are not uniform (Table 2). These differences along with vari-

TABLE 1

Coronary Angiographic Atherosclerosis Trials

Study	Treatment	Number	Duration	Type of Patients
Group A: Lipid-modifying Therapies: Visual Assessment				
NHLBI (1984)	R) placebo@ 1) cholestyramine@	57 59	5 years	type II hyperlipoproteinemia, 82% NYHA I, mean age 46 years
CLAS (1987)	R) placebo@ 1) colestipol/niacin@	82 80	2 years	post-CABG, TC between 4.8–9.1 mmol/L, mean age 54 years
POSCH (1990)	R) usual care@ 1) partial ileal bypass surgery@	333 363	3 years	post-MI, TC ≥ 5.7 mmol/L, mean age 51 years
Group B: Lipid-modifying Therapies: Quantitative Coronary Angiography				
FATS (1990)	R) conventional@ 1_1) lovastatin/colestipol@ 1_2) niacin/colestipol@	46 38 36	2.5 years	apolipoprotein B ≥125 mg/dL, 1 lesion ≥50% family history of CAD, 67% angina, mean age 47 years
SCOR (1990)	R_2) placebo/resin@ 1) colestipol/niacin/lovastatin@	32 40	2 years	familial hypercholesterolemia: tendon xanthomas LDL ≥5.2 and TG ≥3.1 mmol/L, mean age 42 years
STARS (1992)	R) usual care 1_1) lipid-lowering diet 1_2) diet/cholestyramine	24 26 24	3 years	TC between 6.0–10.0 mmol/L, mean age 51 years
SCRIP (1994)	R) usual care 1) multiple risk-factor reduction	127 119	4 years	coronary artery disease mean age 56 years
HARP (1994)	R) placebo@ 1) mulitple drug therapy	39 40	2.5 years	mild CAD, TC between 4.7–6.5 mmol/L, mean age 58 years

TABLE 1 (Continued)

Study		Treatment	Number	Duration	Type of Patients
Statin Monotherapy: Quantitative Coronary Angiography					
MARS	R)	placebo@	124	2 years	TC between 4.9–7.6 mmol/L, men and women
(1993)	I)	lovastatin	123		mean age 58 years
CCAIT	R)	placebo@	153	2 years	TC between 5.7–7.8 mmol/L,
(1994)	I)	lovastatin	146		mean age 52 years
MAAS	R)	placebo@	167	4 years	TC between 5.5–7.8 mmol/L, men and women
(1994)	I)	simvastatin	178		mean age 55 years
REGRESS	R)	placebo@	330	2 years	CAD, TC between 4.0–8.0 mmol/L, men
	i)	pravastatin	323		mean age 56 years
Lifestyle Changes: Quantitative Coronary Angiography					
Lifestyle	R)	usual care	19	1 year	no lipid-modifying drugs,
(1990)	I)	lifestyle changes	22		mean age 58 years
STARS-2	R)	usual care	24	3 years	TC between 6.0–10.0 mmol/L,
(1992)	I)	lipid-lowering diet	26		mean age 51 years
Heidelberg	R)	usual care	52	1 year	stable angina,
(1992)	I)	lifestyle changes	40		mean age 53 years

R indicates reference group; I, Index Group;@, dietary counseling; TC, total cholesterol; TG, triglycerides; Number, patients with angiographic follow-up.

TABLE 2

Definitions of Progression and Regression of CAD in Coronary Angiographic Atherosclerosis Trials

Study	Definition
Lipid-Modifying Therapies: Visual Assessment	
NHLBI	definite progression: ≥1 lesion with definite progression and no lesion with regression
	probable progression: ≥1 lesion with probable progression and no lesion with regression or definite progression
	probable regression: ≥1 lesion with probably regression and no lesion with definite regression or any progression
	definite regression: ≥1 lesion with definite regression and no progression
	mixed response: regression and progression: lesion progression and regression in the same patient, whether definite or probable.
	no change: no lesion observed as changed by at least 2 panels
CLAS	CLAS consensus global change score: 0 indicates no change; 1, definitely discernable; 2, moderate; 3 extreme; −, regression; +, progression
POSCH	CLAS consensus global change score: 0 indicates no change; 1, definitely discernable; 2, moderate; 3 extreme; −, regression; +, progression

Study	Definition
Lipid-Modifying Therapies: Quantitative Coronary Angiography	
FATS	progression: 10% increase in percentage diameter stenosis; regression: 10% decrease
SCOR	progression: 10% increase in percentage area stenosis; regression: 10% decrease
STARS	progression: loss of ≥0.17 mm in mean absolute width; regression: gain of ≥0.17 mm
SCRIP	progression: a decrease of >0.2 mm in minimal luminal diameter; regression: increase of >0.2 mm
HARP	progression: a increase of >7.8% in percentage diameter stenosis; regression: decrease of >7.8%

Study	Definition
Statin Monotherapy: Quantitative Coronary Angiography	
MARS	progression: increase ≥12% in diameter percentage stenosis; regression: decrease ≥12%
	CLAS consensus global change score: 0, no change; 1, definitely discernable; 2, moderate; 3, extreme; −, regression, +, progression
CCAIT	progression: a decrease of >0.4 mm in minimal luminal diameter; regression: increase of > 0.4 mm
MAAS	progression: a increase of >15% in percentage diameter stenosis; regression: decrease of >15%
REGRESS	progression: a decrease of >0.4 mm in minimal luminal diameter; regression: increase >0.4 mm

TABLE 2 (Continued)

Study	Definition
Lifestyle Changes: Quantiative Coronary Angiography	
Lifestyle	change in percentage diameter stenosis as a continuous measure; + indicates progression, −, regression
STARS-2	progression: loss of ≥0.17 mm in mean absolute width; regression: gain of ≥0.17 mm
Heidelberg	progression: decrease in minimal luminal diameter of ≥.18 mm; regression: increase of ≥0.18 mm

ations in the specific patient population studied explain the reported differences in the number of patients with progression or regression.

Treatment Effects on Lipid Profile

The treatment effect of the lipid-modifying intervention on total cholesterol, low-density lipoproteins, high-density lipoproteins, and triglycerides is presented in Table 3. Overall the reduction in total cholesterol was 23%, LDL-C 30%, and triglycerides 6%, whereas HDL-C increased by 8%. The lipid changes in the life-style trials were, as may be expected, more modest, but still significant. The effects of monotherapy with a statin (group C) on triglycerides were less, with an 11% reduction, compared with the trials that used a combination of lipid-lowering drugs (group B), where a 22% reduction was achieved.

Treatment Effect on Progression and Regression

The treatment effect on the number of patients who demonstrated progression or regression of coronary atherosclerosis is shown in Table 4 and 5. The reduction of the number of patients with progression was significant in almost all of the individual trials and in the four trial groups. The overall relative risk of progression was 0.72 for the treatment group. The increase in the number of patients with regression was also significant in all four groups. The overall rate ratio of regression was 1.84.

TABLE 3

Lipid Results: Treatment Effects.

Study	Number	TC	LDL-C	HDL-C	TG
Group A: Lipid-Modifying Therapies: Visual Assessment					
NHLBI	116	−16%	−21%	7%	2%
CLAS	162	−22%	−38%	35%	−17%
POSCH*	734	−31%	−35%	6%	16%
ALL	**1012**	**−28%**	**−34%**	**11%**	**9%**
Group B: Lipid-Modifying Therapies: Quantitative Coronary Angiography					
FATS	120	−25%	−32%	17%	−33%
SCOR	72	−23%	−27%	25%	−25%
STARS	74	−18%	−23%	−1%	−11%
SCRIP	245	−14%	−26%	6%	−19%
HARP	79	−28%	−41%	13%	−21%
All	**590**	**−20%**	**−30%**	**11%**	**−22%**
Group C: Statin Monotherapy: Quantitative Coronary Angiography					
MARS	247	230%	237%	7%	224%
CCAIT	331	−22%	−27%	4%	−4%
MAAS	373	−22%	−32%	10%	−17%
REGRESS	653	−20%	−29%	10%	−7%
All	**1604**	**−22%**	**−31%**	**8%**	**−11%**
Group D: Lifestyle Changes: Quantitative Coronary Angiography					
Lifestyle	41	−19%	−31%	0%	31%
STARS-2	50	−16%	−13%	1%	−21%
Heidelberg	113	−10%	−11%	2%	−7%
All	**204**	**−13%**	**−15%**	**1%**	**−3%**
Overall	**3360**	**−23%**	**−30%**	**8%**	**−6%**

TC indicates cholesterol; LDL-C low-density lipoprotein cholesterol; HDL-C, high-density lipoprotein cholesterol; TG, triglycerides; *, POSCH data at 5 years follow-up.

TABLE 4

Angiographic Results: Progression of Coronary Atherosclerosis.

Study		Number of patients Progression / Total	Rate	Relative risk (95% CI)	
Group A: Lipid-modifying Therapies: Visual Assessment					
NHLBI	R	28/57	49%	0.66	(0.42, 1.03)
	I	19/59	32%		
CLAS	R	50/80	61%	0.64	(0.46, 0.88)
	I	32/82	39%		
POSCH	R	138/333	41%	0.68	(0.55, 0.84)
	I	102/363	28%		
All				**0.67**	**(0.57, 0.78)**
Group B: Lipid-modifying Therapies: Quantitative Coronary Angiography					
FATS	R	21/46	46%	0.50	(0.30, 0.85)
	$I_{1\&2}$	17/74	23%		
SCOR	R	13/32	41%	0.50	(0.23, 1.04)
	I	8/40	20%		
STARS	R	11/24	46%	0.31	(0.14, 0.69)
	$I_{1\&2}$	7/50	14%		
SCRIP 0.2 mm	R	63/127	50%	1.02	(0.79, 1.31)
	I	60/119	50%		
HARP	R	13/39	33%	0.98	(0.52, 1.83)
	I	13/40	33%		
All				**0.77**	**(0.63, 0.94)**
Group C: Statin Monotherapy: Quantitative Coronary Angiography					
MARS	R	51/124	41%	0.71	(0.50, 1.01)
	I	36/123	29%		
CCAIT	R	76/153	50%	0.66	(0.50, 0.88)
	I	48/146	33%		
MAAS	R	54/167	32%	0.71	(0.50, 1.00)
	I	41/137	23%		
REGRESS	R	140/327	43%	0.86	(0.71, 1.04)
	I	115/314	37%		
All				**0.76**	**(0.69, 0.87)**
Group D: Lifestyle Changes: Quantitative Coronary Angiography					
Lifestyle	R	10/19	53%	0.35	(0.13, 0.92)
	I	4/22	18%		
STARS-2	R	11/24	46%	0.34	(0.12, 0.91)
	I_1	4/26	15%		
Heidelberg	I	25/52	48%	0.47	(0.25, 0.89)
	R	9/40	23%		
All				**0.40**	**(0.26, 0.63)**
Overall				**0.72**	**(0.66, 0.78)**

R indicates reference group; I, index group; 95% CI, 95% confidence interval.

TABLE 5

Angiographic Results: Progression of Coronary Atherosclerosis.

Study		Number of patients Regression / Total	Rate	Relative risk (95% CI)	
Lipid-modifying Therapies: Visual Assessment					
NHLBI	R	4/57	7%	0.97	(0.25, 3.68)
	I	4/59	7%		
CLAS	R	2/80	2%	6.67	(1.55,28.89)
	I	13/80	16%		
POSCH	R	24/333	7%	1.26	(0.76, 1.90)
	I	33/363	9%		
All				**1.57**	**(1.02, 2.40)**
Lipid-modifying Therapies: Quantitative Coronary Angiography					
FATS	R	5/46	11%	3.20	(1.34, 7.82)
	I$_{1\&2}$	26/74	35%		
SCOR	R	4/32	13%	2.60	(0.94, 7.20)
	I	13/40	33%		
STARS	R	1/24	4%	8.64	(1.22, 61.0)
	I$_{1\&2}$	18/50	36%		
SCRIP 0.2 mm	R	13/127	10%	1.97	(1.05, 3.69)
	I	24/119	20%		
HARP	R	7/39	18%	0.70	(0.24, 2.01)
	I	5/40	13%		
All				**2.03**	**(1.58, 3.35)**
Statin Monotherapy: Quantitative Coronary Angiography					
MARS	R	15/124	12%	1.88	(1.06, 3.35)
	I	28/123	23%		
CCAIT	R	10/153	7%	1.47	(0.67, 3.20)
	I	14/156	10%		
MAAS	R	20/167	12%	1.55	(0.93, 2.59)
	I	33/178	19%		
REGRESS	R	30/327	9%	1.88	(1.23, 2.85)
	I	54/314	17%		
All				**1.73**	**(1.33, 2.26)**
Lifestyle Changes: Quantitative Coronary Angiography					
Lifestyle	R	8/19	42%	1.90	(1.11, 3.41)
	I	18/22	82%		
STARS	R	1/24	4%	9.24	(1.28, 66.8)
	I$_1$	10/26	38%		
Heidelberg	R	9/52	17%	1.88	(0.89, 3.95)
	I	13/40	33%		
All				**2.35**	**(1.54, 3.58)**
Overall				**1.84**	**(1.54, 2.19)**

R indicates reference group; I, index group; 95% CI, 95% confidence interval.

Treatment Effects on Cardiac Events

The treatment effects on cardiac mortality and nonfatal myocardial infarction and for all cardiac events including cardiac mortality, nonfatal myocardial infarction, revascularization procedures, or hospitalization for unstable angina are shown in Tables 6 and 7. Treatment induced an overall reduction in cardiac mortality and nonfatal myocardial infarction with a relative risk of 0.78, as well as in all cardiac events with a relative risk of 0.66.

TABLE 6

Cardiac Mortality and Nonfatal Myocardial Infarction.

Study		Number of patients Event / Total	Rate	Relative risk	(95% CI)
Lipid-Modifying Therapies: Quantitative Coronary Angiography					
NHLBI	R	12/72	17%	0.68	(0.29, 1.55)
	I	8/71	11%		
CLAS	R	5/94	5%	0.20	(0.02, 1.68)
	I	1/94	1%		
POSCH*	R	42/417	10%	0.99	(0.66, 1.49)
	I	42/421	10%		
FATS	R	0/52	0%	@2%	(−8%, 5%)
	I$_{1\&2}$	2/94	2%		
SCOR	R	1/49	2%	@−2%	(−6%, 2%)
	I	0/48	0%		
STARS	R	5/28	18%	0.34	(0.09, 1.30)
	I$_{1\&2}$	3/50	6%		
SCRIP	R	13/155	8%	0.49	(0.19, 1.25)
	I	6/145	4%		
HARP	R	1/40	5%	2.05	(0.19, 21.7)
	I	2/39	3%		
CCAIT	R	7/166	4%	1.01	(0.36, 2.81)
	I	7/165	4%		
MAAS	R	16/188	9%	0.85	(0.43, 1.70)
	I	14/193	7%		
REGRESS	R	19/434	4%	0.61	(0.30, 1.24)
	I	12/450	3%		
STARS2	R	5/28	18%	0.42	(0.09, 1.96)
	I	2/27	7%		
Heidelberg	R	3/57	5%	0.83	(0.14, 4.74)
	I	2/46	4%		
Overall				**0.78**	**(0.60, 1.00)**

R indicates reference group; I, Index group; 95% CI, 95% confidence interval;
*POSCH data at 3 years follow-up, @: risk difference.

TABLE 7

All Cardiac Events.

Study		Number of patients Event / Total	Rate	Relative risk (95% CI)	
NHLBI	R	12/72	17%	0.68	(0.29, 1.55)
	I	8/71	11%		
CLAS	R	22/94	23%	0.96	(0.57, 1.61)
	I	21/94	22%		
FATS	R	11/52	21%	0.25%	(0.09, 0.68)
	I$_{1\&2}$	5/94	5%		
SCOR	R	1/49	2%	@−2%	(−6%, 2%)
	I	0/48	0%		
STARS	R	10/28	36%	0.21	(0.07, 0.61)
	I$_{1\&2}$	4/50	8%		
SCRIP	R	34/155	22%	0.63	(0.38, 1.04)
	I	20/145	14%		
HARP	R	4/40	10%	1.03	(0.28, 3.82)
	I	4/40	10%		
MARS	R	31/124	25%	0.72	(0.44, 1.16)
	I	22/123	18%		
CCAIT	R	18/166	11%	0.78	(0.40, 1.52)
	I	14/165	9%		
MAAS	R	50/188	27%	0.78	(0.54, 1.12)
	I	40/193	21%		
REGRESS	R	93/434	21%	0.58	(0.43, 0.79)
	I	56/450	12%		
STARS2	R	9/28	32%	0.35	(0.11, 1.14)
	I	3/27	11%		
Heidelberg	R	4/57	7%	1.55	(0.44, 5.44)
	I	5/46	11%		
Overall				**0.66**	**(0.56, 0.78)**

R indicates reference group; I, Index group; 95% CI, 95% confidence interval; @, risk difference; POSH, not reported.

Treatment Effects on Focal and Diffuse Coronary Atherosclerosis

Quantitative coronary angiography allows the assessment of both the changes in focal (minimum lumen diameter, or percent diameter stenosis) and diffuse coronary atherosclerosis (mean lumen diameter). Progression of diffuse coronary atherosclerosis is frequently not noted or underestimated because coronary angiography, particularly when visually evaluated, is an unreliable technique

TABLE 8

Changes in QCA Measurements per Year

Study	Group	Number of patients	Increase MLD (mm / year)	Increase DS (% / year)	Increase MD (mm / year)
Group B: Lipid-modifying Therapies					
FATS	R	46	−0.020	0.8	
(2.5 yrs)	I[1]	38	0.005	0.3	
	I[2]	36	0.014	0.4	
STARS	R	24	−0.077	1.9	−0.067
(3 yrs)	I[1]	26	0.010	−0.4	0.001
	I[2]	24	0.039	−0.6	0.034
SCRIP	R	127	−0.046	0.7	−0.016
(4 yrs)	I	119	−0.024	0.5	−0.015
HARP	R	39	−0.068	1.0	
(2.5 yrs)	I	40	−0.048	0.8	
All	**R**		**−0.048**	**0.9**	**−0.024**
	I		**−0.010**	**0.3**	**−0.006**
Group C: Statin Monotherapy					
MARS	R	124	−0.030	1.1	
(2 yrs)	I	123	−0.015	0.8	
CCAIT	R	153	−0.045	1.5	
(2 yrs)	I	146	−0.025	0.9	
MAAS	R	167	−0.033	0.9	−0.020
(4 yrs)	I	178	−0.010	0.3	−0.005
REGRESS	R	330	−0.050		−0.045
(2 yrs)	I	323	−0.030		−0.015
All	**R**		**−0.042**	**1.2**	**−0.037**
	I		**−0.022**	**0.6**	**−0.011**
Group D: Lifestyle Changes:					
Lifestyle	R	19		3.4	
(1 yr)	I	22		−2.2	
STARS-2	R	24	−0.077	1.9	−0.067
(3 yrs)	I[1]	26	0.010	−0.4	0.001
Heidelberg	R	52	−0.130	3.0	
(1 yr)	I	40	−0.010	−1.0	
All	**R**		**−0.113**	**2.8**	**−0.067**
	I		**−0.002**	**−1.1**	**0.001**
Overall	**R**		**−0.047**	**1.2**	**−0.034**
	I		**−0.019**	**0.4**	**−0.010**

R indicates reference group; I, index group, #, not reported; MLD, minimum lumen diameter, DS, percentage diameter stenosis, MD, mean lumen diameter.

for the detection of diffuse disease. However, the introduction of quantitative coronary angiography allows the accurate measurement of changes caused by diffuse atherosclerosis. The STARS,[10] SCRIP,[11] MAAS,[15] and REGRESS[16] trials have clearly demonstrated that diffuse changes do occur and can be slowed by lipid-lowering therapy (Table 8). Results from the MAAS-trial[15] demonstrated that lipid-lowering intervention effectively decreased the progression of diffuse coronary atherosclerosis both in "diseased" and "normal" coronary segments.

The overall effect of treatment on the progression of coronary atherosclerosis is small (Table 8). Overall treatment slows progression of coronary atherosclerosis. The minimal lumen diameter decreases by 0.047 mm per year in the placebo group versus 0.019 in the treatment group. The diameter stenosis increased 1.2% per year in the placebo group and 0.4% in the treatment group. The mean luminal diameter (a measure of diffuse disease) decreased by 0.034 mm per year in the placebo group and by 0.01 mm per year in the treatment group.

Conclusion

The use of coronary angiography as an end point for a trial studying progression or regression of coronary atherosclerosis is attractive. First, it is a safe, widely available method of studying changes in a vessel lumen in humans. Second, an angiographic trial needs fewer patients and the study duration can be shorter, yet yield sufficient statistical power compared to a trial with clinical end points.

However, serial angiography to study progression/regression only provides a surrogate end point, albeit useful. Slowing of progression or frank regression of a lesion is not necessarily linked with a lesser occurrence of coronary events. However, the pooled results of the angiographic trials provide sufficient evidence to show that slowing of progression or frank regression was associated with an improved prognosis. In the 3230 patients included in this review, the overall relative risk for progression of coronary atherosclerosis was 0.72 and for regression 1.84. Alternatively stated, progression was reduced with 28% and the incidence of regression, although in absolute terms not as frequent as progression, was almost doubled. The induced angiographic changes in an individual patient are relatively small and exert only a minimal effect on the functional significance of a lesion. It is noteworthy that lipid-lowering interventions not only beneficially change focal lesions, but this effect is also apparent on diffuse disease both of the diseased coronary segments as well as the "normal" coronary segments. These beneficial anatomic changes were associated with a reduced occurrence of cardiac death or nonfatal myocardial infarction and less cardiac events including death, nonfatal myocardial infarction or revascularization procedures. Comprehensive life-style changes produced remarkable beneficial effects on the progression of coronary atherosclerosis. Although the number of patients studied was

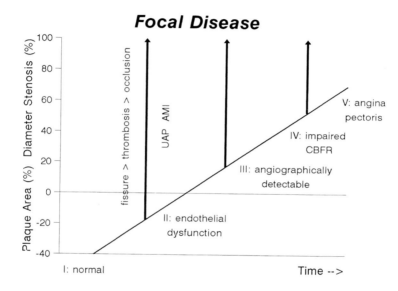

FIGURE 1. *Diagram illustrating the possible natural course of focal atherosclerotic plaque progression, plaque fissure, thrombosis, and ensuing clinical results.* **Phase 1:** *no abnormalities, the endothelium is normal.* **Phase 2:** *a focal atherosclerotic plaque is present, but the internal elastic lamina is <40% occupied by atheroma, and because of remodeling does not encroach upon the lumen, making this lesion angiographically undetectable. However, plaque rupture and ensuing acute coronary syndrome may occur.* **Phase 3:** *The plaque occupies ≥40% of the area of the internal lamina elastica, remodeling falls short and the lesion encroaches upon the lumen making this lesion angiographically visible. Clinically this lesion is silent, but plaque rupture and ensuing acute coronary syndrome may occur.* **Phase 4:** *Plaque growth occurs, which may still be clinically silent; the coronary blood flow reserve (CBFR) is impaired and plaque rupture may occur.* **Phase 5:** *Plaque growth to an obstruction of >50% causes angina pectoris; plaque rupture may occur. The gradually increasing severity of the lesion induces collaterals which exert protection in the case of plaque rupture and occlusive thrombosis.*

small, and the duration of the studies short so that generalization of these results is preliminary, the results are encouraging and warrant further study.

The natural course of progression of focal and diffuse coronary atherosclerosis is presented in Figures 1 and 2. Progression of both focal and diffuse disease may be beneficially changed by lipid-modifying interventions.

Therapeutic modulation of the atherosclerotic process appears possible. However, until now, this has been demonstrated in secondary prevention trials, mainly in men, and unfortunately in a few women at high risk of future coronary events. Studies are needed to show that modulation of the atherosclerotic process is also pos-

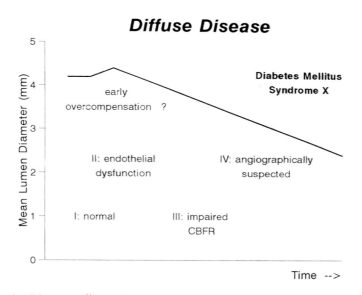

Diffuse Disease

FIGURE 2: *Diagram illustrating the possible natural course of diffuse atherosclerotic plaque progression.* **Phase 1:** *Normal wall, normal endothelium.* **Phase 2:** *Intimal wall abnormalities, undetected by angiography. Endothelial dysfunction may be present as can be demonstrated by abnormal vasoconstrictor response to acetylcholine.* **Phase 3:** *Progression of diffuse disease, still angiographically undetected, may cause endothelial dysfunction and impaired coronary blood flow. This may cause angina: syndrome X, or may be associated with diabetes mellitus.* **Phase 4:** *Further progression of diffuse disease results in the presence of abnormally small caliber epicardial vessels, raising a high-suspicion "angiographically" diffuse disease. Endothelial dysfunction and impaired coronary blood flow are more pronounced. This is often seen in syndrome X and diabetes mellitus.*

sible in "normal" patients. Progression of disease is slowed and most striking is the fact that the disease process can be stabilized in the majority of patients. Although the ultimate goal of an intervention would be regression of the lesion, so far, this has only been accomplished in a small number of patients. However, the majority of the patients would settle for stabilization of their coronary artery disease, a goal that now appears to be within reach.

References

1. Sytkowski PA, Kannel WB, D'Agostino RB. Changes in risk factors and the decline in mortality from cardiovascular disease. The Framingham Heart Study. *N Engl J Med* 1990;322;1635–1641.
2. Ross R. The pathogenesis of atherosclerosis: A prospective for the 1990's. *Nature* 1993;362:801–809.
3. Gibbons GH, Dzau VJ. The emerging concept of vascular remodeling. *N Engl J Med* 1994;330:1431–1438.
4. de Feyter PJ, Serruys PW, Oliver M, et al. Quantitative coronary angiography to measure progression or regression of coronary atherosclerosis: Value, limitations and implications for clinical trials. *Circulation* 1991;84:412–423.
5. Brensike JF, Levy RI, Kelsey SF, et al. Effects of therapy with cholestyramine on progression of coronary arteriosclerosis: Results of the NHLBI Type II Coronary Intervention Study. *Circulation* 1984;69: 313–324.
6. Blankenhorn DH, Nessim SA, Johnson RL, et al. Beneficial effects of combined colestipol-niacin therapy on coronary atherosclerosis and coronary venous bypass grafts. *JAMA* 1987;257:3233–3240.
7. Buchwald H, Varco RL, Matts JP, et al. Effect of partial ileal bypass surgery on mortality and morbidity from coronary heart disease in patients with hypercholesterolemia. Report of the Program on the Surgical Control of the Hyperlipidemias (POSCH). *N Engl J Med* 1990;323: 946–955.
8. Brown G, Albers JJ, Fischer LD, et al. Regression of coronary artery disease as a result of intensive lipid lowering therapy in men with high levels of apolipoprotein B. *N Engl J Med* 1990;323;1289–1298.
9. Kane JP, Malloy MJ, Ports TA, et al. Regression of coronary atherosclerosis during treatment of familial hypercholesterolemia with combined drug regimes. *JAMA* 1990;264:3007–3012.
10. Watts GF, Lewis B, Brunt JNH, et al. Effects on coronary artery disease of lipid-lowering diet, or diet plus cholestyramine, in the St Thomas' atherosclerosis regression study (STARS). *Lancet* 1992:339: 563–569.
11. Haskell WL, Alderman EL, Fair JM, et al. Effects of intensive multiple risk factor reduction on coronary atherosclerosis and clinical cardiac events in men and women with coronary artery disease. The Stanford coronary risk intervention project (SCRIP). *Circulation* 1994;89: 975–990.
12. Sacks FM, Pasternak RC, Gibson CM, et al. for the Harvard Atherosclerosis reversibility project (HARP) Group. Effect on coronary ather-

osclerosis of decrease in plasma cholesterol concentrations in normo-cholesterolaemic patients. *Lancet* 1994;344:1182–1186.

13. Blankenhorn DH, Azen SP, Kramsch DM, et al. Coronary angiographic changes with lovastatin therapy. The monitored atherosclerosis regression study (MARS). *Ann Intern Med* 1993;119:969–976.

14. Waters D, Higginson L, Gladstone P, et al. for the CCAIT study group. Effects of monotherapy with an HMG-CoA reductase inhibitor on the progression of coronary atherosclerosis as assessed by serial quantitative arteriography. The Canadian Coronary Atherosclerosis Intervention Trial. *Circulation* 1994;89:959–968.

15. Effect of simvastatin on coronary atheroma. the Multicentre Anti-Atheroma Study (MAAS). The Maas Investigators. *Lancet* 1994;344:633–638.

16. Jukema JW, Bruschke AVG, van Bowen AJ, et al. Effects of lipe lowering by pravastin on progression and regression of coronary artery disease in symptomatic men with normal to moderately elevated serum cholesterol levels. The Regression growth Valuation Statin Study (REGRESS). *Circulation* 1995;91:2528–2540.

17. Ornish D, Brown SE, Schwerwitz LW, et al. Can lifestyle changes reverse coronary heart disease? *Lancet* 1990;336:129–133.

18. Schuler G, Hambrecht R, Schlierf G, et al. Regular physical exercise and low-fat diet. Effects on progression of coronary disease. *Circulation* 1992;86:1–11.

Chapter 25

Carotid and Femoro-Iliac Disease as Models for the Use of Newer Imaging Techniques

Robert Byington, PhD

Introduction

B-mode ultrasonography emerged during the 1980s as an alternative to angiography to quantify atherosclerotic lesions and their progression in research settings. This chapter describes the use of B-mode ultrasonography in epidemiologic studies and clinical trials. Because most of the work to date has been in the study of carotid artery disease, the carotid arteries form the focus for discussion. However, the femoral arteries will also be discussed, although in lesser detail.

Rationale for the Use of B-Mode Ultrasonography

When a clinical trial or an epidemiologic study of coronary heart disease is being designed, there is usually a great deal of discussion regarding the selection of the outcome measure, or end point, of interest. Obviously, having a clinical end point, such as the incidence of a fatal or nonfatal coronary event, would be a good choice because ultimately, this is what we wish to see reduced. However, studies or trials with clinical outcomes tend to need to be large, long, and expensive.

Another outcome modality that has been successfully and more frequently used in recent years is the angiographic study of

From: Fuster V, (ed.) *Syndromes of Atherosclerosis: Correlations of Clinical Imaging and Pathology.* Armonk, NY: Futura Publishing Company, Inc.: © 1996.

coronary patients. This type of study has a number of positive characteristics. For example, the sample size of such a study can be much smaller than an events study, and such a study can apply to any organ. Angiographic studies also come closer to measuring atherosclerosis itself, rather than a clinical sequelae of the underlying disease. Finally, and from a clinical point of view, angiographic studies allow the calculation of the degree of stenosis, which conceptually is an outcome that is between the disease in the arterial wall and an overt clinical event.

However, as good as angiographic studies are, they have a number of obvious disadvantages. First, this method is necessarily invasive. As such, angiographic studies are generally restricted to population groups that require the procedure clinically, such as coronary patients. Therefore, this method is inappropriate for population groups free of clinical disease. Even among coronary patients, the very invasiveness of the method prevents its multiple use over time, so clinical trials with an angiographic outcome usually only have two measurements, one at the beginning of the trial and one at the end. Finally, because it measures lumen diameter, angiography is still not measuring atherosclerosis itself, but again a sequelae of atherosclerosis.

Figure 1 presents a possible cross-sectional depiction of the progression of arterial atherosclerosis based on the experimental evidence of Glagov and coworkers.[1] The hallmark of this depiction is the compensatory dilatation of the artery. As the artery becomes more diseased, the artery expands or compensates to maintain lumen area. The figure shows that voluminous wall changes occur early (overcompensation) with little lumen encroachment. In fact, in stenoses <40%, the lumen area is only marginally different than the nondiseased lumen. However, in stenoses >40% there is an acceleration of the decline in lumen area.

The implications of this scenario are important for those who are interested in understanding and combating early atherosclerosis. Atherosclerosis is a disease of the arterial wall, and significant lumen encroachment is apparent only after the artery has experienced tremendous mural changes. Angiography, which measures lumen encroachment, is therefore an inadequate tool to use in the study of early atherosclerosis.

With the capability of measuring the intimal-medial thickness in the arterial wall, B-mode ultrasonography meets these challenges. Because it can be used to study early atherosclerosis and the massive mural changes associated with early atherosclerosis, B-mode ultrasonography is conceptually superior to angiography.

B-mode imaging offers several other advantages over angiog-

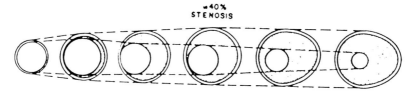

FIGURE 1. *Diagrammatic representation of a possible sequence of change in atherosclerotic arteries. Reprinted with permission from Reference 1.*

raphy: it is noninvasive, risk free, and less expensive than angiography. These characteristics allow the possibility of multiple serial measurements, which would subsequently allow not only an estimation of the progression of disease, but also a description of the pattern of progression. For example, is the progression of atherosclerosis linear or nonlinear? Also, multiple measurements permit reductions in variability and sample size, and actually permit the development of better measures of monitoring reliability. For example, duplicate examinations taken during a study are easily used to measure the degree of reproducibility of the measurements. Finally, these characteristics also allow the possibility of studying populations free of clinical disease, and from a public health point of view, primary prevention is an important consideration in developing research questions and study designs.

For the reasons listed above, since the mid-1980s, many investigators have invested a good proportion of their research time and energy towards the development of epidemiologic studies and clinical trials using B-mode ultrasonographic outcome measures.

Ultrasonographic Outcome Measures

Measuring Intimal Medial Thickness

The Asymptomatic Carotid Artery Progression Study (ACAPS) can serve as a model on how carotid B-mode measurements can be made.[2,3] Analogous methods were used in the Pravastatin, Lipids, and Atherosclerosis in the Carotids (PLAC II) Trial.[4,5] In ACAPS, sonographers in the four clinical centers and B-mode image readers in the Central Reading Center were required to complete a 3-month training and certification program before acquiring data on ACAPS participants. These individuals were trained to be able to distinguish the following arterial wall interfaces: lumen-intima, media-adventitia, and adventitia-periadventitia. From these interfaces, intimal medial thicknesses (IMT) were calculated and used as a measure of atherosclerosis. After a careful circumferential scan of the neck, sonographers used a high-resolution 10-MHz ultrasound system to obtain longitudinal B-mode images of the arterial wall boundaries in each of 12 defined carotid segments (Figure 2). The walls that were scanned were the near and far wall of the common, bifurcation, and internal carotids, on the right and left side of the neck.

The primary objective of the sonographers in the clinical centers was to image and record on super-VHS videotape the maximum IMT in each of the 12 segments. The videotapes were then mailed to the Central Reading Center, where the images were analyzed by readers who were unaware of treatment group assignment. As part of this image analysis, the maximum IMT (in millimeters) of each segment was computed by the use of cross-hair locations placed on the wall boundaries to a precision of 0.05 mm.

Participants underwent nine B-mode examinations during the 3-year course of the trial: twice at baseline, once every 6 months thereafter, and twice again at the final clinic visit. The purpose of the double scans at baseline and at the end was twofold. First, the double scans provided a measure of the reliability of the mean maximum IMT outcome measure (described below). To this end, the overall as well as inter- and intrasonographer and reader variabilities were estimated. Second, the double scans provided a statistical method for reducing the interperson variability of the outcome measure.

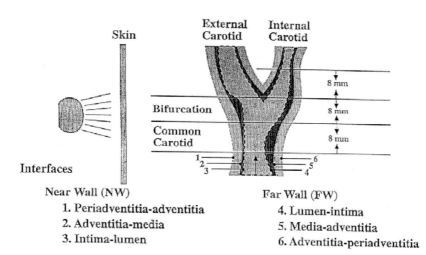

FIGURE 2. *Diagrammatic representation of carotid artery with sample landmarks and interfaces for B-mode imaging.*

B-Mode Outcome Measures

For each participant at each clinic visit in ACAPS, summary measures of the amount of atherosclerosis were simply estimated. The principal summary measure, the mean maximum IMT, was the mean of the 12 maximum IMT measurements described above. This value is less variable than any single measurement, and permits reductions in sample size while still representing a measure of the individual's total atherosclerotic burden. Another summary measure that was used was the single maximum thickness, which was the greatest value of the 12 maximum IMT measurements.

The primary ultrasound outcome measure in ACAPS and PLAC II was the change over time of the mean maximum IMT. Figure 3 illustrates how this outcome measure was estimated for one of the PLAC II participants. A least squares regression line was estimated through the available B-mode examinations. It is noted that this individual was missing data for the 30-month clinic visit. An estimate of IMT change was still made with the available data, but when the mean treatment group rate of change was estimated, this person's rate was weighted less. This highlights the advantage of multiple B-mode examinations performed over follow-up: any available data contribute something to the estimation of the rate of change. This is in contrast to the typical angiography trial that only has mea-

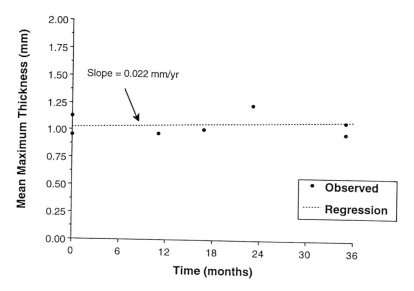

FIGURE 3. *Observed intimal-medial thickness versus regression slope over 3 years of follow-up (participant X).*

surements at the beginning and end of the trial. Any person without a final angiogram (because of death, refusal, or being lost to follow-up) is lost to the analysis.

Atherosclerotic disease progression and regression are thus derived from the serial IMT data. A positive change over 3 years (ie, an increase in IMT) denotes disease "progression;" a negative change (ie, a decrease in IMT) denotes disease "regression."

The measurements and outcome measures presented here for the carotid ateriess have recently been extended to the femoral arteries.[6] The IMT in the femoral arteries are easily measured and followed, using the same principles described above. The results of a clinical trial using the progression of femoral IMT as a secondary outcome measure is described below.[7]

Finally, it should be noted that different combinations and permutations of the above have been used in other studies. For example, some investigators have restricted their measurements to the common carotid artery. Other investigators have taken measurements from only the far wall.[8,9]

Correlates of B-Mode Measurements

The question arises that if we are ultimately interested in studying and reducing the incidence of coronary disease, is it worthwhile examining the carotid arteries? In fact, to many investigators, carotid artery investigation implies that the incidence of stroke is the primary focus of interest. If the study of cerebrovascular disease in general and stroke in particular are inherently important, a response to the question is that we are interested in reducing the sequelae of atherosclerosis, regardless of which vascular bed is troublesome. However, people who experience or die from an atherosclerotic event are more likely to experience or die of a coronary event, which explains the prominence given to heart disease.

Given that we wish to study atherosclerosis itself, B-mode ultrasonography is easy to use in an epidemiologic setting for the reasons described above. In addition, and as may be expected, atherosclerotic disease in the carotid arteries as measured by ultrasonography is correlated with the disease in other vascular beds.

Pathologically, carotid artery atherosclerosis was correlated with coronary artery atherosclerosis as long ago as 1960. In that year, Young and co-workers[10] presented correlations of the degree of atherosclerosis determined at autopsy among coronary and cerebral vascular beds in 95 people. Among the coronary arteries, correlation coefficients were in the range of about 0.1 to 0.5, a moderate level of correlation. For example, the correlation coefficient for the amount of atherosclerosis between the left main and the circumflex artery was 0.4 for the 49 autopsies of people between the ages of 70 and 79. Between the coronary and cerebral vessels, however, approximately the same range of correlation was observed. Therefore, for example, in the same 49 cases, the correlation coefficient for the amount of atherosclerosis between the circumflex and the carotid artery was 0.6, and between the left main and the carotid artery it was 0.3.

In 1986, arterial examination by ultrasound advanced via a study by Pignoli and coworkers[11] who concluded that measurements of IMT by B-mode did not differ significantly from IMT measurements obtained by dissection. This paved the way for cross-sectional and prospective epidemiologic studies, and for clinical trials, the results of which are only becoming available now.

Craven and coworkers[12] were among the first to demonstrate that carotid artery disease measured by ultrasound correlated with angiographic evidence of coronary artery disease. In fact, in their analysis the greatest predictor of the degree of coronary disease was carotid atherosclerosis.

The Salonen group[13] in Finland were the first to demonstrate cross sectionally that increased carotid IMT measured by ultrasound was related to the traditional risk factors for clinical coronary events. For example, and as shown in Figure 4, they reported in 1988 that there was a positive correlation between low-density lipoprotein (LDL) cholesterol and increasing carotid artery disease. Subsequently, carotid artery disease as measured by ultrasound has been cross-sectionally associated with smoking,[14,15] hypertensionm,[15] diabetes,[16] and preexisting clinical vascular disease.[16]

Regarding the measurement of femoral artery disease by ultrasound, the Salonen group[17] reported in 1993 a comparison of the factors cross-sectionally associated with increased carotid IMT and increased femoral IMT. Whereas there was some agreement (eg, smoking and fibrinogen levels were associated with increased thickness in both beds), there were some differences in predictors, as noted in Table 1. For example, whereas LDL and systolic blood pressure appeared to be good predictors of increased carotid IMT, they were poor predictors of increased femoral IMT. Conversely, triglyceride levels were good predictors of femoral IMT, but poor predictors of carotid IMT.

The reports noted above are a sample of the recent reports

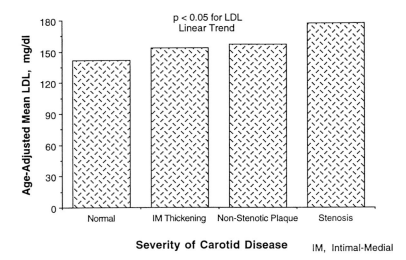

FIGURE 4. *Association between low density lipoprotein (ldl) and carotid atherosclerosis as detected by B-mode. Adapted with permission from Reference 13.*

TABLE 1

Cross-sectional, Age-adjusted Correlation Coefficients Between Arterial Mean Maximum Intimal-Medial Thicknesses (IMT) and the Main Coronary Risk Factors[17]

	Carotid IMT* (mm)	Femoral IMT (mm)
Years of Smoking	0.245[†]	0.413[†]
Serum LDL (mmol/l)	0.158[†]	0.064
Plasma Fibrinogen (g/l)	0.212[†]	0.320[†]
Systolic Blood Pressure (mm Hg)	0.111[†]	−0.010
History of CHD (yes vs no)	0.146[†]	−0.030
Serum Triglycerides (mmol/l)	0.059	0.116[†]
Current Number of Cigarettes/day	0.156[†]	0.326[†]
Serum Apo A-I (g/l)	−0.006	−0.168[†]
Days Since Quit Smoking	−0.099	−0.146[†]

*Includes the common carotid and the bifurcation.
[†]P <0.05
LDL indicates low density lipoprotein; CHD, coronary heart disease.

demonstrating cross-sectionally that increased carotid and femoral IMTs are associated with disease in other vascular beds and with traditional cardiovascular risk factors. The next logical step in validating the method was the demonstration that increased IMT was predictive of subsequent events. This was first reported by Salonen in 1991.[18] In that report, as baseline carotid artery morphology increased from normal to intimal-medial thickening to stenosis, the relative risk of an acute myocardial infarction in men increased eightfold.

In 1993, the Salonen group also reported which baseline characteristics were the strongest predictors of a 2-year increase in the IMT of the common carotid arteries of 126 middle-aged men.[17] As noted in Table 2, age, serum LDL levels, smoking status, thrombocytic aggregability, serum copper, and blood hemoglobin levels were all positively associated with increased IMT progression; serum selenium was negatively associated with increased IMT progression.

Taken together, the findings outlined in this section underscore the general correlations that have been observed of atherosclerotic disease among the various vascular beds. They also underscore the general correlations that have been observed between traditional cardiovascular risk factors and subsequent increased IMT. The next question that was raised was: if a risk factor, such as LDL-cholesterol, could be reduced, would this result in a diminution of the IMT progression rate? Answers to this question were recently given in a number of clinical trials that used B-mode ultrasonography to measure IMT progression, three of which are discussed here.

TABLE 2

Biological Predictors of the Two-Year Progression of the Intimal-Medial Thickness of the Common Carotid Artery[17]

	Standardized Regression Coefficient	P Value
Age (years)	0.28	0.0003
Serum LDL (mmol/l)	0.26	0.0012
Nicotine excretion (mg/l)	0.25	0.0011
Thrombocyte aggregability (mV/sec)	0.25	0.0014
Serum Copper (> vs <17.6 μmoL/l)	0.24	0.0030
Serum Selenium (> vs <1.4 μmoL/l)	−0.20	0.0094
Blood Hemoglobin (> vs <147 g/L)	0.15	0.0375

LDL indicates low density lipoprotein.

Results of Three Recent Clinical Trials Using IMT Progression as the Primary Outcome Measure

The Asymptomatic Carotid Atherosclerosis Progression Study

The Asymptomatic Carotid Atherosclerosis Progression Study (ACAPS) was a randomized, double-masked, placebo-controlled, multicenter clinical trial to determine the effects of the lovastatin and minidose warfarin on the 3-year progression of atherosclerosis in the carotid arteries of 919 men and women, 40 to 79 years of age. The progression of atherosclerosis was defined as the progression of the mean maximum IMT, as described above. The design of the trial is described in detail elsewhere.[2]

Briefly, all participants were asymptomatic, but at high risk of developing clinical cardiovascular disease with LDL cholesterol levels between the 60th and 90th percentile values for the United States population. These were levels below the treatment levels recommended in 1988 (the year the trial was designed) by the National Cholesterol Education Program (NCEP).[19] The trial used a factorial design and the participants were randomized to one of four treatment groups: active lovastatin/active warfarin (LW); active lovastatin/warfarin placebo (LP); lovastatin placebo/active warfarin (PW); and lovastatin placebo/warfarin placebo (PP). Lovastatin, an hepatic hydroxymethyl glutarl coenzyme A (HMG CoA) reductase inhibitor, was selected as one of the interventions because of the expectation that its potent lipid-lowering effect would translate into a reduction of atherosclerosis. Warfarin was selected as the other intervention because of its anticoagulant property, which was felt to complement independently the lipid-lowering effect of lovastatin. It was hypothesized that both agents would alter the progression of atherosclerosis, but through different pathways.

Although it was required that the ACAPS participants be free of clinical disease at entry, they were required to have evidence of early carotid artery atherosclerosis as measured by B-mode ultrasonography. At baseline, the mean maximum IMT was 1.32 mm for the PP group, and 1.33 mm for the LP group. For reference, investigators from the large Atherosclerosis Risk In Communities (ARIC) cohort study recently reported that the average IMT for a typical middle-aged American is 0.60 mm, or about one half that observed for ACAPS.[20] Thus, it could be argued that ACAPS was not a primary prevention trial, but rather a secondary prevention trial.

The effect of lovastatin on the mean maximum IMT progression has been reported.[3] A statistically significant interaction (P = 0.04) was detected for this outcome measure: the observed effect of the lovastatin and warfarin combination on progression was less than the effect of lovastatin alone. For this reason, progression data from the four individual treatment groups were compared, rather than the marginals of the factorial design.

Figure 5 shows the progression of the cross-sectional mean maximum IMTs for the LP and PP groups. The curves have been aligned so that the baseline values coincide. It is noted in the figure that that the curves for the LP and PP are almost superimposable for the first year of follow-up. After the 12-month visit, the curves diverge with the lovastatin curve going downwards and the placebo curve going upwards. Overall, the annualized progression rate for the PP group was 0.006 mm per year, whereas the rate for the LP group was −0.009 mm per year, with the negative rate denoting regression. This difference in the rates, the primary ACAPS hypothesis, was statistically significant (P = 0.001, Bonferroni-adjusted, Table 3).

The observed 6- to 12-month delay in the treatment effect on progression was unexpected and previously unreported. However, it is consistent with 1- to 2-year treatment lags on the reduction in clinical events previously reported in the early lipid-lowering trials.[21,22]

ACAPS was the first trial to demonstrate the benefit of lipid-lowering treatment in asymptomatic people with LDL cholesterol

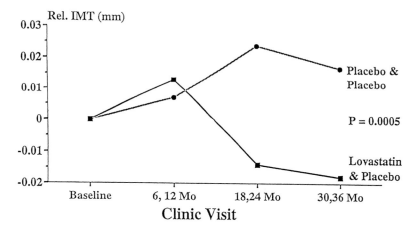

FIGURE 5. *Graph showing cross-sectional relative intimal-medial thicknesses (IMT) for the ACAPS lovastatin and placebo groups, excluding participants on warfarin. Adapted with permission from Reference 3.*

TABLE 3

Progression Rates for the Mean Maximum Intimal-Medial
Thickness by ACAPS Treatment Group[3]

	Mean (± Standard Error) Progression Rates (mm/year)	P - Value*
Active Lovastatin + Placebo Warfarin	−0.009 ± 0.003	0.001
Active Lovastatin + Active Warfarin	−0.003 ± 0.003	0.06
Placebo Lovastatin + Placebo Warfarin	0.004 ± 0.003	—

*Difference from double placebo based upon Bonferroni-adjusted analysis of covariance, with clinical center and baseline value as covariates.

below the recommended NCEP treatment levels. With respect to using ultrasonography as method for monitoring disease progression, ACAPS was the first trial to demonstrate the validity and statistical efficiency of B-mode ultrasonography in a multicenter setting.

The Pravastatin, Lipids, and Atherosclerosis in the Carotid Arteries Study

The Pravastatin, Lipids, and Atherosclerosis in the Carotid Arteries (PLAC II) study was a randomized, double-masked, placebo-controlled, single-center clinical trial to determine the effects of the lipid-lowering agent pravastatin on the 3-year progression of atherosclerosis in the carotid arteries of 151 coronary patients. PLAC II and ACAPS were run concurrently. Pravastatin, like the lovastatin used in ACAPS, is an HMG CoA reductase inhibitor. The primary outcome measure was again defined as the progression of the mean maximum IMT in the 12 carotid walls, as described above. Because of the uncertainty of where the drug would have its greatest and least effects, three ultrasonographic secondary outcome measures were identified at the beginning of the trial. One of these was the 3-year IMT progression rate in the 4 walls of the common carotid. The design of the trial is described elsewhere.[4]

Briefly, all participants were required to have a history of clinical myocardial infarction or angiographic evidence of at least 50% stenosis in one coronary artery. Like ACAPS, participants were also required to have an LDL cholesterol value between the 60th and

90th percentile for the United States population. Finally, and again like ACAPS, all participants were required to have evidence of early carotid atherosclerosis, as measured by B-mode.

The effect of pravastatin on the mean maximum IMT progression has been previously reported.[5] Overall, there was a nonsignificant 12% reduction in IMT progression associated with pravastatin use (0.059 mm per year for the pravastatin participants compared with 0.068 mm per year for the placebo participants). However, there was a statistically significant 35% reduction in progression in the common carotid artery (0.046 mm per year for the pravastatin participants compared with 0.030 mm year for the placebo participants, $P = 0.03$).

PLAC II and ACAPS

It is interesting to compare and contrast the design features and results of ACAPS and PLAC II. Both trials used almost identical primary B-mode outcome measures, although slightly different protocols because the reading centers were different. Both trials used similar agents and both effected reductions in progression attributable to the drugs. The required sample sizes, however, were very different: 919 participants in ACAPS compared with 151 in PLAC II. The primary reason for this was the assumption made during the design stages of these trials that the coronary patients in PLAC II would be on a "faster track" of progression, simply because they already had exhibited clinical disease. This expected greater progression thus translated itself into a lower required sample size for PLAC II. It is to be noted that at the conclusions of these trials, this assumption was confirmed. Among the placebo participants in both trials, the PLAC II participants had a 10-fold greater annualized carotid IMT progression rate: 0.068 mm per year in PLAC II compared with 0.006 mm per year in ACAPS.

The Kuopio Atherosclerosis Prevention Study

The Kuopio Atherosclerosis Prevention Study (KAPS) was a placebo-controlled primary prevention trial that tested whether lipid lowering (using pravastatin again) would effect a reduction in the rate of atherosclerosis development in 447 hypercholesterolemic men.[7] The primary end point for the trial was the progression of the IMT of the far walls of the bifurcation and common carotid arteries combined. A secondary end point was the progression of the IMT in the femoral arteries.

For the primary end point, the IMT progression rate in the pravastatin group was 28.6% lower than the rate in the placebo group ($P < 0.05$). Similarly, the IMT progression rate in the femoral arteries among the pravastatin participants was 26.3% lower than the rate in the placebo group ($P < 0.05$). When the common and bifurcation arteries were analyzed separately, there was a 64.0% reduction in the common artery alone, and a <3% reduction in the bifurcation artery.

Overall Interpretation of the Results of The Three Clinical Trials

ACAPS, PLAC II, and KAPS each demonstrated that IMT progression could be halted and possibly reversed by lipid-lowering therapy. The PLAC II and KAPS data also suggested that treatment effects apply to greater and lesser extents in various vascular beds. The common carotid, the bifurcation, and the femoral arteries are similar, although not identical tissue types. The ultimate message, however, is that the natural history of atherosclerotic progression, as measured by B-mode ultrasonography, can be altered by risk factor modification.

Conclusions

With proper standardization, B-mode imaging represents a valuable research tool for the noninvasive assessment of carotid and femoral atherosclerosis.[9] Rigorous training and standardization are essential to any project, particularly multicenter studies. Variability in the scanning and the reading of images contributes to the imprecision of the technique, although the use of duplicate examinations at baseline and at the completion of the trial, together with interim examinations and the use of a summary outcome measure, can reduce the intraindividual variability.

Because of the inevitable variability and because the recently completed cohort studies and trials have been of relatively short duration (3 years is a short period of time over the course of a lifetime), it is difficult to comment at this time on the progression patterns in individuals. The changes in progression in group mean data are smaller than the resolution for individual participants. Two large-scale, long-term, population-based cohort studies, the Atherosclerosis Risk in Communities Study[15] and the Cardiovascular Health Study[16], are collecting B-mode ultrasound data and will eventually be able to better describe the progression of atherosclerosis, in individuals and in population subgroups.

B-mode ultrasonographic imaging of the carotid and femoral arteries is a valid and reproducible method for assessing early atherosclerotic lesions. The technique can also be used to describe atherosclerotic progression in the arterial walls, and is thus valid for testing possible antiatherogenic modalities.

References

1. Glagov S, Weisenberg E, Zarins CK, et al. Compensatory enlargement of human atherosclerotic coronary arteries. *N Engl J Med* 1987;316: 1371–1375.
2. The ACAPS Group: Rationale and design for the Asymptomatic Carotid Artery Plaque Study (ACAPS). *Controlled Clin Trials* 1992;13:293–314.
3. Furberg CD, Adams HP, Applegate WB, et al. Effect of lovastatin on early carotid atherosclerosis and cardiovascular events. *Circulation* 1994; 90:1679–1687.
4. Crouse JR, Byington RP, Bond MG, et al. Pravastatin, lipids, and atherosclerosis in the carotid arteries—Design features of a clinical trial with carotid atherosclerosis outcome. *Controlled Clin Trials* 1992;13:495–506.
5. Crouse JR, Byington RP, Bond MG, et al. Pravastatin, lipids, and atherosclerosis in the carotid arteries (plac ii)—A clinical trial with atherosclerosis outcome. *Am J Cardiol* 1995;75:455–459.
6. Joensuu T, Salonen R, Winblad I, et al. Determinants of femoral and carotid artery atherosclerosis. *J Intern Med* 1994;236:79–84.
7. Salonen R, Nyyssönen K, Porkkala E, et al. KAPS—The effects of pravastatin on atherosclerotic progression in carotid and femoral arteries. *Circulation* 1994;90(suppl I):I–127.
8. Wikstrand J, Wendelhag I. Methodological considerations of ultrasound investigation of intima-media thickness and lumen diameter. *J Intern Med* 1994;236:555–559.
9. Furberg CD, Byington RP, Craven TE. Lessons learned from clinical trials with ultrasound endpoints. *J Intern Med* 1994;236:575–580.
10. Young W, Gofman JW, Tandy R, et al. The quantification of atherosclerosis. III. The extent of correlation of degree of correlation of atherosclerosis within and between the coronary and cerebral vascular beds. *Am J Cardiol* 1960;6:300–308.
11. Pignoli P, Tremoli E, Poli A, et al. Intimal plus medial thickness of the arterial wall—A direct measurement with ultrasound imaging. *Circulation* 1986;74:1399–1406.
12. Craven TE, Ryu J, Espeland MA, et al. Evaluation of the associations between carotid artery atherosclerosis and coronary artery stenosis—A case-control study. *Circulation* 1990;82:1230–1242.
13. Salonen R, Seppanen K, Rauramaa R, et al. Prevalence of Carotid Atherosclerosis and Serum Cholesterol Levels in Eastern Finland. *Arteriosclerosis* 1988;8:788–792.
14. Tell GS, Howard G, McKinney WM, et al. Cigarette smoking cessation and extracranial carotid atherosclerosis. *JAMA* 1989;261:1178–1180.
15. Heiss G, Sharrett AR, Barnes R, et al. Carotid atherosclerosis measured

by B-mode ultrasound in populations: Associations with cardiovascular risk factors in the ARIC Study. *Am J Epidemiol* 1991;134:250–256.

16. O'Leary DH, Polak JF, Kronmal RA, et al. Distribution and correlates of sonographically detected carotid artery disease in the Cardiovascular Health Study. *Stroke* 1992;23:1752–1760.

17. Salonen JT, Salonen R. Ultrasound b-mode imaging in observational studies of atherosclerotic progression. *Circulation* 1993;87(suppl II):II-56–II-65.

18. Salonen R: Risk factors for ultrasonographically assessed common carotid atherosclerosis—A cross-sectional and longitudinal population-based study in eastern Finnish men. *University of Kuopio (Finland) Community Health Original Report*. 1991:64–65.

19. Report of the National Cholesterol Education Program Expert Panel on Detection, Evaluation, and Treatment of High Blood Cholesterol in Adults. *Arch Intern Med* 1988;148:36–69.

20. Howard G, Sharett AR, Heiss G, et al. Carotid artery intimal-medial thickness distribution in general populations as evaluated by B-mode ultrasound. *Stroke* 1993;24:1297–1304.

21. Lipid Research Clinics Program. The Lipid Research Clinics Coronary Primary Prevention Trial results. I. Reduction in the incidence of coronary heart disease. *JAMA* 1984;251:351–364.

22. Frick MH, Elo O, Haapa K, et al. Helsinki Heart Study—Primary prevention trial with gemfibrozil in middle-aged men with dyslipidemia: Safety of treatment, changes in risk factors, and incidence of coronary heart disease. *N Engl J Med* 1987;317:1237–1245.

Chapter 26

Coronary Angiographic Changes, Lipid-Lowering Therapy, and their Relationship to Clinical Cardiac Events

B. Greg Brown, MD, PhD, Xue-Qiao Zhao, MD, Drew Poulin, BS, and John J. Albers, PhD

Introduction

The first goal of therapy for ischemic heart disease (IHD) is to improve the symptoms of arterial obstruction in which the blood supply is inadequate for the peak myocardial oxygen demands. Current medical management relieves these symptoms by favorably altering the oxygen supply-demand imbalance. Relief of symptoms may also be achieved through more direct structural and/or physiological changes favorably affecting the diminished vascular flow reserve. Among these, regression has been debated as a possible mechanism for symptom relief. This chapter reviews evidence for the promotion of regression by lipid lowering.

The second goal of therapy in IHD is to prevent the anticipated progression to a clinical event such as sudden death, myocardial infarction, or worsening angina requiring bypass surgery or angioplasty. We now appreciate that most clinical events are precipitated

Supported in part by NIH Grants R01 HL 19451, P01 HL 30086, and R01 HL 42419 from the National Heart, Lung and Blood Institute, and in part by a grant from the John L. Locke, Jr. Charitable Trust, Seattle, WA.

This chapter is a substantially modified and abbreviated version of a previous publication.[30]

From: Fuster V, (ed.) *Syndromes of Atherosclerosis: Correlations of Clinical Imaging and Pathology.* Armonk, NY: Futura Publishing Company, Inc.: © 1996.

by an episode of plaque disruption. Data are presented in this chapter that indicate a linkage between lipid lowering and stabilization of plaque structure.

Regression and Progression of Coronary Lumen Obstruction

The recanalization of a previously obstructed coronary artery, and the improvement of ordinary lesions are occasionally observed in a later arteriogram. Thus, the critical question is not *does regression happen in patients* (because it does), but, *can repression be promoted with sufficiently great magnitude and frequency to favorably alter the clinical course of the disease?* The emerging evidence regarding this question is extremely encouraging.

Experimental Observations

The fact that atherosclerosis can regress with lipid lowering has been shown in studies in cholesterol-fed primates.[1–5] Such "atherogenic" diets increase coronary artery collagen (3×), elastin (4×), and cholesterol (7×, mostly esterified). Cholesterol esters are among the more mobile of the plaque lipids; they are transported to the intima by plasma lipoproteins accumulating first in foam cells and as interstitial droplets.[4] Eventually, foam cells may undergo necrosis and release their lipid content. Cholesterol gradually accumulates deep in the intima as ester droplets and monohydrate crystals. When the animals are changed to a vegetarian "regression" diet, serum cholesterol returns to normal (140 mg/dL), and the arterial lipid and connective tissue changes partially regress over 20–40 months. Collagen content does not decrease much from its peak value (−20%), but elastin (−50%) and cholesterol (−60%, mostly esterified) do; and the plaques shrink.[2,4]

Evidence of Regression in Patients

Regression in patients has been indirectly defined in terms of arteriographic lumen improvement and may occur in several ways. Plaque lipid may be depleted,[4] and to a lesser extent, so may its connective tissues.[3,5] Lysis of fully occlusive thrombi or of mural thrombi is commonly seen. Remodeling of the underlying vascular architecture or relaxation of excess vasomotor tone may improve lumen size independently of changes in plaque size.[6] The importance of endothelial dysfunction as a basis for abnormal vasomotor and thrombogenic states, and the relationship(s) of therapy to functional recovery are becoming clarified in many of these processes.[7]

Beginning in 1984, a series of randomized clinical arteriographic trials (Tables 1 and 2) has documented the magnitude and frequency of, as well as the conditions under which regression can occur in patients. These trials include the National Heart, Lung and Blood Institute, Type II Study,[8] the Cholesterol-Lowering Atherosclerosis Study;[9,13] the Program of Surgical Control of the Hyperlipidemia;[10] the Lifestyle Heart Trial;[11] the Familial Atherosclerosis Treatment Study;[12] the University of California San Francisco SCOR Study;[14] the St. Thomas Atherosclerosis Regression Study;[15] the Stanford Coronary Risk Intervention Project;[16] and the Heidelberg Trial.[17]

More recently, a series of trials have examined the effect of monotherapy with one of the hepatic hydroxymethyl glutaryl coenzyme A (HMG-CoA) reductase inhibitors on atherosclerosis, as assessed quantitatively from the coronary arteriogram or from percutaneous B-mode ultrasound of the carotid bifurcation. These include the Monitored Atherosclerosis Regression Study;[18] the Canadian Coronary Atherosclerosis Intervention Trial;[19] the Pravastatin Limitation of Atherosclerosis in the Coronary Arteries Study;[20] and the Multicentre Anti-Atheroma Study.[21]

Of interest, in only about half of these trials was there an entry requirement for even modest hyperlipidemia. Despite the heterogeneity among these studies in clinical presentation, lipid entry requirements, treatment regimens, and methods for arteriographic analysis, the results (Table 1 and 2) are surprisingly consistent. The control group in each study had minimal (<10%) low-density lipoprotein cholesterol (LDL-C) reduction in virtually all cases and no change in high-density lipoprotein cholesterol (HDL-C). The LDL-C responses were substantial in all treated groups; HDL-C also rose when niacin was used. Each study demonstrated an arterial treatment benefit. As a generalization, less than one twelfth of the control group patients were judged to have improvement in arterial obstruction ("regression") during the study period. In contrast, more than one fourth of treated patients improved (a three- to fourfold increase). Furthermore, averaged estimates of coronary disease severity, per patient, worsened (progressed) by about 3% stenosis among the controls, while improving (regressing) by 1% to 2% stenosis among the treated patients. In nearly every study the frequency of clinical cardiovascular events decreased substantially with therapy, although because of their small sizes, the reductions achieved statistical significance in only 5 of the 13 trials.

TABLE 1

Summary Descriptions for Fifteen Reported Arteriographic Lipid-Lowering Trials: Lipid Response to Treatments

Study+	N	Entry Req'ts	Control Regimen**	Treatment Regimen	Treatment Response		Years
					LDL	HDL	
Combination Therapy Studies:							
CLAS	188	CABG	D (−)	D + R + N	−43%	+37%	2
POSCH	838	MI, CHOL	D	D + PIB ± R	−42%	+5%	9.7
LIFESTYLE	48	CAD	U	V + M + E	−37%	−3%	1
FATS (N+C)	146	CAD, APO B	D ± R	D + R + N	−32%	+43%	2.5
FATS (L+C)	146	CAD, APO B	D ± R	D + R + L	−46%	+15%	2.5
CLAS II	138	CABG	D	D + R + N	−40%	+37%	4
UC-SCOR	97	FH	U	D + R + N ± L	−39%	+25%	2
STARS (D+R)	90	CAD, CHOL	U	D + R	−36%	−4%	3
SCRIP	300	CAD	U	D + (R/N/LF) + E, BP	−22%	+12%	4
HEIDELBERG	113	CAD	U	D + Ex	−8%	+3%	1
HARP	91	CAD "NL" Lipids	D ± R	P ± N ± R ± F	−41%	+13%	2.5
Monotherapy Studies:							
NHLBI	143	CAD, LDL	D	D + R	−31%	+8%	5
STARS (D)	90	CAD, CHOL	U	D	−16%	0%	3
MARS	270	CAD	D	D + L	−38%	+9%	2
CCAIT	331	CAD, CHOL	D	D + L	−29%	+7%	2
PLAC I	408	CAD, LDL	D	D + P	−28%	+9%	3
MAAS	381	CAD	D	D + S	−31%	+9%	4
REGRESS	885	CAD	D	D + P	−29%	+10%	2

+See text for the details and full name of these studies. **Mean LDL-c response to control regimen: −7% mean HDL-c response: 0%. **CAD** indicates coronary artery disease; **LDL,** low density lipoprotein > 90th percentile; **CABG,** coronary artery bypass graft surgery; **MI,** myocardial infarction; **apo B,** apolipoprotein B ≤125 mg/dl; **FH,** familial hypercholesterolemia; **CHOL,** cholesterol >220 mg/dl; **D,** diet; **U,** usual care; **R,** resin (colestipol or cholestyramine); **N,** nicotinic acid; **PIB,** partial ileal bypass; **V,** vegetarian diet <10% fat; **M,** relaxation techniques; **Ex,** exercise program, **L,** lovastatin; **S,** simvastatin, **C,** colestipol, **F,** fibrate-type drugs; **BP,** blood pressure therapy.

TABLE 2

Summary of Arteriographic Outcomes, Treatment Lipid Response, and Frequencies or Reported Clinical Events in Fifteen Lipid-Lowering Coronary Arteriographic Trials.

Study[+]	Control Patients				Changes Among Treated Patients				% "EVENT"**
	Prog'n	Reg'n	Δ %S‡	Δ MLD (mm)	Prog'n	Reg'n	Δ%S(P)*	Δ MLD (P)*	Red'n
Combination Therapy Studies:									
CLAS	61%	2%	—	—	39%	16%	—	—	25%
POSCH (10-year)	65%	6%	—	—	37%	14%	—	—	35% (62%[Y])§
LIFESTYLE	32%	32%	+3.4%	—	14%	41%	−2.2 (.001)†	—	0 vs 1 (↑)
FATS (N+C)	46%	11%	+2.1%	−0.05	25%	39%	−0.9 (.005)	+0.035 (0.005)	80%§
FATS (L+C)	46%	11%	+2.1%	−0.05	22%	32%	−0.7 (.02)	+0.012 (0.06)	70%
CLAS II	83%	6%	—	—	30%	18%	—	—	43%
UC-SCOR	41%	13%	+0.8%	—	20%	33%	−1.5 (.04)	—	1 vs 0
STARS (D+R)	46%	4%	+5.8%	−0.23	12%	33%	−1.9 (.01)	+0.12 (0.001)	89%§
SCRIP	50%	10%	+3.2%	−0.20	50%	20%	+1.2 (.02)	−0.08 (.003)	50%
HEIDELBERG	42%	4%	+3.0%	−0.13	20%	30%	−1.0 (.05)†	0.00 (0.05)	−27%(↑)
HARP	38%	15%	+2.4%	−0.17	33%	13%	+2.1 (NS)	−0.12 (NS)	33%
Monotherapy Studies:									
NHLBI	49%	7%	—	—	32%	7%	—	—	33%
STARS (D)	46%	4%	+5.8%	−0.23	15%	38%	−1.1 (NS)	+0.03 (0.05)	69% §
MARS	41%	12%	+2.2%	−0.06	29%	23%	+1.6% (0.2)	−0.03 (0.2)	29%
CCAIT	50%	7%	+2.9%	−0.09	33%	10%	+1.7% (0.04)	−0.05 (0.01)	22%
PLAC I	38%	14%	+3.4	−0.15	26%	14%	+2.1% (0.13)	−0.09 (0.04)	13% (54%[X])
MAAS	32%	12%	3.6%	−0.13	23%	19%	1.0 (0.006)	−0.04 (0.007)	22%
REGRESS	NA	NA	NA	NA	NA	NA	NA	−0.03 (0.001)	39%§

[+]See text for the details, abbreviations, and full name of these studies. Progression and regression are variably defined, per patient, in each study. **Events are variably defined in these studies; in general, the frequency of cardiovascular events (death, MI, unstable ischemia requiring revascularization or hospitalization, or both) in control and treated groups are compared using the sometimes sketchy details and definitions provided. ‡Δ(%S) is usually reported as the average change in percent stenosis over all the lesions measured per patient. A positive (+) value represents "progression"; (−), "regression". *P-value for comparison of Δ%S or ΔMLD in control vs. treated groups. †Statistical comparison in Lifestyle uses a lesion-based method. §Studies for which the reduction in cardiovascular clinical events was statistically significant. ↑ An increase of −27% reduction means 27% increase (NS). [X]54% reduction in CHD death and non-fatal MI. [Y]62% reduction in coronary bypass surgery.

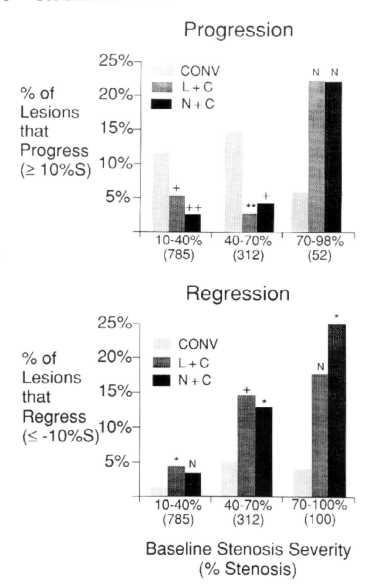

FIGURE 1. *Frequency of definite lesion progression and regression in FATS[12] expressed as the percentage of lesions that change in severity by a measured 10% stenosis or more. Lesions (n=1197) from 120 patients are subgrouped by baseline severity into mild (10% to 40%S), moderate (40% to 70%S), and severe (70% to 100%S). x^2 statistical comparisons vs. control group (CONV) frequency: *P<0.05; †P < 0.02; N=not significant. L indicates lovastatin 20–40 mg twice daily; N, niacin 1–1.5 gm four times daily; C, colestipol 10 gm three times daily with meals.*

Regression Among Lesions

As seen in Figure 1, the likelihood that a given lesion will regress was surprisingly low. In the Familial Atherosclerosis Treatment Study (FATS), only 5% of control group and 12% of treated group lesions were seen as improved by the criterion amount of ≤10% diameter stenosis (%S), which we consider definite regression with our method. Thus, very few lesions undergo natural or spontaneous regression. This number can be increased significantly by lipid-lowering therapy; nevertheless, a large majority of lesions are unaltered by therapies that can be characterized as intensive and that result in marked alterations in the lipid and lipoprotein profile. Paradoxically, these regimens are commonly associated with substantial reductions in clinical event rate. We will return to this apparent paradox below.

Retarding Progression of Coronary Artery Disease

Data supporting the idea that lipid-lowering therapy can effectively retard progression of atherosclerotic arterial obstruction are summarized in Tables 1 and 2 and Figure 1. Again, despite the diversity of these trials, the evidence for reduced disease progression with therapy is surprisingly consistent. Over one half of the control group, but only one fourth of treated patients, were judged to have worsening arterial obstruction during the study periods.

Preventing Plaque Disruption and Clinical Events

Prevention of Clinical Events

The Lipid Research Clinics-Coronary Primary Prevention Trial[22] and the Helsinki Heart Trial,[23] each with only modest LDL-C change achieved significant reductions in total cardiac events, but not mortality. Additional evidence that clinical events, cardiovascular death, confirmed infarction, and medically refractory progressive or unstable ischemia requiring bypass or angioplasty are decreased by lipid-lowering therapy is presented in Table 1. It is thus clear from these data that clinical cardiovascular events are reduced by lipid-lowering therapy. The amount of risk reduction seems incongruous with the average 1%S to 2%S regression in lesion severity and with the fact that only about 12% of all intensively treated lesions actually regress. To understand this, we must understand the series of events in the plaque that turn a stable quiescent lesion into an unstable ischemia-provoking culprit lesion.

Determinants of Plaque Disruption

Two evolving insights have altered our understanding of the precipitation of clinical coronary events. First, mild and moderate coronary lesions (<70% stenosis) may abruptly progress to severe obstruction, with resulting unstable angina, myocardial infarction, or death. In fact, a majority of clinical events occur under these circumstances.[24,25] Specifically, when the lesion precipitating a myocardial infarction has, by chance, been visualized on a recent angiogram, its pre-infarct severity averages 50% stenosis, and it will not usually possess features indicating that it will soon become occluded.[24,25] A second insight is that for the great majority of ischemic coronary events, a culprit lesion can be identified with one or more of the following morphological features at histologic examination: 1) a fissured, torn, or vented fibrous cap;[26-28] 2) mural thrombus adherent at the site of the fissure;[29] 3) bleeding into a large core lipid region;[28] and 4) severe arterial obstruction secondary to the aggregate mass of expanded plaque and thrombus. Thus, the histologic findings of a large lipid pool, and of an abundance of lipid-laden foam cells in a thinned fibrous cap and in the shoulder region of the atheroma each predispose to plaque fissuring and to subsequent plaque disruption, hemorrhage, and coronary events. Based on experimental studies, we propose that this small subpopulation of such fatty lesions accounts for most of the 12% frequency of lesion regression with therapy.

Prevention of Plaque Disruption

Reduction of plasma LDL might be expected to reduce the likelihood of fissuring because of the experimentally demonstrated favorable effects of LDL reduction on the above predictors.[4] A consequence of such protection against fissuring would be a decline in the frequency of abrupt progression to clinical events among patients in whom LDL has been therapeutically reduced. Indeed, this has been the case. Analysis of the 13 coronary events among the 146 FATS[12] patients reveals that all were associated with a culprit coronary lesion in the distribution of worsening ischemia that had progressed substantially in severity from the baseline stenosis measurement to that at the time of the event. Furthermore, the progression of mild and moderately narrowed lesions to clinical events was virtually abolished by intensive lipid-lowering therapy (Figure 2). Eight of nine clinical events among the conventionally treated patients arose from lesions <65% stenosis at baseline; the eight associated episodes of plaque disruption occurred among a pool of 414 mild or moderate lesions. Only 1 of 683 such lesions progressed to an event in the 2 groups of patients who were treated intensively ($P < 0.005$, per patient or per lesion). Thus, reduction in clinical events is strongly linked with stabilization of mild and moderate coronary lesions.

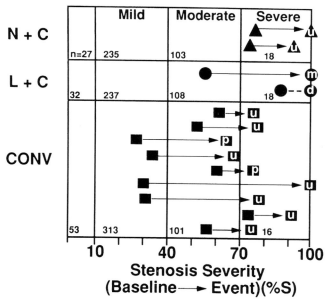

FIGURE 2. *Lesion changes associated with the 13 coronary events as measured from 1316 lesions in FATS patients. Among lesions exposed to intensive lipid-lowering therapy, only 1 of 638 mild or moderate lesions at baseline among 74 such patients progressed to a clinical event, and 8 of 414 such lesions among 46 conventionally treated patients did so (P<0.005). N indicates niacin; C, colestipol; L, lovastatin; CONV, conventional therapy; U, unstable angina event; M, myocardial infarction; D, death; P, progressive angina; %S, percent diameter stenosis. The number in each panel represents the number of lesions at risk at baseline in each subgroup.*

Summary

Lipid-lowering therapy, as assessed by angiography, appears to benefit the arterial disease process. For example, in FATS, the frequency of definite ($\geq$10%S) progression, per lesion at risk, was reduced by 75% among mild and moderate lesions, which form the great preponderance of the lesion population. Furthermore, among patients treated intensively, regression frequency is doubled in mild and moderate lesion subgroups, and quadrupled in the severe lesion subgroup. Clinical events were reduced by 73% in FATS; this was entirely due to a reduction in the likelihood that a mildly or moderately diseased arterial segment would undergo abrupt and substantial progression to a severe lesion at the time of the clinical event. It has been shown that the process of plaque fissuring leading to plaque disruption and thrombosis and to clinical coronary events is predicted by the size of the core lipid pool, and the abundance of lipid-laden macrophages in the fibrous cap of the atheroma. Experimentally, lipid-lowering therapy virtually abolishes lipid-laden intimal macrophages and more slowly depletes core cholesteryl ester deposits. Thus, the composite of data presented here supports the idea that lipid-lowering therapy selectively depletes (regresses) that relatively small subgroup of the lesion population containing a large lipid core and abundant intimal macrophages. By doing so, the lipid-rich lesions, which are most vulnerable to fissuring, are stabilized and the clinical event risk is accordingly decreased.

Acknowledgments

We are grateful for the efforts of Robert Kelly in preparing this manuscript.

References

1. Wissler RW, Vesselinovitch D. Can atherosclerotic plaques regress? Anatomic and biochemical evidence from non-human animal models. *Am J Cardiol* 1990;65:33–40.
2. Armstrong ML, Megan MB. Lipid depletion in atheromatous coronary arteries in rhesus monkeys after regression diets. *Circ Res* 1972;30:675–680.
3. Clarkson TB, Bond MG, Bullock BC, Marzetta CA: A study of atherosclerosis regression in Macaca mulatta. IV. Changes in coronary arteries from animals with atherosclerosis induced for 19 months and then regressed for 24 or 48 months at plasma cholesterol concentrations of 300 or 200 mg/dl. *Exp Mol Pathol* 1981;34:345–368.

4. Small DM, Bond MG, Waugh D, et al. Physiochemical and histological changes in the arterial wall of non-human primates during progression and regression of atherosclerosis. *J Clin Invest* 1984;73;1590–1605.
5. Armstrong MC, Megan MG. Arterial fibrous protein in cynomolygous monkeys after atherogenic and regression diets. *Circ Res* 1975;36:256–261.
6. Glagov S, Weisenberg E, Zarins CK, et al. Compensatory enlargement of human atherosclerotic coronary arteries. *N Engl J Med* 1987;316:1371–1375.
7. Harrison DG, Armstrong ML, Freeman PC, et al. Restoration of endothelium-dependent relaxation by dictory treatment of atherosclerosis. *J Clin Invest* 1987;80:808–811.
8. Brensike JF, Levy RI, Kelsey SF, et al. Effects of therapy with cholestyramine on progression of coronary arteriosclerosis: Results of the NHLBI Type II Coronary Intervention Study. *Circulation* 1984;69: 313–324.
9. Blankenhorn DH, Nessim SA, Johnson RL, et al. Beneficial effects of colestipol niacin therapy on coronary atherosclerosis and coronary venous bypass grafts. *JAMA* 1987;257:3233–3240.
10. Buchwald H, Varco RL, Matts JP, et al. Effect of partial ileal bypass on mortality and morbidity from coronary heart disease in patients with hypercholesterolemia. Report of the Program on Surgical Control of the Hyperlipidermias (POSCH). *N Engl J Med* 1990;323:946–945.
11. Ornish D, et al. Can lifestyle changes reverse coronary heart disease? *Lancet* 1990;336:129–133.
12. Brown BG, Albers JJ, Fisher LD, et al. Regression of coronary artery disease as a result of intensive lipid-lowering therapy in men with high levels of apolipoprotein B. *N Engl J Med* 1990;323:1289–1298.
13. Cashin-Hemphill L, Mack WJ, Pogoda MJ, et al. Beneficial effects of colestipol-niacin on coronary atherosclerosis. *JAMA* 1990;264:3013–3017.
14. Kane JP, Malloy MJ, Ports TA, et al. Regression of coronary atherosclerosis during treatment of familial hypercholesterolemia with combined drug regimens. *JAMA* 1990;264:3007.
15. Watts GF, Lewis B, Brunt JNH, et al. Effects on coronary artery disease of lipid-lowering diet, or diet plus cholestyramine in the St. Thomas' Atherosclerosis Regression Study (STARS). *Lancet* 1992;339: 563–569.
16. Haskell WL, Alderman E, Fain JM, et al. Effects of intensive multiple risk factor reduction on coronary atherosclerosis and clinical cardiac events in men and women with coronary atherosclerosis: The Stanford Coronary Risk Intervention Project (SCRIP). *Circulation* 1994;89:975–990.
17. Schuler G, Hambrecht R, Schlierf G, et al. Regular physical exercise and low fat diet: Effects on progression of coronary artery disease. *Circulation* 1992;86:1–11.
18. Blankenhorn DH, Azen SP, Kramsch DM, et al. Coronary angiographic changes with lovastatin therapy: The Monitored Atherosclerosis Regression Study (MARS). *Ann Intern Med* 1993;119:967–976.
19. Waters D, Higginson L, Gladstone P, et al. Effects of monotherapy with an HMG-CoA reductace inhibitor on the progression of coronary atherosclerosis as assessed by serial quantitative arteriography: The Canadian Coronary Atherosclerosis Intervention Trial. *Circulation* 1994;89:959–968.

20. Pitt B, Mancini GBJ, Ellis SG, et al. Pravastatin Limitation of Atherosclerosis in the Coronary Arteries (PLAC I). *J Am Coll Cardiol* 1994;(suppl):131A. Abstract.
21. The MAAS Investigators. Effect of simvastatin on coronary atheroma: The Multicentre Anti-Atheroma Study (MAAS). *Lancet* 1994;344:633–638.
22. The Lipid Research Clinics Program. The lipid research clinics coronary primary prevention trial results: I. Reduction in incidence of coronary heart disease. *JAMA* 1984;251:351–364.
23. Manninen V, Elo MO, Frick MH, et al. Lipid alterations and decline in the incidence of coronary heart disease in the Helsinki Heart Study. *JAMA* 1988;260:641–651.
24. Ambrose JA, Tannenbaum MA, Alexopoulos D, et al. Angiographic progression of coronary artery disease and the development of myocardial infarction. *J Am Coll Cardiol* 1988;12:56–62.
25. Brown BG, Gallery CA, Badger RS, et al. Incomplete lysis of thrombus in the moderate underlying atherosclerotic lesion during intracoronary infusion of streptokinase for acute myocardial infarction: Quantitative angiographic observations. *Circulation* 1986;73:653–661.
26. Constantinides P. Plaque fissures in human coronary thrombosis. *J Athero Res* 1966;61:1–17.
27. Lendon CL, Davies MJ, Born GVR, et al. Atherosclerotic plaque caps are locally weakened when macrophage density is increased. *Atherosclerosis* 1991;87:87–90.
28. Richardson PD, Davies Mj, Born GVR. Influence of plaque configuration and stress distribution on fissuring of coronary atherosclerotic plaques. *Lancet* 1989;iii:941–944.
29. Davies MJ, Richardson PD, Woolf N, et al. Risk of thrombosis in human atherosclerosis plaques: Role of extracellular lipid, macrophage, and smooth muscle cell content. *Br Heart J* 1993;69:377–381.
30. Brown BG, Zhao X-Q, Sacco DE, et al. Lipid lowering and plaque regression. New insights into prevention of plaque disruption and clinical events in coronary disease. *Circulation* 1993;87:1781–1791.

Panel Discussion IV

Atherosclerotic Disease Progression and Regression

Dr. Valentin Fuster: There are now a number of trials published and others that are going to be published with different lipid-lowering agents. And it seems to me that you can decrease by 30% the LDL level with two different agents, but the impact is different. The question I'm asking to Dr. Brown is whether you suggest that in terms of benefit, it is not only the cholesterol-lowering or -modifying effects of these agents, it may be something else like an antithrombotic effect or a prothrombotic effect that may influence the results of one agent to the other.

Dr. B. Greg Brown: My guess is that the variation among studies is an artifact of relatively small sample size. And so what we are seeing here is a collection of results, some of which appear a little lower and some that appear a little higher, but finally if done in larger numbers would show that the best predictor is LDL lowering. And you can take a few examples, the PLAC-I Study had about a 55% reduction in clinical events over the course of 3 years. The ACAP study, which was I think a 4-year study, had about a 65% [reduction]. The HARP study, had a modest 32% benefit. And the MARS and CCAIT had about a 25% reduction in clinical event rate. So my guess is that they are all centering around what would be predicted with a 30% LDL lowering; while the lipid-lowering drugs or STATINS were different in various studies, the beneficial results did not significantly differ. A final point is that these studies are not all the same length, and it often takes 1 to 2 years before the control group and the treated group begin to diverge. So, the longer studies would be expected to show a greater benefit. In fact, that has been the case. So I think we have to be very skeptical about allegations of differences between the different drugs.

Dr. Fuster: Let's think for a moment. In the PLAC-I and the PLAC-II studies there was a very impressive benefit compared with the MARS study. The lipid-lowering agents or statins were different, but the benefit of follow-up and the reduction or the alteration

483

in LDL cholesterol and HDL cholesterol were similar. And I'm asking myself, the question is, are the different agents doing something else?

Dr. Brown: I think it's a legitimate question and my guess [is] it's going to come out, maybe not to be real difference.

Discussant A from the Audience: I think one thing that is not paid attention to in these studies is that the lipid disorders that you are treating are different. VLDL problems versus LDL problems versus combined LDL and VLDL problems. The Four S Study, the best study to date, shows certainly more striking findings in patients with pure LDL elevation. You have to match the drug to the lipid disorder. I think it's very important to know who you're treating. A familial hypercholesterolemia, obviously the statin is going to do well. In other situations, such as in VLDL, probably niacin is going to do better. You need to aim the treatment to the disease that you are treating metabolically.

Dr. James H. Chesebro: I agree it would not be smart trying to also raise HDL. Don't you have the feeling that it's also quite important to target that aspect of it, as well as lowering the LDL, which is the most emphasized?

Dr. Brown: Surely in many of these trials the multivariate analysis has shown HDL modification to be predictive of benefit in addition to LDL; in FATS, a 20% LDL lowering was as effective as a 20% increase in HDL. We are currently just starting a trial, a 2 1/2-year trial, in patients whose principal abnormality is low HDL, 35 or less, with normal levels of LDL and with coronary heart disease. The intervention there is niacin and symvastatin, so we are treating both sides of the ratio and perhaps won't know which had the greatest effect in that study. I think that the low HDL group is understudied and needs to be treated more aggressively.

Discussant B from the Audience: I would like to hear comments on whether there is a differential effect of lipid lowering with reference to the size of the lesion.

Dr. Brown: At the moment, there is a bit of confusion there because in the FATS study we showed that the most severe lesions showed regression while, for instance, in the CCAIT Trial it was shown that the less severe lesions showed regression. So, at this moment I really don't know where we stand. It seems to me that not only the severity of the lesion plays a role, but apparently, the quantity or characteristics are also important.

Chapter 27

A New View of Restenosis

Edward R. O'Brien, MD
and Stephen M. Schwartz, MD, PhD

Introduction

Any search through the tables of contents of cardiology journals will show numerous articles dealing with the problem of restenosis. These articles, especially those dealing with experimental studies, equate intimal hyperplasia with restenosis. Put another way, most investigators believe that neointimal formation is the principal cause of lumen narrowing in atherosclerosis and restenosis,[1-4] an equation that often leads to use of the terms restenosis and intimal hyperplasia synonymously. The result is, that of numerous experimental studies of restenosis, all but a few measure intimal mass, and only a very few take the time to measure changes in lumen size. Numerous studies even report successful therapies for restenosis with no data indicating whether the therapy successfully maintained the dilation produced by the angioplasty catheter.

To a considerable extent, this view is derived from Ross' *response-to-injury hypothesis,* an explanation for the origins of atherosclerosis, and more recently from various experimental models of arterial injury.[1,5-10] According to this hypothesis, injury to the vessel wall results in a reparative response that originates in the media and primarily involves smooth muscle cell proliferation. A similar result occurs in animal models, in which a normal or artificially altered artery wall is traumatized, resulting in cellular proliferation and formation of a new lesion. Accordingly, a tremendous amount of effort has been focused on antiproliferative therapies directed against smooth muscle cell replication. To date, these an-

From: Fuster V, (ed.) *Syndromes of Atherosclerosis: Correlations of Clinical Imaging and Pathology.* Armonk, NY: Futura Publishing Company, Inc.: © 1996.

tiproliferative therapies have not been proven to be of clinical benefit, which may suggest that our current understanding of the biology of restenosis is misleading.[11–16] In this chapter, we attempt to provide a new model based on a combination of clinical data in humans as well as new insights from animal models.

What Happens with the Initial Interventional Procedure?

Clinicians and investigators who are not cardiologists, as well as lay people often assume that angioplasty debulks the atherosclerotic lesion. Of course, this view is incorrect. A variety of data based on histologic and imaging studies suggest that plaque compression, disruption with fracture and dissection of the intima and media, and stretching of the more normal portions of the media are all involved.[17–24]

With recent advances in intravascular ultrasound (IVUS), it is now possible to study the consequences of balloon dilatation of the arterial wall. For example, Losordo et al[25] used IVUS immediately before and after angioplasty in 40 patients who underwent iliac artery balloon dilatation to study changes in plaque and vessel lumen during the intervention.[25] Over 70% of the increase in luminal area immediately postangioplasty was contained within the plaque fracture—the so-called neolumen. Plaque cross-sectional area actually decreased by approximately one third because of compression, whereas total artery cross-sectional area stretched only minimally (approximately 5%) with the dilatation. It should be noted that measurements were made immediately postdilatation; therefore, the relative contribution of plaque fracture, compression, and stretch over a longer period remains unknown.

Perhaps, however, the simplest point to make about the initial procedure in humans is that the catheter dilates an already stenotic vessel. The object of the procedure is to maintain that dilatation. In contrast, as we will discuss below, the object of animal studies is to create a stenotic vessel.

The Biology of Restenosis

Understanding the Intima

It is essential to realize that the formation of an intima is part of the normal ontogeny of the artery wall (eg, spontaneous closure of the ductus arteriosus, and formation of diffuse intimal hyperplasia).[26–28] A simple intima consisting of a few layers of smooth muscle cells forms very early in postnatal human coronary arteries.[28–29] How the intima develops as an early structure is somewhat speculative, yet, it is surprising how old (eg, 1913) and lengthy this literature is.[27] Deficiencies in the integrity of the internal elastic lamina and a family history of coronary artery disease are two of the variables that are thought to be associated with early intimal thickening. Understanding how these lesions develop may help clarify current concepts of the pathogenesis of adult atherosclerosis. For example, much attention is focused on describing lipids in the established plaque, however, if a preformed intima is a requirement for lipids to enter the vessel wall and wreak havoc, it is illogical to invoke lipids as an initiating factor when at best they may only be contributing to an ongoing process.[1]

The Uniqueness of the Intima and the Role of Replication

Moss[30] and Benditt[31] were the first of several investigators to culture human intimal cells and find that plaque smooth muscle cells have a shortened life span relative to normal medial cells. Therefore, since most of the evidence for smooth muscle replication in vivo is derived from in vitro studies, it is only fair to point out that normal plaque is hypoproliferative, not hyperproliferative. Consistent with this point of view, studies of replication of human atherosclerotic plaque-derived smooth muscle cells have consistently shown very low levels, not significantly higher than those in the normal wall.[32–34] In contrast, morphometric studies suggest that lesion growth may be very rapid during the first few months of life.[28] This early intimal thickening may be especially important because studies of expression of an X-chromosome-linked gene suggest that atherosclerotic lesions in human females express only one or the other allele.[35] Because X-linked genes are randomly inactivated, these observations imply that monoclonal smooth muscle replication is an important part of lesion formation and may occur at an early stage before any sort of diffuse injury process has elicited replication of random cells within the vessel wall. Whether these monoclonal cells differ in other ways from normal smooth muscle cells is unclear, but may be of importance to animal models of arterial injury.

Pharmacology of Neointimal Formation: The Importance of Growth Factors

Current theories suggest that growth factors that are derived from autocrine, paracrine, or endocrine systems have an important influence on neointimal formation.[36] The rat carotid artery balloon injury model is the most extensively studied animal model of the pharmacology of neointimal formation. When this vessel undergoes balloon angioplasty, a response characterized by three waves of change and formation of a neointima result. Figure 1 depicts the three waves. The first wave is replication in the injured media. This begins within 24 hours and can last for a few days. At the end of that time, perhaps beginning on the second day, smooth muscle cells cross the internal elastic lamina and form the first intima, a neointima. We call this the second wave. We do not know how long intimal migration continues. Finally, once smooth muscle cells have migrated into the intima, they continue to divide for some time. It is these several generations of neointimal replication, a third wave, that account for the bulk of neointimal mass. Continued neointimal proliferation (fourth wave or restimulation) resulting from the influence of such mitogens as angiotensin II (AII) or transforming growth factor-β (TGF-β), may be important to the chronic accumulation of neointimal mass.[37] Most of the experimental data on molecules controlling the three waves has focused on three agonists: fibroblast growth factor (FGF), AII, and platelet-derived growth factor (PDGF).

The role of FGF is well established. Reidy and colleagues[38] have shown that FGF can stimulate the first and second waves. Antibodies to FGF can largely abolish first and second waves. Interestingly, FGF may not be able to stimulate the vessel wall, even when given via the adventitia, unless the vessel is first injured. FGF is a weak mitogen when infused in the third wave.

Unlike FGF, AII can stimulate DNA synthesis in the media of uninjured vessels.[37] We have not tried to use AII to stimulate first wave or second wave; however, Dup 753, an AII receptor-blocking agent, blocks both first wave and second wave. Converting enzyme inhibitors (CEI) appear to block migration.[39] AII does restimulate cell replication in the third wave, but there are no data on the ability of Dup 753 or CEI to block normal third-wave replication. AII and other low-molecular weight vasoactive factors may be particularly important because of the frequent use of antihypertensive and afterload-reducing drugs in cardiac patients undergoing angioplasty.

A great deal of effort has focused on AII since the reports that neointimal formation is inhibited by CEI.[39-42] Excitement about

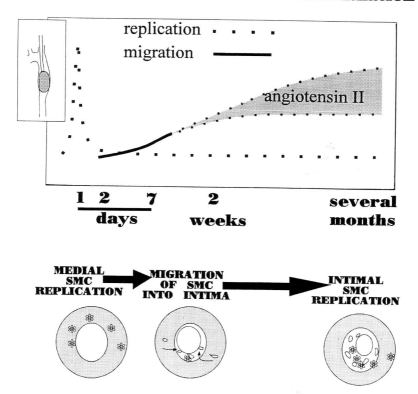

FIGURE 1. *Balloon injury to the rat carotid artery produces medial smooth muscle cell (SMC) proliferation (first wave). This is followed by migration of smooth muscle cells across the internal elastic lamina (second wave), and formation of a neointima. Intimal smooth muscle cell replication lasts a few weeks (third wave); however, in the presence of angiotensin II, the intima remains hyperproliferative (fourth wave or restimulation).*

AII, however, has diminished because of the apparent failure of clinical trials of CEI to block restenosis in humans.[16] CEI also failed to inhibit lesion formation in swine.[43] Moreover, several inconsistencies in the experimental data have begun to appear. For example, blocking studies with Dup 753 are problematic, because it is not clear that at the concentrations used, that this antagonist is limited to AT1 receptors, and doses effective against the neointima may be much higher than antihypertensive doses[41,42,44] (Grove and Speth, unpublished data). Similarly, CEI studies should be considered with caution, because the high doses used may mean that this peptidase inhibitor acted on other substrates.[39–42,45–46] Of particular interest, angiotensin-converting enzyme (ACE) is responsible for processing and activating kinins. The binding affinity (K_m/K_{cat}) of ACE for bradykinin is 10 times higher than for AII[46]. The recent observation that the inhibitory effects of CEI can be ablated by a bradykinin antagonist outlines the importance of bradykinin to the response to injury.[42] Finally, human arteries have a second enzyme able to activate angiotensin. This enzyme, chymase, is not inhibited by ACE inhibitors.[47]

Despite all the attention focused on PDGF, there is little evidence that this molecule is mitogenic in vivo—at least in the rat model. We know, for example, that PDGF has very little mitogenic effect in the first wave, but does appear to increase the numbers of cells that cross the internal elastic lamina.[1,48] Other molecules, including FGF, also stimulate migration[49] and the relative contributions of different molecules remain to be explored. PDGF has no detectable effect on replication in the third wave, but overexpression of PDGF-A chain is prominent in areas of the neointima that show elevated replication.[50] In contrast, PDGF is a consistent mitogen for smooth muscle in vitro, but is only a weak mitogen in vivo.[48] Finally, PDGF transfected in vivo as an oncogene appears to be mitogenic in swine.[51] This result, however, is confusing because transfected PDGF is expressed inside the cell as is its viral homologue v-*sis*, a simian sarcoma virus. The relevance of a transforming gene to a mechanism based on release of a protein from platelets is not necessarily clear. These data cast some doubt on the validity of in vitro assays of smooth muscle growth control.

Luminal Narrowing vs. Wall Thickening

The response-to-injury hypothesis of Ross is based on assumptions that formation of a neointimal mass implies that the mass intrudes into the lumen rather than increases wall thickness. It is intriguing to note that a similar hypothesis, ie, that vascular injury results in an increase in vascular mass that restricts the lumen in the presence of vasoconstrictors, is also a fundamental part of contemporary studies of the hypertensive microvasculature.[52–54]

We know that balloon injury to a rat does cause a neointima to form and does narrow the vessel, but the experimental data supporting the assumption that intimal mass obstructs the lumen of large vessels is confusing. Glagov,[55] for example, noted that human vessels can undergo massive accumulations of atherosclerotic plaque without narrowing the lumen. Instead, the wall compensates for the lesion by remodeling and dilating to permit a normal level of blood flow. Compensatory structural change is a normal response that allows the vessel to maintain normal levels of blood flow and wall stress, and can be seen in small muscular arteries as well as in large elastic arteries.[56–57] However, when a lesion reaches a critical mass (eg, about 40% of the internal elastic lamina area), the ability to compensate is lost, and further increases in lesion mass lead to decreases in lumen diameter. Therefore, because animal models generally involve vessels with an initially normal lumen, the processes involved in experimental narrowing may be very different from those that lead to restenosis in human atherosclerosis when lumen encroachment is usually >60% to begin with.

Proliferation In Human Restenotic Coronary Artery Lesions: Towards A General Understanding of the Problem

At this point, the source of confusion about restenosis should be obvious. The most obvious question is whether the sequence of events, the three waves, seen in animal models occurs postangioplasty in the human atherosclerotic vessel.

We have detailed knowledge of animal models in different species that proceed through a stereotypic set of proliferative and migration events in a known time course.[5–10] Unfortunately, little is known about the proliferative profile of human restenotic coronary artery lesions. To begin with, it is important to note that most studies that have described proliferation in human restenotic coronary arteries have not used an objective measurement of replication. For example, Nobuyoshi et al. examined the histologic findings in 39 dilated lesions from 20 patients who had undergone ante-mortem coronary angioplasty. The extent of intimal proliferation, defined by the presence of stellate-shaped cells of the so-called synthetic smooth muscle cell phenotype, was significantly greater in lesions with evidence of medial or adventitial tears compared with those without tears or tears limited to the intima (Nobuyoshi et al, unpublished data). Therefore, on the basis of these histologic findings, it was assumed that cells with this morphology had recently proliferated. Unfortunately, these proliferative-like stellate cells are also commonly seen in primary atherosclerotic coronary artery lesions that have never been exposed to an interventional device.[58–59] Moreover, very similar cells can be seen even in the subendothelium of nonatherosclerotic intima.[60–61]

Thus, stellate cells appear to be a normal component of the vessel wall. Their apparent increase in number may represent either a phenotypic switch of preexisting cells or a change in the sampling of cells already in the wall as a result of the redistribution of cell types secondary to the dilatation. It is conceivable that primary coronary atherectomy specimens may include more of the superficial luminal layer—which typically is the fibrous cap. With subsequent restenotic biopsies, deeper layers of the plaque may be removed. One must therefore be careful not to assume that differences in histology between primary and restenotic coronary atherectomy specimens, which may have been long-standing and preceded the initial procedure, are necessarily due to a difference in vessel wall biology that occurred with the so-called restenotic process. These differences may simply represent the results of sampling different arterial layers.

Recently, we have used immunocytochemical labeling for the proliferating cell nuclear antigen (PCNA) to determine the proliferative profile of 100 restenotic coronary atherectomy specimens.[62] PCNA is regulated at both the pre- and posttranscriptional levels, and the protein is expressed during S-phase (as well as G1 and G2) of the cell cycle.[63] To our surprise, the vast majority of the restenotic specimens (74%) had no evidence of PCNA labeling. The majority of the remaining specimens had only a modest number of PCNA-positive cells per slide (typically <50 cells per slide). Based on the mean number of nuclei per slide, the vast majority of these specimens had $\leq$1% of all cells labeled PCNA-positive. PCNA labeling was detected over a wide time interval after the initial procedure (eg, 1 day to 390 days), with no obvious proliferative peak. There was no difference in the proliferative profile of restenotic specimens collected in the first 3 months, 4 to 6 months, 7 to 9 months, or more than 9 months after the initial interventional procedure (Spearman rank correlation coefficient = 0.081, P = 0.43). Furthermore, only 12 of 30 specimens obtained within 60 days of the initial coronary interventional procedure had one or more PCNA-positive nucleus per slide (including 9 specimens collected within 6 days of the initial procedure, only 3 of which had immunolabeling of 1, 7, and 20 cells per slide, respectively). In support of these findings, a recent preliminary study using in vitro bromodeoxyuridine labeling also found low levels of proliferation in restenotic atherectomy specimens.[64]

Conversely, Pickering et al[65] have found different proliferation profiles in restenotic atherectomy tissue. These investigators found that all restenotic coronary and peripheral arterial specimens had surprisingly high percentages of cells that were considered PCNA-positive as measured by either immunocytochemistry (15.2% ± 13.6%), or in situ hybridization (20.6% ± 18.2%). However, only 4 of the 19 restenotic atherectomy specimens reported by Pickering and colleagues were obtained from coronary artery lesions and none were obtained within 1 month of the initial interventional procedure (eg, 1.6, 5.2, 6.1, and 7.9 months). (In unpublished studies, we too have found PCNA labeling to be higher and more frequent in peripheral atherectomy specimens.) Moreover, the labeling indices reported by Pickering et al[66] seem exceptionally high, (eg, as high as 59% of cells being PCNA-positive), and resemble those of malignant neoplasms. Furthermore, unlike the present study that used intestinal crypt epithelium, the Pickering study lacked a reference tissue with a known replication rate, thereby making the subjective interpretation of PCNA positivity difficult. Nonetheless, it is unlikely that mean PCNA labeling indices of 15% to 20% are physically possible in atherosclerotic coronary arteries where small changes in vessel wall mass can result in dramatic changes in residual luminal diameter.

Certainly, PCNA immunolabeling requires careful interpretation. While we found low levels of replication in restenotic coronary atherectomy tissue, Gordon et al[67], using the same methodology, found PCNA immunolabeling of rapidly stenosing human arteriovenous hemodialysis arteriovenous fistulas to be high. This suggests that PCNA immunolabeling is capable of adequately detecting proliferation when it is present. Finally, one criticism of anti-PCNA labeling relative to other proliferative measurements is that it is likely to be oversensitive in detecting proliferative cells because PCNA is expressed through a broader period of cell-cycle traverse.[34] Therefore, if anti-PCNA antibodies are overlabeling proliferating cells, the degree of proliferation in these atherectomy specimens may actually be lower than the already minimal levels that we have measured.

Clinical data might give us an idea of when proliferation should occur. With most of our knowledge from animal models based on the first 2 weeks or perhaps 4 weeks after injury, it is likely that these models are not mimicking the more prolonged biological processes that might be causing clinical renarrowing. We do not know that this early proliferative response is even needed for restenosis. For example, although proliferation is detected very early after experimental arterial injury, it is curious to note the absence of a more widespread reaction to injury in any or every segment of human coronary arteries that a guide catheter, angioplasty balloon, or other interventional device have traversed. While there are reports of iatrogenic lesions that arise after an initial manipulation of an artery, Nguyen et al[68] as well as others suggest that this is generally not the case.[69-70]. Follow-up coronary angiography of 140 lesions dilated 6 to 30 months prior to restudy found a 31% restenosis rate (>50% loss of initial gain). New lesions (defined by the emergence of a new >20% lesion more than 2 cm from the angioplasty site at a previously normal arterial segment), and progression of an existing lesion (defined by a further decrease of >20% in luminal diameter in a previously diseased segment that was not dilated) were studied in 94 patients. New or progressive lesions occurred in 35% of patients, with a similar frequency in arteries that did or did not undergo angioplasty, (10% vs. 15%, P=NS), or in patients that did or did not succumb to restenosis (29% vs. 40%, P=NS). Therefore, given the robust reaction to balloon dilatation in virgin animal arteries, one must question the relevance of such models to clinical restenosis.[5]

What is Restenosis?

If smooth muscle cell proliferation is not the dominant biological event in restenosis, what is? First, one cannot discount the role of proliferation and must recognize that low levels of proliferation, especially of cells other than smooth muscle cells, may have profound effects on plaque mass. Only a very small number of doublings would be required to replace the plaque mass removed during angioplasty or even atherectomy. Moreover, that replication might be in the most superficial part of the lesion. We need to be concerned that the atherectomy catheter used to biopsy lesions may abrade the surface, wiping off superficial replicating cells. We need also be aware that a replicative event could be extremely transient. While our study included numerous atherectomies from the first few days after a primary procedure, patients coming for repeat angioplasty (atherectomy) this soon may not be the patients undergoing replication.

Second, the smooth muscle cell may not be the only replicative cell in restenosis. This is particularly true of the endothelial cells that are involved in the formation of the plaque's vasa vasorum. We have recently found vasa vasorum to be more common in restenotic compared to primary specimens. Although proliferation is infrequent in the plaque, when present it is strongly related to the presence of these microvessels. Furthermore, focal areas of proliferation have surprisingly high percentages of proliferating endothelial cells (eg, approximately 10% to 15% of all endothelial cells being PCNA immuno-positive).[62] Therefore, understanding plaque angiogenesis might help clarify how lesions progress.

Third, there is renewed interest in intramural coagulation with thrombin being a potential critical mitogen and vasoconstrictor involved in remodeling events.[71–72] Knowledge that advanced atherosclerotic plaques show evidence of repeated thrombotic/coagulative events is an old observation in the study of atherosclerosis.[73] Hatton and colleagues showed that thrombin activity remains elevated for weeks after injury in balloon-injured animal vessels; in contrast, the platelet response is over in 1 to 2 days.[74–75] Indirect evidence implies that thrombin is functioning in vivo after balloon injury. We showed that the pattern of gene expression for the PDGF-receptors and PDGF-A chain after balloon injury in vivo closely follows the pattern seen when cultured smooth muscle cells are treated with thrombin[76]. Other growth factors and vasoactive molecules do not reproduce this pattern. Activation by thrombin might also explain the synthesis of PDGF-B chain by endothelial cells and by macrophage within advanced atherosclerotic plaques.[77–78] A thrombin pathway is of special interest because many other pathways may be activated via proteolytic activity, and thrombin may activate or deactivate other molecules implicated in thrombin's response to injury, including plasmin and bradykinin.[42,79] Moreover, there is evidence that nonproteolytic domains of thrombin have their own activities, and the protease itself may have different substrate specificities depending on occupation of the exosite, binding to thrombomodulin, or perhaps binding to as yet undefined protease nexins within the vessel wall.[80–81]

Fourth, as suggested above, restenosis may not be stenotic at all. When the usual animal model undergoes angioplasty, the result is an increase in wall mass and a loss of lumen—at least partly due to the increase in intimal mass. We can call this stenosis (Figure 2). However, if an angioplastied vessel simply heals, even with an intima formation, the result would be a return to the original narrowed lumen. We can call this restenosis (Figure 2).

Figure 2 compares the simple animal model of response to balloon injury with the events in human angioplasty. The distinction between stenosis (loss of lumen due to new mass) and restenosis (loss of the added lumen gained during angioplasty) is clear. Our ability to determine the extent of true stenosis in humans has been enhanced by the development of IVUS. Unlike angiography, IVUS can image the full cross-sectional thickness of the vessel wall. In addition, it can be performed serially, before and after an interventional procedure in vivo, to determine the mechanisms by which the intervention enlarged the vessel lumen. Recent preliminary information on vessel wall dimensions with IVUS before and after balloon dilatation, as well as crude measurements of vessel wall

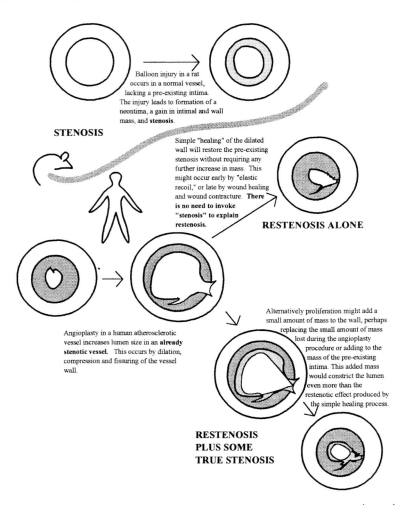

FIGURE 2. *Comparison of pathways leading to stenosis in animal models or restenosis after angioplasty in human atherosclerotic lesions.*

composition, are intriguing. Mintz et al[82] report that increases in plaque area with restenosis are actually small (eg, 5% to 7%).[82] The clinical significance of this small increase in plaque mass in an artery that is already severely diseased is unknown. The authors speculate that intimal hyperplasia may not be a dominant factor in the restenotic lesion, and that instead, chronic recoil may account for most of the progressive luminal narrowing. The idea of chronic recoil is startlingly similar to the observations of normal blood vessels responding to decreases in blood flow described as remodeling by Langille et al[56] and by Folkow et al.[57] Interestingly, Heagerty and coworkers[83] have shown that microvascular remodeling, as seen in hypertension, can occur by remodeling without changes in cell number. Furthermore, given the modest and relatively infrequent proliferation that we have detected by PCNA immunolabeling in restenotic coronary atherectomy specimens, this imaging data can be taken as complementary evidence that proliferation is only one of several important events in the biology of restenosis.

Fifth, restenosis could also be the result of early recoil in the first few hours after angioplasty, followed by small additional changes due to contraction or hyperplasia over a period of several weeks. Some interesting data is emerging on the timing of luminal loss. Kuntz et al[84] have used a continuous regression model to examine the results of quantitative follow-up coronary angiographic studies on patients who have undergone either angioplasty, directional atherectomy, or stenting. Luminal diameter was measured immediately before and after coronary intervention in 524 consecutive lesions. Three- to 6-month follow-up angiography was obtained in 91% of patients. Restenosis was found to depend solely on the residual stenosis immediately after the procedure, regardless of the device employed. Moreover, the loss index (late loss divided by acute gain), a measurement that corrects for differences in acute gain, was not significantly different for all three types of intervention. This result is surprising, as one would expect from animal models that atherectomy, being more invasive, and stenting, being more intrusive, would result in more intimal hyperplasia. Therefore, what this study highlights is the importance of achieving the largest acute luminal gain possible—the so-called "bigger is better hypothesis."[85]

Early and Late Recoil

The mechanisms that result in loss of acute gain are often lumped together into the term recoil. Recoil may be something as simple as the elastic properties of the artery resulting in return of the artery to its preprocedural dimensions. Alternatively, it may refer to more complex events, such as active vasospasm or wound contraction.

Vasospasm after angioplasty may be caused by acute and dramatic increases in vessel wall blood flow immediately postintervention, and high tissue levels of vasoconstrictive substances.[86–87] Earlier reports suggest that balloon angioplasty routinely caused severe smooth muscle cell injury, thereby disabling the artery into a state of paralysis.[88–91] Studies by Fischell et al[92] using a perfused whole-vessel ex vivo model indicate that severe arterial stretching is required before smooth muscle vasoconstriction is impaired. On the basis of geometric models, medial stretching of critically stenosed human coronary arteries in vivo is probably only modest (eg, 15% to 40%) and not sufficient to cause severe smooth muscle injury and hence arterial paralysis. In fact, the same authors used quantitative coronary arteriography and documented the routine occurrence of vasospasm at, and distal to, the site of dilatation in 10 patients post-coronary angioplasty.[93] Furthermore, Nobuyoshi et al[94] performed angiography on 185 patients 24-hours postballoon angioplasty, and found restenosis (>50% loss of gain in absolute diameter) already present in 14% of patients. Undoubtedly, this form of restenosis was caused by mechanical recoil, spasm, or possibly even platelet deposition and organized mural thrombus accumulation. However, given that recoil can be documented with intravascular ultrasound immediately on balloon deflation of combined balloon ultrasound imaging catheters, it is likely that recoil is an instantaneous event.[95] Therefore, beyond acute recoil, restenosis appears to be a more drawn-out process occurring over the next 1 to 6 months (Figure 3).[94,96]

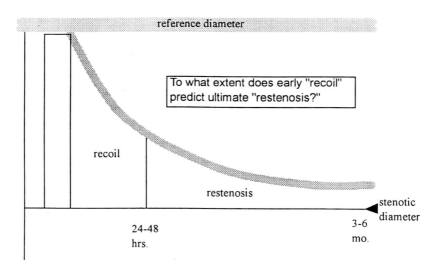

FIGURE 3. *Proposed time course of arterial recoil and remodeling after coronary angioplasty (PTCA) and directional atherectomy (DCA). Data from serial angiographic studies suggest that there is a substantial incidence of restenosis as early as 24 hours post-PTCA, but not DCA. Later, after 1 month, there is a progressive increase in the percentage of patients who develop restenosis, with little difference in the PTCA and DCA groups at 6 months.*

Confusingly, the term late recoil is often used to describe loss of lumen without evidence of intimal hyperplasia. While serial histologic studies would probably require autopsy material, it is at least possible that this late recoil represents contraction of the wound material formed early after injury, much as any wound heals.

Summary

While it may be easiest to think of restenosis in terms of the well-understood animal models of the arterial response to injury and the formation of neointima, a much more important issue may be the final diameter of the lumen. For example, Glagov's observations suggest that there may be a critical amount of intimal mass that prevents the vessel wall from undergoing normal, flow-dependent dilatation and thus maintenance of a proper lumen size. Therefore, it is intriguing to consider ways that a unique pharmacology, as well as a critical mass of intima, may contribute to progressive narrowing of the lumen in atherosclerosis and restenosis. Other processes, such as connective tissue synthesis, injury by oxygen-free-radicals, spasm, and calcification, are certainly worthy of further evaluation. Some or all of these events may depend on the expression of plaque-specific molecules—including certain molecules that might be selectively overexpressed in restenotic lesions.[97] Ideally, with parallel advances in the molecular biology and imaging of the vessel wall, a more comprehensive understanding of restenosis and atherogenesis will unfold.

Acknowledgments

The authors wish to express their appreciation for thoughtful discussions with fellow cardiologists at the University of Washington, and to Holly Kabinoff for editorial assistance with preparation of the manuscript.

References

1. Ross R. The pathogenesis of atherosclerosis: A perspective for the 1990s. *Nature* 1993;362:801–813.
2. Austin GE, Ratliff NB, Hollman J, et al. Intimal proliferation of smooth muscle cells as an explanation for recurrent coronary stenosis after percutaneous transluminal coronary angioplasty. *J Am Coll Cardiol* 1985;6:369–375.
3. Essed CE, Vandenbrand M, Becker AE. Transluminal coronary angioplasty and early restenosis: Fibrocellular occlusion after wall laceration. *Br Heart J* 1983;49:393–396.

4. Giraldo AA, Esposo OM, Meis JM. Intimal hyperplasia as a cause of restenosis after percutaneous transluminal coronary angioplasty. *Arch Pathol Lab Med* 1985;109:173–175.
5. Clowes AW, Clowes MM, Reidy MA. Kinetics of cellular proliferation after arterial injury. I. Smooth muscle growth in the absence of endothelium. *Lab Invest* 1983;49:327–333.
6. Clowes AW, Clowes MM, Reidy MA. Kinetics of cellular proliferation after arterial injury. III. Endothelial and smooth muscle growth in chronically denuded vessels. *Lab Invest* 1986;54:295–303.
7. Sarembock IJ, Laveau PJ, Sigal SL, et al. Influence of inflation pressure and balloon size on the development of intimal hyperplasia after balloon angioplasty: A study in the atherosclerotic rabbit. *Circulation* 1989;80:1029–1040.
8. Hanke H, Strohschneider T, Oberhoff M, et al. Time course of smooth muscle cell proliferation in the intima and media of arteries following experimental angioplasty. *Circ Res* 1990;67:651–659.
9. Steele PM, Chesebro JH, Stanson AW, et al. Balloon angioplasty: Natural history of the pathophysiological response to injury in a pig model. *Circ Res* 1985;57:105–112.
10. Schwartz RS, Murphy JG, Edwards WD, et al. Restenosis after balloon angioplasty: A practical proliferative model in porcine coronary arteries. *Circulation* 1990;82:2190–2200.
11. Schwartz L, Bourassa MG, Lesperance J, et al. Aspirin and dipyridamole in the prevention of restenosis after percutaneous transluminal coronary angioplasty. *N Engl J Med* 1988;318:1714–1719.
12. Ellis SG, Roubin GS, Wilentz J, et al. Effect of 18- and 24-hour heparin administration for prevention of restenosis after uncomplicated coronary angioplasty. *Am Heart J* 1989;117:777–782.
13. Grigg LE, Kay TWH, Valentine PA, et al. Determinants of restenosis and lack of effect of dietary supplementation with eicosapentenoic acid on the incidence of coronary artery restenosis after angioplasty. *J Am Coll Cardiol* 1989;13:665–672.
14. Corcos T, David PR, Val PG, et al. Failure of diltiazem to prevent restenosis after percutaneous transluminal coronary angioplasty. *Am Heart J* 1985;109:926–931.
15. Pepine CJ, Hirschfield JW, MacDonald RG, et al. A controlled trial of corticosteroids to prevent restenosis after coronary angioplasty. *Circulation* 1990;81:1753–1761.
16. MERCATOR Study Group. Does the new angiotensin-converting enzyme inhibitor cilazapril prevent restenosis after percutaneous transluminal coronary angioplasty? *Circulation* 1992;86:100–110.
17. Dotter CT, Judkins MP. Transluminal treatment of atherosclerotic obstructions: Description of new technique and a preliminary report of its application. *Circulation* 1964;30:654–670.
18. Gruentzig AR, Myler RK, Hanna EH, et al. Restenosis after balloon angioplasty. *Circulation* 1977;84(suppl II):II-55–II-56.
19. Lee G, Ikeda RM, Joye JA, et al. Evaluation of transluminal angioplasty of chronic coronary artery stenosis. *Circulation* 1980;61:77–83.
20. Block PC, Myler RK, Stertzer S, et al. Morphology after transluminal angioplasty in human beings. *N Engl J Med* 1981;305:382–385.
21. Castaneda-Zuniga WR, Formanek A, Tadavarthy M, et al. The mechanism of balloon angioplasty. *Radiology* 1980;135:565–571.

22. Baughman KL, Pasternak RC, Fallon JT, et al. Transluminal coronary angioplasty of postmortem human hearts. *Am J Cardiol* 1981;48:1044–1047.
23. Waller BF. Pathology of transluminal balloon angioplasty used in the treatment of coronary heart disease. *Human Pathol* 1987;18:476–484.
24. Mizuno K, Jurita A, Imazeki N. Pathologic findings after percutaneous transluminal coronary angioplasty. *Br Heart J* 1984;52:588–590.
25. Losordo DW, Rosenfield K, Pieczek A, et al. How does angioplasty work? Serial analysis of human iliac arteries using intravascular ultrasound. *Circulation* 1992;86:1845–1858.
26. Slomp J, Van Munsteren JC, Poelmann RE, et al. Formation of intimal cushions in the ductus arteriosus as a model for vascular intimal thickening. An immunohistochemical study of changes in extracellular matrix components. *Atherosclerosis* 1992;93:25–39.
27. Davies H. Atherogenesis and the coronary arteries of childhood. *Int J Cardiol* 1990;28:283–292.
28. Sims FH, Gavin JB, Vanderwee MA. The intima of human coronary arteries. *Am Heart J* 1989;118:32–38.
29. Velican C, Velican D. The precursors of coronary atherosclerotic plaques in subjects up to 40 years old. *Atherosclerosis* 1980;37:33–46.
30. Moss NS, Benditt EP. Human atherosclerotic plaque cells and leiomyoma cells: Comparison of in vitro growth characteristics. *Am J Pathol* 1975;78:175–190.
31. Ross R, Wight TN, Strandness E, et al. Human atherosclerosis II. Cell constitution and characteristics of advanced lesions of the superficial femoral artery. *Am J Pathol* 1984;114:79–93.
32. Spagnoli LG, Pietra GG, Villaschi S, et al. Morphometric analysis of gap junctions in regenerating arterial endothelium. *Lab Invest* 1982;46:139–148.
33. Villaschi S, Spagnoli LG. Autoradiographic and ultrastructural studies on the human fibroatheromatous plaque. *Atherosclerosis* 1983;48:95–100.
34. Gordon D, Reidy MA, Benditt EP, et al. Cell proliferation in human coronary arteries. *Proc Natl Acad Sci USA* 1990;87:4600–4604.
35. Benditt EP, Benditt JM. Evidence for a monoclonal origin of human atherosclerotic plaques. *Proc Natl Acad Sci USA* 1973;70:1753–1756.
36. Jackson CL, Schwartz SM. Pharmacology of smooth muscle cell replication. *Hypertension* 1992;20:713–736.
37. Daemen MJAP, Lombardi DM, Bosman FT, et al. Angiotensin II induces smooth muscle cell proliferation in the normal and injured arterial wall. *Circ Res* 1991;68:450–456.
38. Edelman ER, Nugent MA, Smith LT, et al. Basic fibroblast growth factor enhances the coupling of intimal hyperplasia and proliferation of vasa vasorum in injured rat arteries. *J Clin Invest* 1992;89:465–473.
39. Prescott M, Webb R, Reidy MA. ACE inhibitors vs. AII, AT1 receptor antagonist: Effects on smooth muscle cell migration and proliferation after balloon catheter injury. *Am J Pathol* 1991;139:1291–1302.
40. Powell J, Clozel J, Muller R, et al. Inhibitors of angiotensin-converting enzyme prevent myointimal proliferation after vascular injury. *Science* 1989;245:186–188.
41. Kauffman RF, Bean JS, Zimmerman KM, et al. Losartan, a nonpeptide AII receptor antagonist, inhibits neointima formation following balloon injury to rat carotid arteries. *Life Sci* 1991;49:PL223–PL228.

42. Farhy RD, Ho KL, Carretero OA, et al. Kinins mediate the antiproliferative effect of ramipril in rat carotid artery. *Biochem Biophys Res Commun* 1992;182:283–288.
43. Lam JYT, Lacoste L, Bourassa MG. Cilazapril and early atherosclerotic changes after balloon injury of porcine carotid arteries. *Circulation* 1992;85:1542–1547.
44. Ohlstein EH, Gellai M, Brooks DP, et al. The antihypertensive effect of the angiotensin II receptor antagonist DuP 753 may not be due solely to angiotensin II receptor antagonism. *J Pharmacol Exp Ther* 1992;262: 595.
45. Dzau VJ, Gibbons GH, Pratt RE. Molecular mechanisms of vascular renin-angiotensin system in myointimal hyperplasia. *Hypertension* 1991;18(4 Suppl):II100–II105.
46. Bunning P, Holmquist B, Riordan JF. Substrate specificity and kinetic characteristics of angiotensin-converting enzyme. *Biochemistry* 1983; 22:103–110.
47. Kaartinen M, Penttila A, Kovanen PT. Mast cells of two types differing in neutral protease composition in the human aortic intima. Demonstration of tryptase- and tryptase/chymase-containing mast cells in normal intimas, fatty streaks, and the shoulder region of atheromas. *Arterioscler Thromb* 1994;14:966–972.
48. Jawien A, Bowen-Pope DF, Lindner V, et al. Platelet-derived growth factor promotes smooth muscle migration and intimal thickening in a rat model of balloon angioplasty. *J Clin Invest* 1992;89:507–511.
49. Olson NE, Chao S, Lindner V, et al. Intimal smooth muscle cell proliferation after balloon catheter injury. The role of basic fibroblast growth factor. *Am J Pathol* 1992;140:1017–1023.
50. Majesky MW, Reidy MA, Bowen-Pope DF, et al. Platelet-derived growth factor (PDGF) ligand and receptor gene expression during repair of arterial injury. *J Cell Biol* 1990;111:2149–2158.
51. Nabel EG, Yang Z, Liptay S, et al. Recombinant platelet-derived growth factor B gene expression in porcine arteries induce intimal hyperplasia in vivo. *J Clin Invest* 1993;91:1822–1829.
52. Schwartz SM, Heimark RL, Majesky MW. Developmental mechanisms underlying pathology of arteries. *Phys Rev* 1990;70:1177–1209.
53. Mulvany MJ. Are vascular abnormalities a primary cause or secondary consequence of hypertension? *Hypertension* 1991;18(3 Suppl):I52–I57.
54. Folkow B. "Structural factor" in primary and secondary hypertension. *Hypertension* 1990;16:89–101.
55. Glagov S, Weisenberg E, Zarins CK, et al. Compensatory enlargement of human atherosclerotic coronary arteries. *N Engl J Med* 1987;316: 1371–1375.
56. Folkow B. Physiological aspects of primary hypertension. *Physiol Rev* 1982;62:347–504.
57. Jamal A, Bendeck M, Langille BL. Structural changes and recovery of function after arterial injury. *Arterioscler Thromb* 1992;12:307–317.
58. Miller MJ, Kuntz RE, Friedrich SP, et al. Frequency and consequences of intimal hyperplasia in specimens retrieved by directional atherectomy of native primary coronary artery stenoses and subsequent restenoses. *Am J Cardiol* 1993;71:652–658.
59. Schnitt SJ, Safian RD, Kuntz RE, et al. Histologic findings in specimens obtained by percutaneous directional coronary atherectomy. *Human Pathol* 1992;23:415–420.

60. Rekhter MD, Andreeva ER, Mironov AA, et al. Three-dimensional cytoarchitecture of normal and atherosclerotic intima of human aorta. *Am J Pathol* 1991;138:569–580.

61. Rekhter MD, Andreeva ER, Andrianova IV, et al. Stellate cells of aortic intima: I. Human and rabbit. *Tissue Cell* 1992;24:689–696.

62. O'Brien ER, Alpers CE, Stewart DK, et al. Proliferation in primary and restenotic coronary atherectomy tissue: Implications for anti-proliferative therapy. *Circ Res* 1993;73:223–231.

63. McCormick D, Hall PA. The complexities of proliferating cell nuclear antigen. *Histopathology* 1992;21:591–594.

64. Leclerc G, Kearney M, Schneider D, et al. Assessment of cell kinetics in human restenotic lesions by in vitro bromodeoxyuridine labeling of excised atherectomy specimens. *Clin Res* 1993;41:343A.

65. Pickering JG, Weir L, Jekanowski J, et al. Proliferative activity in peripheral and coronary atherosclerotic plaque among patients undergoing percutaneous revascularization. *J Clin Invest* 1993;91:1469–1480.

66. Garcia RL, Coltrera MD, Gown AM. Analysis of proliferative grade using anti-PCNA/cycin monoclonal antibodies in fixed, embedded tissues: Comparison with flow cytometric analysis. *Am J Pathol* 1989;134:733–739.

67. Rekhter M, Nicholls S, Ferguson M, et al. Cell proliferation in human arteriovenous fistulas used for hemodialysis. *Arterioscler Thrombosis* 1993;13:609–617.

68. Nguyen KPV, Shaw RE, Myler RK, et al. Does percutaneous transluminal coronary angioplasty accelerate atherosclerotic lesions?. *Catheterization Cardiovasc Diagn* 1990;21:1–6.

69. Waller BF, Pinkerton CA, Foster LN. Morphologic evidence of accelerated left main coronary artery stenosis: A late complication of percutaneous transluminal balloon angioplasty of the proximal left anterior descending coronary artery. *J Am Coll Cardiol* 1987;9:1019–1023.

70. Cequiera A, Bonan R, Crepeau J, et al. Restenosis and progression of coronary atherosclerosis after coronary angioplasty. *J Am Coll Cardiol* 1988;12:49–55.

71. Schwartz RS, Holmes DRJ, Topol EJ. The restenosis paradigm revisited: An alternative proposal for cellular mechanisms. *J Am Coll Cardiol* 1992;20:1284–1293.

72. Wilcox JN. Thrombin and other potential mechanisms underlying restenosis. *Circulation* 1991;84:432–435.

73. Ross R, Masuda J, Raines EW. Cellular interactions, growth factors, and smooth muscle proliferation in atherogenesis. *Ann NY Acad Sci* 1990a;598:102–112.

74. Reidy MA. Proliferation of smooth muscle cells at sites distant from vascular injury. *Arteriosclerosis* 1990;10:298–305.

75. Hatton MW, Moar SL, Richardson M. De-endothelialization in vivo initiates a thrombogenic reaction at the rabbit aorta surface. *Am J Pathol* 1989;135:499–508.

76. Okazaki H, Majesky MW, Harker LA, et al. Regulation of platelet-derived growth factor ligand and receptor gene expression by α-thrombin in vascular smooth muscle cells. *Circ Res* 1992;71:1285–1293.

77. Wilcox JN, Smith KM, Williams LT, et al. Platelet-derived growth factor mRNA detection in human atherosclerotic plaques by in situ hybridization. *J Clin Invest* 1988;82:1134–1143.

78. Ross R, Masuda J, Raines EW, et al. Localization of PDGF-B protein

in macrophages in all phases of atherogenesis. *Science* 1990b;248:1009–1012.

79. Clowes AW, Clowes M, Kirkman T, et al. Heparin inhibits the expression of tissue-type plasminogen activator by SMC in injured rat carotid artery. *Circ Res* 1992;70:1128–1136.

80. Carney DH, Mann R, Redin WR, et al. Enhancement of incisional wound healing and neovascularization in normal rats by thrombin and synthetic thrombin receptor-activating peptides. *J Clin Invest* 1992;89:1469–1477.

81. Bar-Shavit R, Benezra M, Eldor A, et al. Thrombin immobilized to extracellular matrix is a potent mitogen for vascular smooth muscle cells: Nonenzymatic mode of action. *Cell Regulation* 1990;1:453–463.

82. Mintz GS, Douek PC, Bonner RF, et al. Intravascular ultrasound comparison of de novo and restenotic coronary artery lesions. *J Am Coll Cardiol* 1993;21:118A.

83. Heagerty AM, Aalkjaer C, Bund SJ, et al. Small artery structure in hypertension. Dual processes of remodeling and growth. *Hypertension* 1993;21:391–397.

84. Kuntz RE, Gibson M, Nobuyoshi M, et al. Generalized model of restenosis after conventional balloon angioplasty, stenting and directional atherectomy. *J Am Coll Cardiol* 1993;21:15–25.

85. Baim DS, Kuntz RE. Why "bigger is better" in coronary intervention. *Cardiovasc Interven* 1993;24–26.

86. Zollikofer CL, Redha FH, Bruhlmann WF, et al. Acute and long-term effects of massive balloon dilation on the aortic wall and vasa vasorum. *Radiology* 1987;164:145–149.

87. Cragg AH, Einzig S, Rysavy JA, et al. The vasa vasorum and angioplasty. *Radiology* 1993;148:75–80.

88. Faxon DP, Weber VJ, Haudenschild C, et al. Acute effects of transluminal angioplasty in three experimental models of atherosclerosis. *Arteriosclerosis* 1982;2:125–133.

89. Sanborn TA, Faxon DP, Haudenschild C, et al. The mechanism of transluminal angioplasty: Evidence for formation of aneurysms in experimental atherosclerosis. *Circulation* 1993;68:1136–1140.

90. Castaneda-Zuniga WR, Laerum R, Rysavy J, et al. Paralysis of arteries by intraluminal balloon dilation. *Radiology* 1982;144:75A.

91. Cosigny PM, Tulenko TN, Nicosia RF. Immediate and long-term effects of angioplasty-balloon dilation on normal rabbit iliac arteries. *Arteriosclerosis* 1986;6:265–276.

92. Fischell TA, Grant G, Johnson DE. Determinants of smooth muscle injury during balloon angioplasty. *Circulation* 1990;82:2170–2184.

93. Fischell TA, Derby G, Tse TM, et al. Coronary artery vasoconstriction routinely occurs after percutaneous transluminal coronary angioplasty. A quantitative arteriographic analysis. *Circulation* 1988;78:1323–1334.

94. Nobuyoshi M, Kimura T, Nosaka H, et al. Restenosis after successful percutaneous transluminal coronary angioplasty: Serial angiographic follow-up of 229 patients. *J Am Coll Cardiol* 1988;12:616–623.

95. Isner JM, Rosenfield K, Losordo DW, et al. Combination balloon-ultrasound imaging catheter for percutaneous transluminal angioplasty. Validation of imaging, analysis of recoil, and identification of plaque fracture. *Circulation* 1991;84:739–754.

96. Serruys PW, Luijten HE, Beatt KJ, et al. Incidence of restenosis after

successful coronary angioplasty: A time-related phenomenon. *Circulation* 1988;77:361–371.

97. Schwartz SM, O'Brien ER, deBlois D, et al. Relevance of smooth muscle replication and development to vascular disease. In: Schwartz SM, Mecham RP, eds. *The Vascular Smooth Muscle Cell*. San Francisco, CA: Academic Press; in press.

Chapter 28

Clinical-Pathobiological Correlations Emerging from the Study of Restenosis Lesions Obtained by Excisional Atherectomy

J. Geoffrey Pickering, MD, PhD, Carol M. Ford, MSc, Marianne Kearney, BS, and Jeffrey M. Isner, MD

Introduction

The advent of percutaneous transluminal coronary angioplasty has had a profound effect on the practice of cardiology over the past two decades. Given the high acute success rate and the low morbidity, it has become an important and widespread means of arterial revascularization. The persistent and frequent problem of restenosis after angioplasty, therefore, is a situation that frustrates cardiologists and patients alike. Indeed there are few other clinical scenarios in which therapeutic success is followed so closely and so frequently by its abrogation.

Much has been learned about the manner in which the vessel wall responds to mechanical injury from animal studies.[1-3] Clinical restenosis is, however, ultimately unique to humans. This uniqueness is due, in part, to the underlying atherosclerotic plaque that animal models can presently, at best, only approximate. In this context, the advent of directional atherectomy[4] has

Supported by a grant from the Medical Research Council of Canada (MT-11715 [JGP]) and the National Heart, Lung, and Blood Institute (HL-40518–05 and HL-02824 [JMI]).

From: Fuster V, (ed.) *Syndromes of Atherosclerosis: Correlations of Clinical Imaging and Pathology.* Armonk, NY: Futura Publishing Company, Inc.: © 1996.

provided an unparalleled opportunity to study the pathobiological features of restenosis lesions and compared these with those of de novo atherosclerosis. The advantages afforded by directional atherectomy include: 1) the acquisition of lesion fragments large enough to be studied histologically; 2) immediate access to fresh vascular tissue that can then be specifically processed to preserve antigens or messenger RNA, or placed in culture for ex vivo experiments; 3) the unique opportunity to study the putative "culprit" lesion in patients with a clinically manifest ischemic syndrome.

Any analysis of atherectomy tissue should take into account that the tissue retrieval process is essentially one of sampling. While concomitant use of intravascular ultrasound may augment the amount of plaque retrieved, histologic analysis of the intact, full-thickness artery will remain in the domain of postmortem analyses. Despite this caveat, much has been learned from the study of atherectomy tissue and several of these advances are discussed here.

Ex Vivo Studies of Atherectomy Tissue: Clues That Restenosis is an Active Process and Biologically Distinct from Atherosclerosis

If atherectomy fragments are placed promptly in the culture environment, cell viability is maintained such that in vitro studies can be performed.[5] Care must be taken in interpreting culture-derived findings, however, because the in vitro environment is clearly different from the in vivo environment. This is particularly important if isolated cells are maintained in culture for prolonged periods. One way to minimize the likelihood of spurious findings is to study intact fragments of atherectomy tissue and to evaluate these in the immediate days after placing in culture. It has been recognized for many years that if segments of arterial media are allowed to adhere to the culture dish, smooth muscle cells (SMCs) will migrate out of the tissue and proliferate.[6] We and others have observed that this SMC outgrowth phenomenon can also occur from explants of atherectomy fragments.[5,7] The rate at which this outgrowth proceeds is different between restenosis and atherosclerosis tissue fragments. We quantified SMC outgrowth from 20 atherosclerosis lesions and 21 restenosis lesions retrieved from peripheral arteries (37 of 41) or venous conduits. Outgrowth of SMCs was significantly more robust from the restenosis lesions. After 5 days ex vivo, SMC outgrowth had begun among 32%±4% of the explant fragments from restenosis tissue and became half-maximal by 5.9±0.6 days. In contrast, among explants from primary lesions, SMC outgrowth had begun among only 9%±5% of the fragments by 5 days and did not reach the half-maximum until 8.7±0.4 days ($P=<0.001$ for both parameters). The rate at which SMCs accumulated around the explant fragments was also substantially higher for restenosis tissue ($P<0.01$).

These studies thus highlighted the SMC and its behavior as a potentially key distinguishing feature between restenosis and atherosclerosis lesions in patients with symptomatic ischemia. Furthermore, a number of possible reasons for the enhanced SMC outgrowth from restenosis tissue could be proposed. One possibility was that the total number of SMCs in restenosis atherectomy tissue may be higher than that in atherosclerosis lesions, thereby yielding a more robust outgrowth. This is supported by morphological assessment of restenotic atherectomy material by a number of investigators who identified a relative abundance of SMCs in restenosis atherectomy lesions.[8–10] In a series of 37 peripheral and coronary atherectomy lesions, we found that the intimal cell density of restenosis tissue was, on average, twice that of de novo atherosclerotic tissue (500±238 vs. 241±197 cells/mm², $P<0.001$) and the majority of these cells were SMCs. The relatively vigorous SMC outgrowth ex vivo is therefore likely to be, in part, a consequence of this difference.

The enhanced outgrowth from restenosis tissue may also reflect intrinsic differences in the growth behavior of SMCs in restenosis tissue. This notion was supported by proliferation studies of subcultured SMCs. Dartsch and co-workers[5] noted that SMCs isolated from restenotic tissue had a shorter doubling time than those derived from atherosclerotic plaque. Similarly, we observed that the thymidine incorporation rate, normalized for total cell number, was 1.3-fold higher in SMCs originating from the restenotic lesions.[7]

Another explanation for the difference in outgrowth rates may lie in differences in the composition of the extracellular matrix. As discussed below, the extracellular matrix of restenotic tissue is histologically distinct from that of atherosclerotic plaque with differences in proteoglycan content[11] and collagen content.[12] The restenotic matrix may therefore be a more favorable milieu for SMC locomotion and facilitate migration of SMCs through it, and ultimately on to the floor of the culture dish. In contrast, the extracellular matrix of atherosclerotic fragments may be less favorable and possibly pose a mechanical impediment to outgrowth.

Histologic Features: Identification of a Focus of Intimal Modeling

Analysis of the morphological features of restenotic tissue retrieved by atherectomy is no doubt subject to variability that will arise from the sampling inherent in the procedure. In spite of this, certain light microscopic features of the excised restenosis tissue have been consistently observed.[8–10,13,14] The most common among these is that of a hypercellular focus of tissue, containing predominantly vascular SMCs within a relatively loose extracellular matrix. This contrasts with the hypocellular and fibrous morphology commonly found in atherosclerotic plaque not subjected to atherectomy.[15]

Hypercellularity in the intima almost certainly reflects a reactive response and we have used the term intimal modeling focus to connote its presence. As recently emphasized by Glagov,[16] at least two morphologically distinguishable patterns can be found in restenosis tissue. The first, which we term IMF type A, is characterized by SMCs that are relatively widely separated from each other, and aligned in seemingly random orientations. The SMCs have an undifferentiated, synthetic appearance and compared with normal medial SMCs the nucleus is larger and the cytoplasm more bulky, often giving a stellate appearance to the cell. The matrix between the cells has a loose appearance and alcian blue staining identifies a predominance of proteoglycans (Figure 1a). The second morphological form of intimal modeling (IMF type B) is characterized by an even higher concentration of SMCs that now partially align with each other, at times resembling arterial media. The intervening matrix is denser and a fibrous appearance may be evident, although still less compact than that of fibrous atherosclerosis (Figure 1b). These two forms probably represent extremes of a continuum of intimal organization and hemodynamic influence may be important in the transition from the loose phase to the more organized stage.[16]

It should be noted that the intimal modeling focus is not unique to restenosis, but is also common in vascular anastomotic sites, dialysis fistulae, and recurrent carotid artery stenoses.[14] All of these conditions represent abnormal vascular conditions leading to an intimal reaction. An intimal modeling focus may also be seen in atherectomy specimens retrieved from arteries not subjected to a prior intervention,[17] possibly reflecting modeling after an intrinsic plaque crisis.[18] Nevertheless, the pattern is much more commonly found in restenotic fragments. Isner and coworkers[19] have observed a restenosis focus in 165 (65%) of 253 restenosis specimens retrieved by directional atherectomy. In contrast, only 31 (7%) of 425 primary specimens, studied as part of the CAVEAT investigation, contained such a focus.[20]

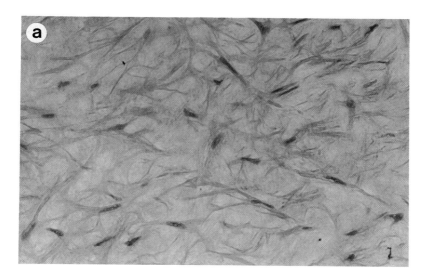

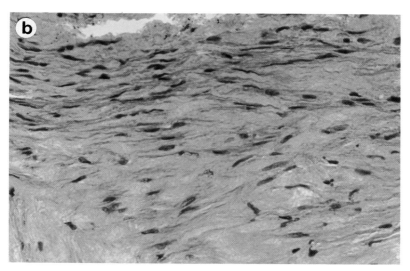

FIGURE 1. *Histologic appearances of an intimal modeling focus (IMF) commonly found in restenosis specimens retrieved by directional atherectomy.* **a:** *Micrograph showing phenotypically modulated smooth muscle cells (SMCs) variably oriented in a loose extracellular marix (IMF type A) in a lesion retrieved 3 months after angioplasty.* **b:** *Micrograph of a restenosis lesion retrieved 4 months after angioplasty showing a more densely cellular region with SMCs oriented parallel to each other (IMF type B).*

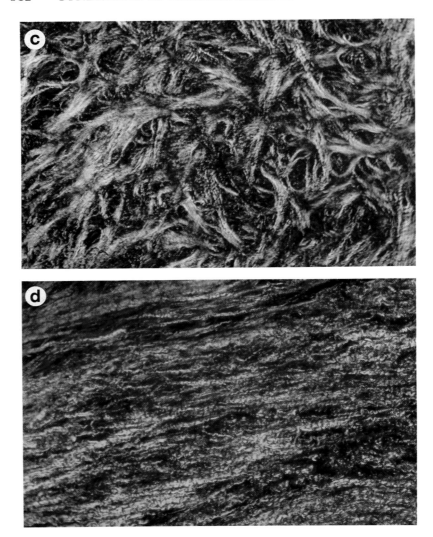

FIGURE 1 *Continued. c:* *Circular polarization photomicrograph of a nearby section to that shown in **a** showing an extensive network of diffusely oriented fibers. **d:** Polarization micrograph of a nearby section to that shown in **b** illustrating aligned, more organized collagen fibers.*

Expression of the Proliferating Cell Nuclear Antigen in Atherectomy Fragments

The proliferating cell nuclear antigen (PCNA) is a nuclear protein that activates DNA polymerase ∂.[21] As such, it is necessary for DNA replication during cell proliferation. When quiescent cells are stimulated to proliferate, there is an increase in PCNA synthesis and the level of PCNA within the nucleus becomes substantially higher.[22,23] The production of antibodies to PCNA has allowed investigators to gauge the proliferative activity of cells immunohistochemically.

Gordon and coworkers[24] used this approach to assess the proliferative status of coronary arteries of hearts explanted from patients undergoing cardiac transplantation. Eleven of fourteen atherosclerotic lesions contained PCNA-positive cells but the proportion of PCNA-positive cells was generally low, ranging from 0% to 4.68%. The relative quiescence of these lesions may reflect an advanced stage of atherosclerosis among the patients with end stage cardiac disease. Katsuda et al[25] studied lesions at the other end of the chronological spectrum, specifically fatty streaks in young adults. In these early atherosclerotic lesions a similarly low level of PCNA-positive cells (<2%) was noted. Directional atherectomy allows for an assessment of PCNA expression in lesions in symptomatic patients and thus a clinical scenario distinct from these extremes. We observed that 5 of 7 atherosclerotic and 8 of 8 restenotic lesions contained PCNA-positive cells.[26] The proportion of PCNA-positive cells was significantly higher in restenotic ($15.2\%\pm13.6\%$) than in primary ($3.6\%\pm3.5\%$) lesions. The high levels in restenosis samples, relative to end-stage atherosclerotic lesions or fatty streaks, were confirmed by analyses of further 22 specimens by in situ hybridization[26] and a more recent assessment of another 33 restenosis atherectomy fragments. Interestingly, the proportion of PCNA-positive cells did not correlate with the length of time between the angioplasty and subsequent atherectomy and positive cells were detected as late as 1 year after angioplasty. This apparent lack of relationship with time from the procedure has also been observed by O'Brien and co-workers.[27] This appears to contrast with animal models in which there is a consistent time course of proliferation.[1,28] This highlights the probable multifactorial nature of the human restenosis process.

It should be noted, that while immunoreactivity to PCNA represents a convenient approach to gauging proliferative activity, the results must be carefully interpreted. Not only is PCNA necessary for DNA replication but it is also required for repair of damaged DNA.[29,30] Whether or not DNA repair is accelerated after vessel injury is not known. Immunodetection of PCNA is also dependent on the tissue fixation protocol.[23,31] We have found that brief exposure to aldehyde fixatives (such as formalin) substantially reduces the sensitivity of detection with the currently available monoclonal antibody.[19] Immunopositivity for PCNA should also be distinguished from measures of DNA synthesis rates, such as incorporation of 5'-bromodeoxyuridine (BrdU) or radiolabeled thymidine. These latter measures identify cells that are in the S-phase (DNA synthesis) of the replicative cycle while the tissue is exposed to the labeled DNA precursor. The presence of PCNA in cycling cells, however, is not restricted to S-phase, but is also found in G_1, and G_2 phases as well as in mitosis.[26,32,33] One comparative analysis revealed that PCNA-positive cells were 8.5 times more abundant than the BrdU-positive cells.[25] Another important consideration is that the half-life of PCNA in human vascular tissue is not known. The protein is, however, considered to be stable.[34] Therefore, use of sensitive techniques to identify PCNA may mark replicating cells as well as a proportion of cells that have replicated at a recent, but as yet unknown, time prior to tissue harvesting. In this context, it is recognized that the intensity and pattern of PCNA staining (eg, diffuse nuclear vs. granular) can vary.[34] We have found that the approach with the least interobserver variation is to denote all cells with a signal localized exclusively in the nucleus as PCNA-positive cells. There must be simultaneous immunostaining of a control tissue, such as tonsil or intestine, and provided the proliferative compartment in the control section is positive and the nonproliferative compartment negative, then all PCNA-positive cells in the atherectomy tissue can be termed proliferating. Others have adopted a more restrictive definition with correspondingly lower rates of PCNA-positivity in atherectomy samples.[27]

Collagen Fibers in Atherectomy Fragments

While activated SMCs are clearly a hallmark of the intimal modeling focus, it is the extracellular matrix that comprises the bulk of the lesion volume. As noted above, this matrix has a loose appearance with an abundance of proteoglycans, including biglycan.[11] Using traditionally histologic stains, collagen fibers are not evident in the early (type A) intimal modeling focus and collagen deposition has generally been considered a late response to angioplasty.[35] However, when SMCs are activated in vitro[36] or by injury in vivo[37,38] enhanced collagen synthesis rates and collagen expression are relatively early phenomena. We therefore considered that traditional light microscopy may be underestimating the amount of collagen in restenosis tissue. This possibility is important from a therapeutic standpoint because the deposition of collagen fibers is generally considered to represent an irreversible stage of tissue remodeling.

To address this we evaluated a series of coronary atherectomy lesions using a specialized microscopy technique based on circularly polarized light.[12] This approach exploits the birefringent properties of collagen fibers that appear bright when stained with picrosirius red and viewed with polarized light.[39] All other structures in the vessel wall, including cells and the remaining extracellular matrix, are not visible and appear dark. When this approach was used to view native atherosclerotic lesions, the dense collagenous bands were identified in a striking fashion. In restenosis lesions, the collagen fibers were thinner than those in de novo lesions and coursed in multiple orientations, but they still constituted an extensive network (Figure 1c). This unique collagen network was exclusively found in intimal modeling foci, and juxtaposition with more densely organized regions often provided a clear demarcation between apparently de novo atherosclerosis and tissue involved in a reactive response. Modeling foci with aligned SMCs (IMF type B) contained thicker fibers that tended to run parallel to the SMC long axis (Figure 1d). Thus, identifiable stages of organization of restenotic tissue may be detectable based on the collagen fabric.

The time point at which collagen fiber deposition is first detectable after angioplasty is not yet defined. Nevertheless, we have found an extensive collagen network within all restenosis lesions studied to date. The notion of collagen deposition as a late phenomenon might therefore be reconsidered and the extent of collagen elaboration after angioplasty and its subsequent organization could have an important impact on the development of restenosis. Approaches to minimize restenosis after angioplasty should consider this robust response.

Evidence That Different Arterial Beds May Respond Differently to Balloon Angioplasty

From this discussion, it is clear that there are quantifiable morphological and immunohistochemical features that identify a reactive process in the vessel wall. Analysis of these features not only provides insight into the pathogenesis of restenosis following angioplasty, but also provides a basis with which to compare the vessel wall response to angioplasty among different arterial beds. It is not known, for example, if peripheral arteries (femoral and popliteal) respond identically to injury as do coronary arteries. The possibility of unique responses is based in part on the embryology of the vessel wall. Whereas the endothelial cells originate from the embryonic vasculature, the SMCs that ultimately surround these channels are derived locally from the parenchyma of the respective organs.[40] Ross[41] has suggested that this may contribute to different responses to agonists among different vasculature beds. Similarly, it might influence the pathobiology of lesion formation. This possibility was raised further by the seemingly disparate frequencies among different reports with which PCNA-positive cells were observed in restenosis tissue. We have noted that PCNA expression, assessed either by immunohistochemistry or by in situ hybridization, is frequently identifiable in peripheral restenosis lesions whereas O'Brien and co-workers[27] noted that only a minority (26%) of coronary restenosis fragments had PCNA-positive cells. As discussed above, some of the differences may be due to differences in technique and counting protocols, however, there is also the possibility that the differences may reflect biological distinctions between coronary and peripheral arteries.

To examine this, we studied 33 restenosis lesions retrieved by directional atherectomy (13 from coronary arteries and 20 from a peripheral bed), either the superficial femoral artery or the popliteal artery. Parameters measured included PCNA-positivity, the frequency with which an intimal modeling focus could be identified, and the fractional area of the sample occupied by an intimal modeling focus. The intimal modeling focus was identified based on the morphological features described above and assessment of collagen network by polarization microscopy to define the borders of the modeling focus. The relative area of intimal modeling focus was determined by digital morphometry.

The results, which are summarized in Table 1, suggest quantitative differences between coronary and peripheral restenosis lesions. While a majority of both coronary and peripheral artery restenosis specimens contained PCNA-positive cells, the number of PCNA-positivity cells per unit area was significantly higher among the peripheral artery samples. Also apparent was a higher prevalence of a type A intimal modeling focus among the peripheral artery specimens and a greater percent area of the excised peripheral artery restenosis lesion was occupied by this focus. These find-

TABLE 1

Characteristics of Restenosis Atherectomy Tissue in Coronary and Peripheral Arterial Beds

	Coronary (n=13)	Peripheral (n=20)
Prevalence of lesions with PCNA-positive cells	11 (85%)	16 (80%)
Density of PCNA-positive cells (cells/mm^2)	8.1±3.3	15.4±6.2*
Lesions with IMF	10 (77%)	16 (80%) %
% Lesion area containing IMF	33.5 ± 6.9	59.6 ± 9.2*

Values denote mean ± standard error of the mean. *$P<0.05$

ings suggest that postangioplasty restenosis in peripheral arteries may not simply be a "scaled-up" version of that in the coronary vasculature. That is, in the peripheral artery with a clinically manifest recurrent stenosis, a disproportionately greater reactive intimal response appears to be present. Conversely, the development of clinically manifest restenosis in coronary arteries may depend to a greater degree on additional responses besides the intimal reaction. Modeling responses in the media or the adventitia could adversely affect lumen size by structural encroachment[42] or by limiting the artery's capacity to dilate appropriately.[43] This is illustrated schematically in Figure 2 that conceptually depicts a remodeling process that leads to a reduction in total arterial cross sectional area. For any given degree of this type of remodeling, less SMC proliferation will be required to produce luminal renarrowing. This type of remodeling, which would not be amenable to study by atherectomy, may play an important accessory role in coronary restenosis and may explain those cases in which anatomic studies disclose no evidence of SMC proliferation.

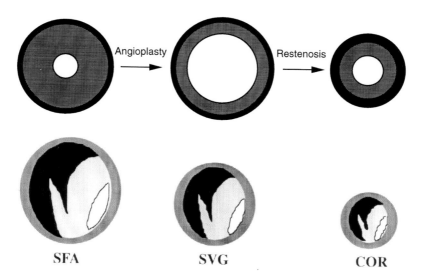

FIGURE 2. **Top:** *Modeling responses of the outer layer(s) of ther artery wall may secondarily renarrow luminal dimensions after angioplasty by loss of compensatory vessel enlargement or by structural changes leading to a net shrinking of the total arterial cross-sectional area.* **Bottom:** *The smaller the native arterial dimensions, the less proliferation is required to produce renarrowing. This may be compounded by any associated remodeling that reduces the cross-sectional area of the vascular segment (as shown in the top panel).*

The native dimensions of the treated artery may also have an impact on both the pathogenesis of restenosis,[16] as well as the sampling bias inherent in directional atherectomy (Figure 2, bottom panel). The smaller the vessel, regardless of the extent to which revascularization is complete, the less proliferation is required, in absolute terms, to produce renarrowing. The more diminutive the contribution of proliferation, the less chance statistically there is that the proliferative foci will be retrieved by atherectomy.

In summary, excisional atherectomy has considerably broadened our understanding of the pathobiology of human restenosis. The process is biologically distinct from atherosclerosis and characterized by reactive changes in the intima that include SMC proliferation and elaboration of a loosely organized collagen matrix. Furthermore, differences in coronary and peripheral restenosis specimens suggest a variability in the basic response to angioplasty among different arterial beds. A greater understanding of the factors influencing these responses will help resolve the vexing problem of restenosis after angioplasty.

References

1. Clowes A, Reidy M, Clowes M. Kinetics of cellular proliferation after arterial injury. I. Smooth muscle growth in the absence of endothelium. *Lab Invest* 1983;49:327–333.
2. Schwartz RS, Huber KC, Murphy JG, et al. Restenosis and the proportional neointimal response to coronary artery injury: Results in a porcine model. *J Am Coll Cardiol* 1992;19:267–274.
3. Schwartz RS, Edwards WD, Bailey KR, et al. Differential neointimal response to coronary artery injury in pigs and dogs. Implications for restenosis models. *Arterioscler Thromb* 1994;14:395–400.
4. Simpson JB, Selmon MR, Robertson GC, et al. Transluminal atherectomy for occlusive peripheral vascular disease. *Am J Cardiol* 1988;61:96G–101G.
5. Dartsch PC, Voisard R, Bauriedel G, et al. Growth characteristics and cytoskeletal organization of cultured smooth muscle cells from human primary stenosing and restenosing lesions. *Arterioslerosis* 1990;10:62–75.
6. Chamley-Campbell J, Campbell G, Ross R. The smooth muscle cell in culture. *Physiol Rev* 1979;59:1–61.
7. Pickering JG, Weir L, Rosenfield K, et al. Smooth muscle cell outgrowth from human atherosclerotic plaque: Implications for the assessment of lesion biology. *J Am Coll Cardiol* 1992;20:1430–1439.
8. Garratt KN, Edwards WD, Kaufmann UP, et al. Differential histopathology of primary atherosclerotic and restenotic lesions in coronary arteries and saphenous vein grafts: Analysis of tissue obtained from 73 patients by directional atherectomy. *J Am Coll Cardiol* 1991;17:442–448.
9. Johnson DE, Hinihara T, Selmon MR, et al. Primary peripheral artery stenoses and restenoses excised by transluminal atherectomy: A histopathologic study. *J Am Coll Cardiol* 1990;15:419–425.

10. Nobuyoshi M, Kimura T, Ohishi H, et al. Restenosis after percutaneous transluminal coronary angioplasty: Pathologic observations in 20 patients. *J Am Coll Cardiol* 1991;17:433–439.
11. Reissen R, Isner JM, Blessing E, et al. Regional differences in the distribution of biglycan and decorin in the extracellular matrix of atherosclerotic and restenotic human coronary arteries. *Am J Pathol* 1994;144:962–974.
12. Pickering JG, Ford CM, Novick R. Collagen elaboration following balloon angioplasty. *J Am Coll Cardiol* 1994;23:235A.
13. Safian RD, Galbfish JS, Erny RE, et al. Coronary atherectomy: Clincial, angiographic and histological findings and observations regarding potential mechanisms. *Circulation* 1990;82:69–79.
14. Schwarcz TH, Yates GN, Ghobrial M, et al. Pathologic characteristics of recurrent carotid artery stenosis. *J Vasc Surg* 1987;5:280–288.
15. Ross R. The pathogenesis of atherosclerosis—an update. *N Engl J Med* 1986;314:488–500.
16. Glagov S. Intimal hyperplasia, vascular modeling, and the resteonsis problem. *Circulation* 1994;89:2888–2891.
17. Orekhov AN, Andreeva ER, Krushinsky AV. Intimal cells and atherosclerosis. Relationship between the number of intimal cells and major manifestations of atherosclerosis in the human aorta. *Am J Pathol* 1986;125:402–415.
18. Iugelman MY, Virmani R, Correa R, et al. Smooth muscle cell abundance and fibroblast growth factors in coronary lesions of patients with nonfatal unstable angina. *Circulation* 1993;88:2493–2500.
19. Isner JM, Kearney M, Bauters C, et al. Use of human tissue specimens obtained by directional atherectomy to study restenosis. *Trends Cardiovasc Med* 1994;4:213–221.
20. Isner JM, Kearney M, Berdan LG. Core pathology lab findings in 425 patients undergoing directional atherectomy for a primary coronary artery stenosis and relation to subsequent outcome: The CAVEAT study. *J Am Coll Cardiol* 1993;21:380A.
21. Bravo R, Frank R, Blundell P, et al. Cyclin/PCNA is the auxiliary protein of DNA polymerase-delta. *Nature* 1987;326:515–517.
22. Baserga R. Growth regulation of the PCNA gene. *J Cell Sci* 1991;98:433–436.
23. Hall P, Levison D, Woods A, et al. Proliferating cell nuclear antigen (PCNA) immunolocalization in paraffin sections: An index of cell proliferation with evidence of deregulated expression in some neoplasms. *J Pathol* 1990;162:285–294.
24. Gordon D, Reidy M, Benditt E, et al. Cell proliferation in human coronary arteries. *Proc Natl Acad Sci USA* 1990;87:4600–4604.
25. Katsuda S, Coltrera MD, Ross R, et al. Human atherosclerosis: IV. Immunocytochemical analysis of cell activation and proliferation in lesions of young adults. *Am J Pathol* 1993;142:1787–1793.
26. Pickering JG, Weir L, Jekanowski J, et al. Proliferative activity in peripheral and coronary atherosclerotic plaque among patients undergoing percutaneous revascularization. *J Clin Invest* 1993;91:1469–1480.
27. O'Brien ER, Alpers CE, Stewart DK, et al. Prolferation in primary and restenotic coronary atherectomy tissue. Implications for antiprolferative therapy. *Circ Res* 1993;73:223–231.
28. Hanke H, Strohschneider T, Oberhoff M, et al. Time course of smooth

muscle cell proliferation in the intima and media of arteries following experimental angioplasty. *Circ Res* 1990;67:651–659.

29. Nishida C, Reinhard P, Linn S. DNA repair synthesis in human fibroblasts requires DNA polymerase Î. *J Biol Chem* 1988;263:501–510.

30. Shivji MKK, Kenny MK, Wood RD. *Cell* 1992;69:367.

31. Galand P, Degraef C. Cyclin/PCNA immunostaining as an alternative to tritiated thymidine pulse labelling for marking S phase cells in paraffin sections from animal and human tissues. *Cell Tissue Kinetics* 1989;22:383–392.

32. Garcia R, Coltrera M, Gown A. Analysis of proliferative grade using anti-PCNA/cyclin monoclonal antibodies in fixed, embedded tissues. Comparison with flow cytometric analysis. *Am J Pathol* 1989;134:733–739.

33. Morris GF, Mathews MB. Regulation of proliferating cell nuclear antigen during the cell cycle. *J Biol Chem* 1989;264:13856–13864.

34. Bravo R, Macdonald-Bravo H. Existence of two populations of cyclin/proliferating cell nuclear antigen during the cell cycle: Association with DNA replication sites. *J Cell Biol* 1987;105:1549–1554.

35. Forrester J, Fishbein M, Helfant R, et al. A paradigm for restenosis based on cell biology: Clues for the development of new preventive therapies. *J Am Coll Cardiol* 1991;17:758–769

36. Ang A, Tachas G, Campbell J, et al. Collagen synthesis by cultured rabbit aortic smooth-muscle cells. Alteration with phenotype. *Biochem J* 1990;265:461–469.

37. Majesky M, Giachelli CM, Reidy MA, et al. Rat carotid neointimal smooth muscle cells reexpress a developmentally regulated mRNA phenotype during repair of arterial injury. *Circ Res* 1992;71:759–768.

38. MacLeod D, Strauss B, De Jong M, et al. Proliferation and extracellular matrix synthesis of smooth muscle cells cultured from coronary atherosclerotic and restenotic lesions. *J Am Coll Cardiol* 1994;23:59–65.

39. Pickering JG, Boughner DR. Fibrosis in the transplanted heart and its relation to donor ischemic time. Assessment with polarized light microscopy and digital image analysis. *Circulation* 1990;81:949–958.

40. Schwartz SM, Campbell GR, Campbell JH. Replication of smooth muscle cells in vascular disease. *Circ Res* 1986;58:427–444.

41. Ross R. The pathogenesis of atherosclerosis: A perspective for the 1990s. *Nature* 1993;362:801–809.

42. Isner JM. Vascular remodeling. Honey, I think I shrunk the artery. *Circulation* 1994;89:2937–2941.

43. Kakuta T, Currier JW, Haudenschild CC, et al. Differences in compensatory vessel enlargement, not intimal formation, account for restenosis after angioplasty in the hypercholesterolemic rabbit model. *Circulation* 1994;89:2809–2815.

Chapter 29

Vein Graft Disease:
A Pathologist's View

Christian C. Haudenschild, MD

Despite the increasing use of arteries as bypass vessels for diseased coronary arteries,[1] saphenous veins are still frequently grafted.[2] Aortocoronary bypass has been performed with so few changes in technique for so long that a number of large follow-up studies covering 10 years and more have been performed. The consensus is that in the long term, saphenous vein grafts continuously and gradually degenerate. Patients are now surviving " . . . beyond the patency of their primary grafts."[3,4] There are multiple etiologies for this vein graft disease: pathological conditions of the vein before grafting, surgical techniques, thrombotic complications, hemodynamic forces, and persistent risk factors for atherosclerosis.

Saphenous vein segments are unlikely to be normal even before they are removed from their original site; they may have focal phlebosclerosis, mild varicosis, some endothelial damage and varying degrees of fibrocellular intimal hyperplasia.[5] Despite the reversed direction of flow, their valves provide an uneven intimal surface, and it is almost impossible to match their caliber with that of the recipient artery. Some further alterations due to surgical techniques cannot be avoided. However, excessive mechanical manipulations, such as the use of a valvulotome, or leak testing by overinflation with saline result in a loss of endothelial cells and irritation of the smooth muscle cells [6] and can be avoided. Indeed, atraumatic removal and careful extracorporeal storage of the grafts under the protection of vasodilators have been successful in preventing unnecessary damage and loss of endothelial cells.[7] Remaining endothelial cells may still show functional impairment, such as diminished production of prostacyclin or endothelium-

From: Fuster V, (ed.) *Syndromes of Atherosclerosis: Correlations of Clinical Imaging and Pathology.* Armonk, NY: Futura Publishing Company, Inc.: © 1996.

derived relaxing factor. The sum of all these micro- and macro-traumata causes a wound-healing response.

In the special case of the vascular wall, this wound-healing response comes primarily from the smooth muscle cells; later in the process, adventitial fibroblasts, adjacent intimal endothelial cells, and blood-borne adhering cells will also become involved. The smooth muscle cells respond with an alteration of their phenotype and with migration and proliferation. Since it was realized that smooth muscle cell migration and proliferation contribute to intimal thickening, substantial efforts have been devoted to antiproliferative strategies attempting to prevent graft closure, restenosis after angioplasty, and atherosclerosis itself, with less than overwhelming success. One must remember that proliferative cellular responses are part of the normal timed mechanisms that are necessary for the proper healing and remodeling of injured vessel walls.[8] At autopsy, successful graft anastomoses with long-term patency show a beautiful fibrocellular bridge between the original vessel walls, with some additional adventitial collagen around the stitches and a cellular intimal cover that is neither hyperplastic nor stenosing, but appears to have been shaped by the local hemodynamic conditions. Another potentially beneficial aspect of smooth muscle cell proliferation is the "arterialization" of a vein graft, a term for the cellular hyperplasia in the tunica media of a grafted vein that increases the cell-to-matrix ratio of the vascular wall and gives the appearance (and presumably the performance) of an artery.

This desired outcome, however, is rare. More typical is the appearance of a patent vein graft shown in Figure 1A, where most of the fibrocellular reaction is in the intima, whereas the original wall of the graft, seen below the internal elastic lamina in this micrograph, retains the typical collagen-rich, sparsely cellular architecture of a vein. In contrast, a coronary artery of similar size, caliber, and

FIGURE 1. *Specimen from a 56-year-old male who had a first bypass 8 years earlier and multiple interventions thereafter.* **A.** *Saphenous vein graft with fibrocellular intimal thickening. Lumen is on top, adventitia on the bottom of the micrograph. Note the single internal elastic lamina (dark line) and the original vein wall (center) consisting mostly of collagen with a few scattered elastic fibers.* **B.** *Atherosclerotic coronary artery (recipient left anterior coronary artery distal of the anastomosis with the vein shown in A) displaying the typical arterial anatomy with (from the top) fibrocellular plaque in the intima, prominent internal elastic lamina (dark line), media rich in normal smooth muscle cells, external elastic lamina, and collagenous adventitia (bottom). A and B: Elastin/van Gieson's stain, ×100.*

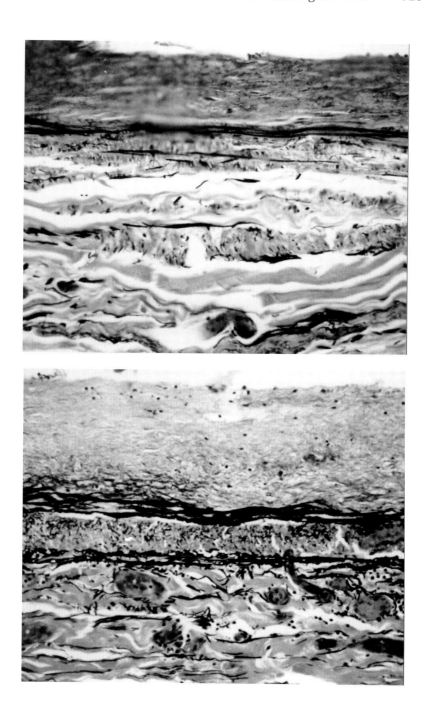

intimal thickening from the same heart, shows the characteristic anatomy of a real musculoelastic artery, consisting of well-defined layers of internal elastic lamina, media rich in smooth muscle cells, external elastic lamina, and collagenous adventitia (Figure 1B).

The proliferative response of the smooth muscle cells is self-limited and turns into a pathogenic mechanism only if the proliferative stimuli are excessive, repetitive, or persistent. In grafts, a specially vulnerable site is the anastomosis, the distal one more so than the proximal one.

Luminal and compliance mismatches and altered hemodynamic forces add to the factors that determine the response of the vein at these sites; the surgical technique and the graft integrity have the most impact on the morphological outcome.[9] The factors and signals that regulate the cellular responses are multiple and similar in arteries and veins, although leukocyte-elaborated cytokines and G-proteins have been reported as having a role in the early pathogenesis of experimental graft intimal hyperplasia.[10,11] In addition to the smooth muscle cells, macrophages participate in the development of vein graft disease as well, especially when poor runoff is combined with hyperlipidemia.[12]

At the anastomosis and along the length of the grafted vein, intimal fbrocellular hyperplasia provides the anatomic basis for plaque formation. Unlike the original vein and artery walls, the intimal thickenings or plaque areas in both the vein and the artery shown in Figure 1 look surprisingly similar. Mautner et al[13] compared the composition of arterial and venous plaques in 1404 vascular segments from 19 men aged 39 to 82 years who survived surgery for more than 1 year. They found that fibrocellular intimal tissues in the intimal thickenings of early vein grafts are gradually replaced by sclerotic tissue, so that after about 7 years, the composition of plaques in

---

FIGURE 2. *Specimen from a 56-year-old male who had a first bypass 8 years earlier and multiple interventions thereafter.* **A.** *Advanced atherosclerosis in a saphenous vein graft to the right coronary artery. Fibrous cap (top) shows a fissure containing a small clot. The bulk of the plaque consists of acellular, atheromatous material with cholesterol clefts (center) and an intraplaque hemorrhage (right). While this venous-complicated plaque is indistinguishable from an arterial one, the original venous wall (bottom) appears as layers of compressed collagen with little elastin.* **B.** *Advanced atheromatous plaque in the same saphenous vein graft, proximal to the position shown in A. S1 indicates a gap where the struts of a first stent were located. The fibrocellular intimal hyperplasia covering the first stent shows an indentation and some fresh thrombus from a second stent (S2). A and B: Elastin/van Gieson's stain ×40.*

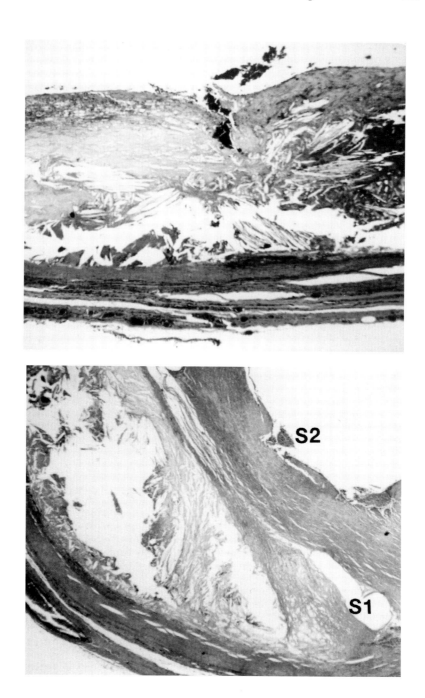

saphenous vein grafts is similar to that in native coronary arteries of the same patients. Thus, while "arterialization" in terms of acquiring the musculoelastic anatomy of an artery is not convincing, the grafted veins certainly behave like the local arteries in terms of the formation of an intimal plaque, and long term, these venous plaques behave exactly like the arterial ones. They develop atheromatous, lipid-rich cores, calcifications, and a fibrous cap that can fissure and lead to intraplaque hemorrhage as shown in Figure 2A. These developments can be silent, or lead to cellular organization of the plaque hematoma with deposition of more tissue mass, or they can be the basis of unstable angina, or lead to instant occlusion, exactly as advanced atherosclerotic plaques in the respective coronary arteries behave.

Treatment of these increasingly appearing atherosclerotic grafts is therefore similar to that of atherosclerotic arteries: regrafting, angioplasty, or stenting. Not surprisingly, the responses to the percutaneous interventions are qualitatively the same for atherosclerotic veins as for atherosclerotic arteries. This is shown in Figure 2B, where the struts of a stent can be seen over a large, lipid-rich plaque in a saphenous vein graft with an overlaying typical fibrocellular intimal hyperplasia; the marks of a second stent that was placed shortly before the patient died can also be seen. While the relatively large lumen diameter vein grafts are favorable for stenting, the restenosis rates for both angioplasty and stenting are higher for vein grafts than for comparable native coronary arteries.[14–16]

Angiographic images of vein grafts with advanced lesions are often difficult to interpret, especially when parts of the original coronary circulation have totally occluded. Figure 3A shows an anastomosis of a saphenous vein graft to the right coronary artery. The recipient artery proximal to the anastomosis occluded, and the

---

FIGURE 3. *Specimen from a 56-year-old male who had a first bypass 8 years earlier and multiple interventions thereafter.* **A.** *Saphenous vein graft (bottom) to the right coronary artery (top). Compare the outer diameter of the graft with that of the totally occluded artery at the asterisk. Small division in scale = 1 mm.* **B.** *Longitudinal profile of the opened graft shows four distinct levels with different lumina (following the direction of flow): a) Severe stenosis due to intimal hyperplasia inside of a stent, with large outer diameter and some metal bent inwards and backwards. The corresponding adventitial hematoma is also seen in Figure 3A left below the asterisk. b) First poststenotic dilatation within the stent, making the metal struts visible. c) Severe stenosis due to a combination of shrinkage and some kinking of the whole venous wall at the end of the stent. d) Second poststenotic dilatation with a thin wall forming a bulb-like lumen. Scale shows millimeters.*

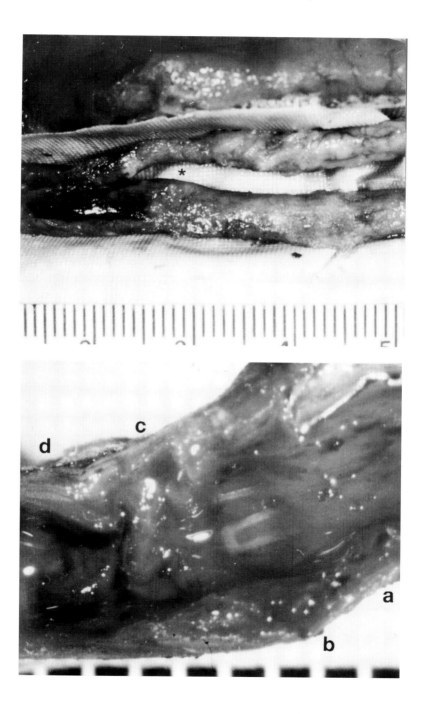

mechanism of occlusion was shrinkage of the entire vessel rather than additional plaque or thrombotic load, as can be suggested by the markedly reduced outer diameter of the artery near the anastomosis. A profile of the graft that had been stented at this position (Figure 3B) demonstrates some additional features of graft atherosclerosis and restenosis, some of which are common with the disease in the original coronary arteries. For example, one of the two most stenotic areas is at the site where the wall is thickest because of a huge fibrofatty plaque augmented by an advanced hyperplasia inside the stent, whereas the other marked stenosis is downstream where the wall is thin and the outer diameter is small because of the shrinkage and a poststent kink in the vessel. Thus, the lumen usually seen by angiography has little relation to the local wall thickness. Part of the stent metal is visible through a thin intimal covering, which would be a desirable result of cell proliferation in response to stent placement. However, there is no explanation why in this case this optimal result is seen side-by-side with an almost occlusive maximal intimal hyperplasia. Perhaps the bending of a piece of metal, indicated by some adventitial hemorrhage and corresponding protrusion of the other side of the deformed metal piece into the lumen, may have contributed to this response. The wider lumen over the visible parts of the stent would then represent a sort of poststenotic dilatation. A more plausible poststenotic dilatation involving the entire wall of the grafted vein, in the absence of a stent, is present downstream from the narrowest stenosis that is caused almost entirely by wall shrinkage and some kinking of the graft. The lumen is largest and the wall is thinnest at this second poststenotic dilatation, demonstrating how much hemodynamic forces can influence the remodeling process in both directions, dilatation and shrinkage, independent of plaque load. This accumulation of a number of possible mechanisms operating in a short stretch of atherosclerotic vein graft is admittedly unusual and is related to multiple interventions in this area. However, it is instructive, because it emphasizes the importance of visualizing the lumen, as well as the entire vessel wall for a better understanding of the multiple mechanisms that ultimately determine the patency of a grafted vein or an artery. Modern techniques including intravascular ultrasound will enable the clinician to see and interpret earlier areas that have, unfortunately, been mostly the pathologist's view of venous graft disease.

References

1. Barner HB. Arterial conduits for coronary bypass. *Coron Artery Dis* 1994;5:799–802.

2. Bryan AJ, Angelini GD. The biology of saphenous vein graft occlusion: Etiology and strategies for prevention. *Curr Opin Cardiol* 1994;9:641–649.
3. Khan SS, Denton T, Matloff JM. Long-term survival after coronary bypass grafting. *Curr Opin Cardiol* 1994;9:692–703.
4. Menkins AH, Carley SD, Clough TM. Reoperation after coronary bypass grafting. *Can Fam Physician* 1993;39:325–332.
5. Charles AK, Gresham GA. Histopathological changes in venous grafts and in varicose and non-varicose veins. *J Clin Pathol* 1993;46:603–606.
6. Sayers RD, Watt PA, Muller S, et al. Endothelial cell injury secondary to surgical preparation of reversed and in situ saphenous vein bypass grafts. *Eur J Uasc Surg* 1992;6:354–361.
7. Haudenschild CC, Quist WC, Gould KE, et al. Protection of endothelium in vessel segments excised for grafting. *Circulation* 1981;64:101–107.
8. Haudenschild CC. Restenosis: Pathophysiologic Considerations. In: Topol EJ, ed. *Textbook of Interventional Cardiology.* Second edition. Philadelphia: W.B.Saunders Co.; 1994:382–399.
9. Quist WC, Haudenschild CC, LoGerfo FW. Qualitative microscopy of implanted vein grafts: Effects of graft integrity on morphologic fate. *J Thorac Cardiovasc Surg* 1992;103:671–677.
10. Hoch JR, Stark VK, Hullett DA, et al. Vein graft intimal hyperplasia: Leukocytes and cytokine gene expression. *Surgery* 1994;116:463–471.
11. Davies MD, Ramkumar V, Gettys TW, et al. The expression and function of G-proteins in experimental intimal hyperplasia. *J Clin Invest* 1994;94:1680–1689.
12. Itoh H, Komori K, Funahashi S, et al. Intimal hyperplasia of experimental autologous vein graft in hyperlipidemic rabbits with poor distal runoff. *Atherosclerosis* 1994;110:259–270.
13. Mautner SL, Mautner GC, Hunsberger SA, et al. Comparison of composition of atherosclerotic plaques in saphenous veins used as aortocoronary bypass conduits with plaques in native coronary arteries in the same men. *Am J Cardiol* 1992;70:1380–1387.
14. Fenton SH, Fischman DL, Savage MP, et al. Long-term angiographic and clinical outcome after implantation of balloon- expandable stents in aortocoronary saphenous vein grafts. *Am J Cardiol* 1994;74:1187–1191.
15. Van Beusekom HM, van der Giessen WJ, van Suylen R, et al. Histology after stenting of human saphenous vein bypass grafts: Observations from surgically excised grafts 3 to 320 days after stent implantation. *J Am Coll Cardiol* 1993;21:45–54.
16. Eeckhout E, Goy JJ, Stauffer JC, et al. Endoluminal stenting of narrowed saphenous vein grafts: Long-term clinical and angiographic follow-up. *Catheterization Cardiovasc Diagn* 1994;31:139–146.

Chapter 30

Aortocoronary Bypass Grafting:
A Clinician's View

James H. Chesebro, MD,
Richard Gallo, MD, Vincenzo Toschi, MD,
Maddalena Lettino, MD,
and Juan J. Badimon, PhD

Introduction

Mural thrombosis and platelet deposition in aortocoronary vein grafts begin intraoperatively as soon as blood begins to flow through the vein graft.[1] This influences occlusion of vein grafts from a matter of days up to 1 year later. Because of this pathophysiology, antithrombotic therapy is started perioperatively with some therapies being started before surgery and others 1–6 hours after the operation via the nasogastric tube. This pathophysiology led to the first convincing results of platelet-inhibitor therapy in coronary bypass operations that documented the importance of perioperative antithrombotic therapy.[2,3] Prior studies that started the same therapy too late, ie, several days after surgery when thrombus had already formed, were unsuccessful.[4] In the first week and early months after surgery, vein graft occlusion is related to thrombosis that is in part caused by vein graft transplantation and trauma, technical problems, associated coronary artery disease with small coronary arteries, low vein-graft blood flow, and systemic factors.[1–3,5–7] Asymptomatic mural thrombosis within vein grafts may be considerable, may be detected by asymmetry of the lumen by angiography or magnetic resonance imaging (MRI), and may only be recognized when it is extensive (Figure 1).

From: Fuster V, (ed.) *Syndromes of Atherosclerosis: Correlations of Clinical Imaging and Pathology*. Armonk, NY: Futura Publishing Company, Inc.: © 1996.

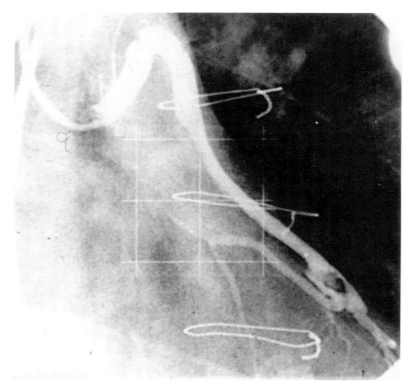

FIGURE 1. *Vein graft angiogram of the left anterior descending coronary artery in asymptomatic patient 8 days after operation. Note the diffuse narrowing of the mid- and distal graft (with hazy irregular borders) and filling defect adjacent to the distal anastomosis that are hallmarks of mural thrombosis.*

Rationale for Antithrombotic Therapy

Perioperative Therapy

Antithrombotic therapy administered perioperatively is critical for preventing mural and occlusive thrombosis of vein grafts because platelet deposition begins intraoperatively as soon as blood flow begins and may relate in part to the presence of tissue factor in the subendothelium of human saphenous veins. (J.T. Fallen, unpublished data)[1,2] In addition, studies in the canine model show that prevention of acute thrombosis in the vein graft markedly reduces subsequent neointimal proliferation 2–3 months later.[9] This concept is also suggested in humans where antithrombotic therapy to reduce acute mural and occlusive thrombosis appears capable of reducing occlusion in the acute phase within the first month after surgery and between 1 month and 1 year later (Figure 2).[2,3,10] Starting therapy before surgery or early after surgery (<24–48 hours) not only helps reduce vein graft occlusion early after surgery, but also 1 year later (Figure 3). Vein graft occlusion is not prevented if therapy is started more than 48 hours after surgery.[5] It appears that the earlier therapy is started after surgery the better.[11-13] Administration of aspirin via the nasogastric tube 1 hour after surgery is safe and effective.[11]

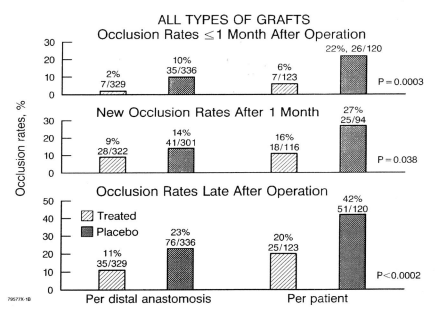

FIGURE 2. *Occlusion rates for all types of vein grafts. The rates are expressed per distal anastomosis and per patient (proportion with at least one occlusion). Occlusion is shown as events occurring within 1 month (95% confidence limits for the per patient difference, 8% to 24%), as new events occurring beyond 1 month (in distal anastomoses and patients without occlusion within 1 month of operation) from angiography performed 1 year later (per patient, P=0.048; 95% confidence limits for the difference, 9% to 22%), and as events at a median of 1 year after operation (95% confidence limits for the per patient difference, 11% to 34%). These subsets include only patients who had angiography within 1 month of operation and again 1 year later. Below each percentage is shown the ratio of distal anastomoses or patients with occlusion to total distal anastomoses or patients. (Reprinted with permission from Reference 4.)*

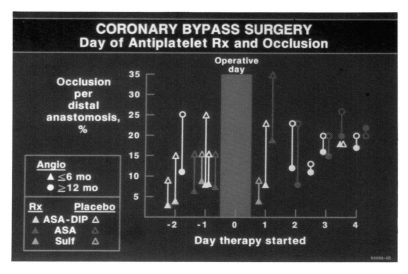

FIGURE 3. *Relationship of vein graft occlusion to the day of starting antiplatelet therapy before (day minus 2 or 1) or after (day 1, 2, 3, or 4) surgery. Studies in which therapy was started before or at least within 48 hours after surgery were the most successful in preventing subsequent vein graft occlusion. The time of angiography is shown by the shape of the symbol (**triangle,** at or before 6 months; **circle,** at 12 months or later). The drugs administered are shown by the type of lines between symbols (**continuous line,** acetylsalicylic acid plus dipyridamole; **dashed line,** acetylsalicylic acid; **dotted line,** sulfinpyrazone; **diagonally dashed line,** ticlopidine). **Open symbols** depict placebo; **closed symbols** depict treatment.*

Perioperative Dipyridamole

Dipyridamole appears to reduce platelet deposition onto artificial surfaces in vivo, but alone does not appear to reduce platelet deposition or mural thrombosis onto deeply injured arteries.[24,25] Thus, dipyridamole decreases platelet activation and maintains the platelet count during cardiopulmonary bypass when experimentally infused during surgery.[26,27]

In patients, dipyridamole maintains platelet counts above 150×10^9 per liter in 71% of patients compared with 28% of control patients when administered orally before surgery and as an infusion at 0.24 mg/kg per hour during surgery. Total chest tube blood loss was reduced from 1550 mL in control patients to 850 mL in dipyridamole-treated patients. Transfusion of packed red cells was reduced from 3.3 units to 1.9 units per patient in the dipyridamole group.[28] However, aspirin alone appears to be equally effective as aspirin plus dipyridamole in reducing the incidence of vein graft occlusion in three trials.[13,15,29,30] However, two of three trials showed a favorable trend towards reduced occlusion with aspirin combined with dipyridamole compared with aspirin alone,[29,30] especially in vein grafts placed into vessels with a lumen diameter ≤1.5 mm.[30]

Intraoperative Aprotinin

Thrombosis and thrombolysis are dynamic and simultaneous processes that may be influenced favorably or adversely by the balance of therapies. Compounds used to block fibrinolysis for decreasing intraoperative blood loss may enhance arterial and vein graft thrombosis.[31] In retrospect, this prothrombotic effect may have been caused by the use of celite rather than kaolin as the stimulant for the activated clotting time (ACT) measurement for monitoring heparin therapy.[32,33] Aprotinin markedly prolongs the ACT when celite is used as the stimulant for initiating clotting rather than kaolin (Figure 4).[32,33]

Aprotinin may have benefits of blood conservation, reduction of reoperation for bleeding, and a reduced effect of cardiopulmonary bypass upon systemic coagulopathy and systemic inflammatory-mediated responses. Risks include a prothrombotic effect when balanced with insufficient heparin, transient renal insuffi-

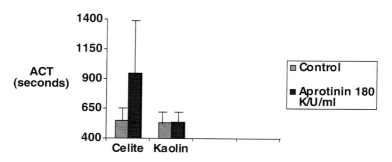

HEPARIN MONITORING BY ACT DURING APROTININ Rx
Effect of Activation System + Aprotinin on ACT

FIGURE 4. *ACT measurements in the presence of aprotinin are artificially prolonged by using celite as the clotting stimulus rather than kaolin. (Reprinted with permission from Wang et. J Thorac Cardiovasc Surg 1992;104:1135.)*

ciency, or allergic responses.[34] When arterial surfaces are very thrombogenetic, even usual amounts of heparin may not counteract the prothromutic effect of aprotinin.[31]

Enhancing Thrombolysis without a Lytic Agent

The dynamic and simultaneous processes of thrombosis and thrombolysis can also be favorably influenced by completely blocking platelet and fibrin deposition of arterial thrombus. Blocking thrombin activity with hirudin causes dissolution of 90% of arterial thrombus when hirudin therapy is administered within 1 hour of deep arterial injury and thrombus formation.[35] We have subsequently extended these studies and also find that blocking thrombin generation (such as with tick anticoagulant peptide [TAP]) also causes a similar degree of thrombus dissolution within 1 hour. These porcine studies have been extended to humans.

In the recombinant hirudin (CGP 39393) angiographic pilot study in unstable angina at rest, an occluded vein graft was the culprit vessel in 10 of 27 hirudin-treated patients with vein grafts.[36,37] Prior to this study, no antithrombotic agent without a thrombolytic agent had been reported to open occluded vein grafts. Recombinant hirudin was administered intravenously over 3–5 days to 10 patients (mean age 65) with totally occluded aortocoronary vein grafts occluded at or near the origin and over several centimeters of length. Five of 10 occluded vein grafts reopened during the infusion of hirudin, and each improved from a total occlusion at baseline to TIMI grade 2 or 3 angiographic flow at the end of the infusion. No thrombolytic agent was infused. In 5 vein grafts that reperfused, quantitation at repeat angiography showed a median luminal cross-sectional area of 3.3 mm², and at the culprit lesion a mean minimal lumen diameter of 0.92 mm. The median activated partial thromboplastin times (aPTT) for each patient during the infusion of hirudin ranged from 62 to 123 seconds. All 5 patients who recanalized with hirudin infusion had successful angioplasty for successful nonsurgical salvage of the vein graft. Thus, infusion of the potent direct antithrombin hirudin to modest aPTTs can block the growth of thrombus and induce endogenous thrombolysis of a considerable volume of thrombus in the aortocoronary vein grafts over 3 to 5 days.[37]

Risks for Vein Graft Occlusion

There is a gradation of risk for aortocoronary vein graft occlusion based on the coronary artery lumen diameter at the vein graft anastomoses (Table 1), intraoperative vein graft blood flow, coro-

TABLE 1

Platelet-Inhibitor Drug Trial in Coronary Artery Surgery:
Risk Factors of Late Occlusion in Individual Grafts

CA lumen diameter (mm)	Dipyridamole-ASA Occl/Total	%	Placebo Occl/Total	%
≤1.0	3/10	30	9/15	60
>1.0≤1.5	8/128	6	39/122	32
>1.5	12/126	9	25/117	21
Total	23/264	9	73/254	29

nary artery endarterectomy, and the final versus the nonfinal anastomoses of sequential vein grafts that anastomose side-to-side in the nonfinal anastomoses and end-to-side for the last anastomoses.[2,4]

Immediate Postoperative Aspirin

Immediate postoperative aspirin improves aortocoronary vein graft patency both early and late after coronary artery bypass graft surgery. Aspirin (324 mg) was administered within 1 hour of surgery via the nasogastric tube and compared with placebo. Vein graft angiography was obtained in 97% of patients, and at 1 week showed occlusion in 1.6% of patients treated with aspirin and 6.2% of those given placebo ($P = 0.004$). Late (1 year) vein graft occlusion was 5.8% in the group receiving aspirin, and 11.6% in the placebo group ($P = 0.01$). There was no significant difference in chest tube blood loss or red cell transfusion requirements. The reoperation rate was 4.8% in the aspirin group and 1% in the placebo group ($P = 0.1$). Thus, immediate postoperative administration of aspirin improves early and late vein graft patency for up to 1 year without greatly enhancing blood loss or transfusion requirements.[11]

Oral Anticoagulants

Oral anticoagulation therapy for the prevention of aortocoronary vein graft occlusion has long been known to be successful. In the first randomized trial, anticoagulation therapy was begun after initiating therapy with platelet inhibition.[38] Recently, oral anticoagulation therapy was started on the day before surgery at a fixed dose for two doses before adjusting to an international normalized ratio (INR) of 2.8–4.0 after surgery. This was nearly as effective as aspirin and dipyridamole, and was as effective as aspirin alone in reducing vein graft occlusion 1 year after surgery.[30] This study also showed the value of continuing therapy for at least a year after surgery.[38] A more extensive discussion for preventing aortocoronary vein bypass graft occlusion has recently been published.[39]

Current Recommendations

Before Surgery

In patients with unstable angina, heparin plus aspirin significantly reduces the incidence of myocardial infarction and death.[40] Patients who present while taking aspirin thus require the addition of heparin. Withdrawal of heparin in patients with unstable angina who are taking heparin without aspirin causes myocardial infarction or recurrent ischemia within hours in approximately 13% of patients, but this is reduced in patients who are also taking aspirin. Thus, patients with unstable angina who are waiting for aortocoronary bypass graft operation should receive continued aspirin (80–160 mg/day) and intravenous heparin (aPTT 60–85 seconds) until at least 3 to 4 hours before surgery.

Perioperative Therapy

Aspirin alone is recommended as routine therapy after coronary bypass operation. Aspirin should be started one hour after operation down the nasogastric tube at a minimum dose of 160 mg/day for loading and thereafter administered at 80–325 mg/day and continued indefinitely.

For patients who have vein graft coronary arteries ≤1.5 mm in diameter, two studies suggest that dipyridamole (225–400 mg/day) in addition to aspirin may be more effective than aspirin alone if dipyridamole (400 mg/day) is administered until 1 to 2 hours before surgery, and aspirin is started within 1 to 2 hours after surgery.[29,30] The main benefit of dipyridamole may be in the perioperative period.

Patients who are at risk because of small coronary artery lumen diameters (≤1.5 mm), low vein-graft blood flow (≤40 mL/min intraoperatively), or a coronary artery endarterectomy may be considered for combined therapy with oral anticoagulation (started on the day before surgery) plus low-dose aspirin at 80–100 mg/day. Combined therapy has been successful in reducing thromboembolism and mortality (especially mortality from vascular causes) as well as major systemic thromboembolism in patients with heart valve replacement, including patients who had concurrent coronary artery bypass graft surgery.[41] The target INR should be 2.5–3.5.

Ticlopidine (250 mg twice daily) is effective in reducing aortocoronary vein graft occlusion both early and late after operation.[16] Because of the side-effect profile of ticlopidine, although it is a very good aspirin substitute, it is only used for those patients who are allergic to or intolerant of aspirin.

Because aspirin may reduce but does not fully prevent deep venous thrombosis, all patients should receive heparin 5,000 units subcutaneously every 12 hours or enoxiparin (low-molecular weight heparin) 30 mg subcutaneously every 12 hours for 2 days or until patients are ambulatory, whichever time period is longer.

At least one internal mammary artery bypass graft should be included in the revascularization procedure (usually to the largest and most significant coronary artery, the left anterior descending coronary artery) because this procedure has the lowest risk of occlusion and greatest longevity for a preserved blood supply which results in a lower mortality.[42] No studies have shown a definite benefit of antiplatelet therapy in patients with internal mammary bypass grafts, but one study did show a trend towards reduction in occlusion.[43] However, aspirin is indicated for patients with coronary artery disease, and thus, for all patients after bypass surgery regardless of type of graft.

Prevention of Late Vein Graft Occlusion

The best prevention of late vein-graft occlusion is maximal reduction of all coronary risk factors and long-term aspirin therapy. Especially important is reduction in low-density lipoprotein (LDL) cholesterol to under 100 mg/dL and an increase in high-density lipoprotein (HDL) cholesterol because these parameters appear to decrease the risk of atherosclerotic plaque disruption. This is suggested by the marked reduction in atherosclerosis, the number of coronary events, and reduced mortality in patients treated with LDL-lowering therapy, HDL-raising therapy, or both.[44–46]

In patients with incomplete correction of risk factors or those who already have one occluded vein graft or appear with new angina after coronary bypass operation, consideration should be given to long-term anticoagulant therapy (INR 2.5–3.5) along with low-dose aspirin at 80 mg/day in order to prevent vein graft occlusion after atherosclerotic plaque disruption. Because plaque disruption in a vein graft leads not only to local occlusion but also to occlusion of the entire graft proximal to the plaque disruption (since vein grafts have no branches and thus are prone to long segments of occlusion), combined anticoagulants plus aspirin may prevent the large amounts of thrombus with occlusion and allow preservation of the vein graft with or without angioplasty. The role of oral anti-coagulant therapy plus aspirin needs short- and long-term study.

References

1. Fuster V, Dewanjee MK, Chesebro JH, et al. Noninvasive radioisotopic technique for detection of platelet deposition in coronary artery bypass grafts in dogs and its reduction with platelet inhibition. *Circulation* 1979;60:1508–1512.
2. Chesebro JH, Clements I, Fuster V, et al. A platelet-inhibitor drug trial in coronary-artery bypass operations: Benefit of perioperative dipyridamole and aspirin therapy on early postoperative vein-graft patency. *N Engl J Med* 1982;307:73–78.
3. Fallon JT. Peripheral vascular disease: A pathologist's view. Presented at the American Heart Association Scientific Conference; January 19–21, 1995; Lake Buena Vista, FL.
4. Chesebro JH, Fuster V, Elveback LR, et al. Effect of dipyridamole and aspirin on late vein-graft patency after coronary bypass operations. *N Engl J Med* 1984;310:209–214.
5. Pantely GA, Goodnight SH Jr, Rahimtoola, et al. Failure of antiplatelet and anticoagulant therapy to improve patency of grafts after coronary-artery bypass. *N Engl J Med* 1979;301:962–966.
6. Grundfest WS, Litvack F, Sherman T, et al. Delineation of peripheral and coronary detail by intraoperative angioscopy. *Ann Surg* 1985;202:394–400.
7. Josa M, Lie JT, Bianco RL, et al. Reduction of thrombosis in canine coronary bypass vein grafts with dipyridamole and aspirin. *Am J Cardiol* 1981;47:1248–1254.
8. Uni KK, Kottke BA, Titus JL, et al. Pathologic changes in aortocoronary saphenous vein grafts. *Am J Cardiol* 1974;34:526–532.
9. Metke MP, Lie JT, Fuster V, et al. Reduction of intimal thickening in canine coronary bypass vein grafts with dipyridamole and aspirin. *Am J Cardiol* 1979;43:1144–1148.
10. Pfiesterer M, Burkart F, Jockers G, et al. Trial of low-dose aspirin plus dipyridamole vs anticoagulants for prevention of aortocoronary vein graft occlusion. *Lancet* 1989;2:1–7.
11. Gavaghan TP, Gebski V, Baron DW. Immediate postoperative aspirin improves vein graft patency early and late after coronary artery bypass surgery. *Circulation* 1991;83:1526–1533.
12. Brown BG, Cukingnan RA, DeRouien T, et al. Improved graft patency in patients treated with platelet-inhibiting therapy after coronary bypass surgery. *Circulation* 1985;72:138–146.
13. Goldman S, Copeland J, Moritz T, et al. Improvement in early saphenous vein graft patency after coronary artery bypass surgery with antiplatelet therapy: Results of a Veterans Administration cooperative study. *Circulation* 1988;77:1324–1332.

14. Baur HR, Van Tassel RA, Pierach CA, et al. Effects of sulfinpyrazone on early graft closure after myocardial infarction. *Am J Cardiol* 1982;49:420–424.
15. Goldman S, Copeland J, Moritz T, et al. Saphenous vein graft patency 1 year after coronary artery bypass surgery and effects of antiplatelet therapy: Results of a Veterans Administration cooperative study. *Circulation* 1989;80:1190–1197.
16. Limer R, David JL, Magotteaux P, et al. Prevention of aortocoronary bypass graft occlusion. *J Thorac Cardiovasc Surg* 1987;94:773–783.
17. Rajah SM, Salter MCP, Donaldson DR, et al. Acetylsalicyclic acid and dipyridamole improve the early patency of aorta-coronary bypass grafts: A double-blind, placebo-controlled, randomized trial. *J Thorac Cardiovasc Surg* 1985;89:373–377.
18. Mayer JE, Lindsay WG, Castaneda W, et al. Influence of aspirin and dipyridamole on patency of coronary artery bypass grafts. *Ann Thorac Surg* 1981;31:204–210.
19. Lorenz RL, Schacky CV, Weber M, et al. Improved aortocoronary bypass patency by low-dose aspirin (100 mg daily). *Lancet* 1984;1:1261–1264.
20. Brooks N, Wright J, Sturridge M, et al. Randomized placebo controlled trial of aspirin and dipyridamole in the prevention of coronary vein graft occlusion. *Br Heart J* 1985;53:201–207.
21. McEnany MT, Salzman EW, Mundth ED, et al. The effect of antithrombotic therapy on patency rate of saphenous vein coronary artery bypass grafts. *J Thorac Cardiovasc Surg* 1982;83:81–89.
22. Sharma GVRK, Khuri SF, Josa M, et al. The effect of antiplatelet therapy on saphenous vein coronary artery bypass graft patency. *Circulation* 1983;68(suppl II):218–221.
23. Chesebro JH, Fuster V. The pathogenesis and prevention of aortocoronary bypass graft occlusion and restenosis after arterial angioplasty: Role of vascular injury and platelet-thrombus deposition. *J Am Coll Cardiol* 1986;8:57B–66B.
24. Lam JYT, Chesebro JH, Steele PM, et al. Antithrombotic therapy for arterial injury by angioplasty: Efficacy of common platelet inhibitors versus thrombin inhibition in pigs. *Circulation* 1991;84:814–820.
25. Pumphrey CW, Fuster V, Dewanjee MK, et al. Comparison of the antithrombotic action of calcium antagonist drugs with dipyridamole in dogs. *Am J Cardiol* 1983;51:591–595.
26. Nuutinen LS, Pihlajanicmi R, Saarcla E, et al. The effect of dipyridamole on the thrombocyte count and bleeding tendency in openheart surgery. *J Thorac Cardiovasc Surg* 1977;74:295–298.
27. Becker RM, Smith MR, Dobell ARC. Effect of platelet inhibition on platelet phenomenon in cardiopulmonary bypass in pigs. *Ann Surg* 1974;179:52–57.
28. Teoh KH, Christakis GT, Weisel RR, et al. Dipyridamole preserved platelets and reduced blood loss after cardiopulmonary bypass. *J Thorac Cardiovasc Surg* 1988;96:332–341.
29. Sanz G, Coello I, Cardona M, et al, and the Grupo Espanol para el Seguimiento del Injerto Coronario (GESIC). Prevention of early aortocoronary bypass occlusion by low-dose aspirin and dipyridamole. *Circulation* 1990;82:765–773.
30. van der Meer J, Hillege HL, Kootstra GJ, et al, for the CABADAS research group of the Interuniversity Cardiology Institute of the Nether-

lands. Prevention of one-year vein-graft occlusion after aortocoronary bypass surgery: A comparison of low-dose aspirin, low-dose aspirin plus dipyridamole, and oral anticoagulants. *Lancet* 1993;324:257–264.

31. Cosgrove DM, Heric B, Lytle BW, et al. Aprotinin therapy for reoperative myocardial revascularization: A placebo-controlled study. *Ann Thorac Surg* 1992;54:1031–1036.

32. Harder MP, Eijsman L, Roozendaal KJ, et al. Aprotinin reduces intraoperative and postoperative blood loss in membrane oxygenator cardiopulmonary bypass. *Ann Thorac Surg* 1991;51:936–941.

33. Wang J-S, Lin C-Y, Hung W-T, et al. In vitro effects of aprotinin on activated clotting time measured with different activators. *J Thorac Cardiovasc Surg* 1992;104:1135–1140.

34. Bidstrup BP, Harrison J, Royston D, et al. Aprotinin therapy in cardiac operations: A report on use in 41 cardiac centers in the United Kingdom. *Ann Thorac Surg* 1993;55:971–976.

35. Wysokinski WE, McBane RD, Hassinger ML, et al. "Dethrombosis": effect of thrombin inhibition on thrombus propagation and maintenance. *Thromb Haemostasis* 1993;69:692. Abstract.

36. Topol EJ, Fuster V, Harrington, RA, et al. Recombinant hirudin for unstable angina pectoris. A multicenter, randomized angiographic trial. *Circulation* 1994;89:1556–1566.

37. Chesebro JH, Rao AK, Schwartz D, et al. Endogenous thrombolysis and recanalization of occluded aortocoronary vein grafts with recombinant hirudin in patients with unstable angina. *Circulation* 1994;90:I–568.

38. Gohlke H, Gohlke-Barwolf C, Sturzenhofecker P, et al. Improved graft patency with anticoagulant therapy after aortocoronary bypass surgery: A prospective randomized study. *Circulation* 1981;64(Suppl II):22–27.

39. Chesebro JH, Meyer BJ, Fernandez-Ortiz A, et al. Antiplatelet drugs. In: Luscher TF, Turina M, eds. *Coronary Artery Graft Disease: Mechanisms and Prevention.* Heidelberg: Springer Publishers; 1994:276–298.

40. Cohen M, Adams PC, Parry G, et al, and the Antithrombotic Therapy in Acute Coronary Syndromes Research Group. Combination antithrombotic therapy in unstable rest angina and non-Q-wave infarction in nonprior aspirin users. Primary endpoints analysis from the ATACS Trial. *Circulation* 1994;1:81–88.

41. Turpie AGG, Gent M, Laupacis A, et al. A comparison of aspirin with placebo in patients treated with warfarin after heart-valve replacement. *N Engl J Med* 1993;329:524–529.

42. Loop FD, Lytle BW, Cosgrove DM, et al. Influence of the internal-mammary-artery graft on 10-year survival and other cardiac events. *N Engl J Med* 1986;314:1–6.

43. Goldman S, Copelan J, Moritz T, et al. Starting aspirin after operation: Effects on early graft patency. *Circulation* 1991;84:520–526.

44. Blankenhorn DH, Nessim SA, Johnson RL. Beneficial effects of combined colestipol-niacin therapy on coronary atherosclerosis and coronary venous bypass graft. *JAMA* 1987;257:3233–3240.

45. Brown G, Albers JJ, Fisher LD, et al. Regression of coronary artery disease as a result of intensive lipid-lowering therapy in men with high levels of apolipoprotein B. *N Engl J Med* 1990;323:1289–1298.

46. Scandinavian Simvastatin Survival Study Group. Randomised trial of cholesterol lowering in 4444 patients with coronary heart disease: The Scandinavian Simvastatin Survival Study (4S). *Lancet* 1994;344:1383–1389.

Panel Discussion V

Post-PTCA Restenosis and Vein Graft Disease

Dr. Valentin Fuster: Dr. Schwartz, Have you been able to look at the cellular composition of atherectomy specimens? Is there evidence from atherectomy of restenosis lesions of a smooth muscle proliferative response? I also wonder if anyone has looked at whether platelet-derived growth factor (PDGF) or thrombin expression also occurs to a greater degree in restenotic plaques?

Dr. Stephen M. Schwartz: If there is much proliferation in atherectomy specimens of plaques, it's hard to find. I am unaware of evidence that PDGF is an in vivo mitogen or that thrombin is an in vivo mitogen. PDGF-AA, which is really the major form of PDGF in plaques, is at best a weak mitogen. In the case of thrombin, the only data I know were an attempt to inhibit smooth muscle proliferation with hirudin, and it failed. In conclusion, as far as I know, if thrombin has a role it's in migration, not in proliferation.

Dr. Fuster: Dr. Schwartz, one can assume a possible proliferation effect after percutaneous transluminal coronary angioplasty (PTCA) injury by PDGF-BB, which is derived from platelets, because if you make an animal thrombotytopenic, there is no proliferation.

Dr. Schwartz: Not quite true. In Michael Reidy's original paper, when he depleted the animals of platelets, he decreased intimal thickening. When we studied recombinant PDGF, we only affected migration. There was no evidence of an effect on proliferation. I think, as of today, that for either PDGF or thrombin the evidence is that whatever they do it may be related to migration. But for proliferation we need other candidates.

Dr. Fuster: What about the work from Russell Ross using a monoclonal antibody in vivo against PDGF?

Dr. Schwartz: That showed no effect on proliferation, only on migration.

Discussant A from the Audience: The finding by Suarez, investigators from Spain, of ultrasound intraplaque lucency predicting restenosis is very interesting. How do you know that's not hemorrhage in the plaque rather than a lipid pool?

Dr. Fuster: These were atherectomy specimens that were also analyzed histologically. If I recall, 100% of the lesions in which atherectomy and intravascular ultrasound suggested a high content of fat developed restenosis. The fibrotic lesions had 40% restenosis. We all know that patients with unstable angina or myocardial infarction, who we assume ruptured a lipid-rich plaque, have a much higher incidence of restenosis, for example, than patients with the stable angina. So the concept is that a lipid-rich plaque with thrombus or predisposing to new thrombus organizes and contributes to restenosis.

Dr. Christopher Zarins: What is the evidence that smooth muscle cell proliferation stops after the regrowth of endothelium, and that this endothelium is functional and not dysfunctional?

Dr. Fuster: Dr. Lina Badimon, working with us, studied pigs in which the surface of the carotid artery was deendothelialized by the "dry air" technique, and then these animals were followed for a period of up to 5 weeks, and killed at various times. We then looked at the coverage of the endothelium and the number of layers of smooth muscle cells and their appearance, whether they were secreting cells or quiescent cells. And the data suggested that when the whole surface is covered, which tends to happen after 2–4 weeks, the smooth muscle cells are much more quiescent. So, we have a correlation of this relationship.

Dr. Schwartz: Going back to atherectomy specimens, the problem with atherectomies is that there are so many questions to ask and so many things to look at. For example, we haven't looked at proteases. Protease is required for second wave migration of smooth muscle cells from the media to the intima. Protease inhibitors will block it. Whether these phenomena, first- and second-wave media replication and migration, are related to restenosis is a really critical question. In the case of angiopeptin, there is substantial evidence that it blocks the first and second wave, yet it didn't do very well in human trials.

Dr. Pickering, your finding that intimal remodeling was much more prominent in peripheral than coronary restenosis is consistent with our data and data from Europe. One of the questions I have is about how we interpret sampling. The sampling in peripheral atherectomies is a lot more abundant than it is in coronaries. So perhaps the difference is a sampling difference rather than a real difference, which, unfortunately you can only get at autopsy.

Dr. J. Geoffrey Pickering: No question. We tried to at least minimize that by expressing everything in terms of specimen area. But the procedure and the proportion of plaque that is extracted in the peripherals and coronaries may not be the same at all.

Discussant B from the Audience: I'm also intrigued by the difference between coronary and peripheral restenosis and wonder if hemodynamic differences may have something to do with that. There are a number of animal models that showed that anastomotic intimal hyperplasia could be substantially inhibited by the addition of a distal AV fistula with an increase in the flow. I wonder if you had any perspective of etiology for these differences?

Dr. Pickering: No. In fact, some of the information Dr. Glagov has proposed would, to my mind, have pointed the other way around. I must say I don't have a good explanation, although I think it's probably key in some way.

Dr. Kenneth Rosenfield: Is the process of reocclusion of synthetic grafts comparable to that of arterial reocclusion?

Dr. Christian C. Haudenschild: I think that's a very good question. Below 3 mm, any thrombotic action becomes critical in terms of the lumen. So, if you have a little bit of thrombus in a 3-mm vessel, that can occlude, but if you have the same amount relative to the wall size in a large-diameter vessel such as the aorta, it doesn't occlude. Now, there is no biomaterial that is totally non-thrombogenic, so you have to always have some thrombosis. That is something that you must take into account with a biomaterial prosthesis supplying a 3-mm artery.

Dr. Schwartz: In my opinion, the concept of restenosis is breaking down into lots of different things. I think stent stenosis is one thing and balloon angioplasty restenosis is another thing. What about anastomosis stenosis?

Dr. Haudenschild: I think it's a remodeling problem. We have almost a controlled experiment when you compare the proximal aorta with the distal coronary anastomosis. In the proximal, you have hemodynamically favorable conditions. You have a large hole and you have a large vessel, and you have enough space to even account for some hyperplasia, which is inevitable with wound healing. And, most of the time you have a nondiseased situation. That can't always be avoided at the coronary arterial anastomosis. They have to take the best there is, and given the size mismatch, the differences in compliance, the angles, the stitches, the much bigger effect of a little hyperplasia on a smaller lumen than on the big lumen proximally, that all combines into a worst-case situation at the distal anastomosis. And then, chances are that the other insults, including bad outflow and hypercholesterolemia, will be the straws that break the camel's back—the beginning of a vicious circle that leads to repeat performances of wound healing and possibly ultimate occlusion.

Dr. Fuster: Since we are already discussing aorto-coronary vein graft pathology, maybe there are a number of issues that we can clarify at this time. I know Dr. Insull has a few questions.

Dr. William Insull: Dr. Chesebro, is there a role for the hirudin as a therapeutic agent for individuals with bypass grafts?

Dr. James H. Chesebro: We don't know. First of all we have to see the outcome of GUSTO and TIMI for patients with acute coronary syndromes. Early after bypass surgery, of course, the risks are bleeding versus thrombosis. I think that for the future I would look to trying to passivate by whatever means the surface of the vein graft more than trying to give significant systemic therapy early after operation, when one could increase the bleeding risk. So, I can't say that I could recommend hirudin. Obviously, there need to be further studies in this regard.

Dr. Insull: How about the option of timed dosing so that you wait, for example, the first 6 hours to let things seal off and then give the hirudin?

Dr. Chesebro: This is possible, but I think we don't know enough yet to recommend that. One of the things we really need to learn about all of these antithrombotic drugs, including hirudin, is the appropriate duration of therapy. Our feeling is beginning to be towards therapy that inhibits the thrombin generation, not just the activity. We find with hirudin that thrombin generation continues, but if we inhibit factor Xa before this in the coagulation system, we can inhibit the generation of thrombin. There is some suggestion from experimental studies that there may be a longer-lasting effect if one is inhibiting thrombin generation. This is still quite theoretical, and needs further documentation. But that's my vision for the future—moving to an earlier stage in the coagulation system. It may even be back to the point of tissue factor. But there's still a lot of work to be done.

Dr. Insull: One further question. Would you recommend vigorous treatment to get LDL down rapidly?

Dr. Chesebro: I would give the usual therapy to get it down, and I would use the American Heart Association recommendation of an LDL below 100. We have had the tendency in the past to advise trying diet first, but so often the patient goes home and gets lost to follow-up, and is never treated. So I think we have to see what type of hyperlipidemia they have, then follow them up to see that they get treated sufficiently, and I think that's the critical role.

Dr. Insull: Should they get maximum dosage, trying to get the LDL under 100 within a couple of weeks or less?

Dr. Chesebro: Pathologically, aside of the early thrombotic process, atherosclerosis of the vein graft is not severe until one gets out to 3 years. So I'm not sure that the very early level is of critical importance. There is some lowering with all of the dietary reductions associated with surgery, as well. But I would say, certainly it is wise to start it in the hospital, so they have it when they go home.

Discussant C from the Audience: I'd like to propose that the fundamental lesion that we're dealing with is a chronic ulcerated plaque that may exist for days, weeks, months, or years, and slowly progress on to stenosis or to resolution. Does anyone have any comments on that?

Dr. Haudenschild: I think that what we've really been discussing in this whole meeting is the problem of progression of disease—of plaque disruption and the recurrence involved in this progression. In patients who have had an acute infarction and then go on for noncardiac surgery, the risk is high in the first 6 months, especially in the first 3 months, and after the first 6 months it's down to a baseline of about 4% to 5% risk from older studies. So I would say it may take as long as 6 months for this plaque to heal fully.

Discussant C from the Audience: But during that period of 6 months, it is a potentially unstable lesion, is that not correct?

Dr. Haudenschild: That's correct. Especially in the early days and early weeks.

Discussant C from the Audience: How would you explain ulcerated plaques without thrombosis?

Dr. Haudenschild: Probably most do have some degree of thrombus. The size of thrombus may be a matter of a number of variables that could be involved. Part of it could be the substrate, part of it could be the size of what's exposed. Part of it could be the hemodynamics—we are dealing with a high shear-low shear situation, and so on. But I would say probably most of these plaques have some degree of thrombus.

Dr. Fuster: In the pig, we may have lots of ulcerations in the distal aorta, at the site of the trifurcation, and never get thrombus because the high flow washes it out. So the hemodynamic component is important, and might explain why an ulcer may not have a thrombus.

Discussant D from the Audience: Diet and exercise might help that?

Dr. Fuster: Who knows? When we feed pigs with a high-cholesterol diet we have ulceration and no thrombus.

This is the end of the symposium. I would like to thank all the participants and certainly the audience. It was a very stimulating meeting with outstanding individuals coming from different disciplines: pathologists, basic investigators, clinicians, surgeons, radiologists, and other imaging experts. I believe imaging is coming along, and it's time to catch up in the living human with what the pathologists have been telling us over the years, and I hope we can work and think all together in an integrated manner. This meeting, which was sponsored by the American Heart Association, in my view was a landmark for achieving this particular purpose. Thank you all.

Index